ALLE ZEIT WACH 1842

H. Tscherne J. Schatzker (Eds.)

Major Fractures of the Pilon, the Talus, and the Calcaneus

Current Concepts of Treatment

With 121 Figures and 42 Tables

Springer-Verlag
Berlin Heidelberg New York
London Paris Tokyo
Hong Kong Barcelona
Budapest

Professor Dr. Harald Tscherne
Unfallchirurgische Klinik
Medizinische Hochschule Hannover
Konstanty-Gutschow-Strasse 8, W-3000 Hannover 61, FRG

Professor Dr. Joseph Schatzker
Sunnybrook Medical Centre, University of Toronto
2075 Bayview Avenue, Toronto, Ontario M4N 3M5, Canada

Library of Congress Cataloging-in-Publication Data
Major fractures of the pilon, the talus, and the calcaneus: current concepts of treatment / H. Tscherne, J. Schatzker (eds.). p. cm.
Includes bibliographical references and index.

ISBN-13: 978-3-642-77731-8 e-ISBN-13: 978-3-642-77729-5
DOI: 10.1007/978-3-642-77729-5

1. Tibia–Fractures. 2. Heel bone–Fractures. 3. Anklebone–Fractures. I. Tscherne, H. (Harald), 1933– . II. Schatzker, Joseph.
[DNLM: 1. Calcaneus–injuries. 2. Fractures–therapy. 3. Talus–injuries. 4. Tibial Fractures–therapy. WE 870 M234]
RD560.M35 1993 617.1'58 – dc20 DNLM/DLC 92-49465

Softcover reprint of the hardcover 1st edition 1993

24/3130-5 4 3 2 1 0 – Printed on acid-free paper

Preface

This book contains the proceedings of an historic symposium, the first joint symposium of the Austrian, German and Swiss Trauma Associations and the Orthopaedic Trauma Association of North America. In an effort to bring European and North American trauma surgeons closer together and foster a free and productive exchange of ideas, these associations chose the meeting of the Austrian, German, and Swiss trauma associations, which was held in Vienna in May of 1991, as the occasion for their first joint session. The Austrian Trauma Association, led by its President, Professor Heinz Kuderna, was the host. The joint symposium of the European and the North American trauma associations, conducted in English, was held concurrently with the regular meeting of the AGS, conducted in German.

In order to explore and compare the current concepts in trauma on the two continents, the organizing committee felt that the discussion should focus on an area full of challenge and controversy. Thus the major fractures of the pilon, the talus, and the os calcis were chosen as the topics of discussion. Each subject was introduced by two keynote speakers, one from Europe and one from North America, who were chosen by their respective trauma associations on the basis of their expertise and distinguished contributions. These presentations were then followed by five or six invited shorter presentations on the subject. At the end of each session, the presenters formed a panel, debated controversial points, and answered questions from the audience. The discussions after the sessions have been omitted from this volume, since the questions and the ensuing discussions were too difficult to transcribe.

The reader will see from this book that the surgical treatment of pilon fractures which are caused by high-energy compressive forces and of open pilon fractures continue to be fraught with many complications. Great advances have been made in the techniques of internal fixation and preoperative planning, as demonstrated in the chapters by

Thomas Rüedi and Jeff Mast. However, all authors have recognized that some of the B types, all of the C types of pilon fractures, and most of the open fractures, show totally unacceptable degrees of soft tissue complications if treated by early reconstruction of the metaphyseal component of the injury. The message of this part of the book is very clear: Open fractures must be irrigated and debrided. The joint should be reconstructed with minimal internal fixation. In order to decrease soft tissue dissection, percutaneous screws should be used. The metaphyseal portion and the soft tissue wounds should be splinted in an external fixator until the soft tissue envelope has been reconstructed and is healed. One of the most important problems in the treatment of high-energy pilon fractures are the soft tissues. If needed, free flap coverage should therefore be done early. Only then can the metaphysis be reconstructed with bone graft and internal fixation as indicated. Larry Bone shows here that even immobilization of the joint in an external fixator for 10 weeks will not result in permanent stiffness.

The surgical treatment of the closed injuries should be delayed until swelling and other soft tissue complications have subsided. This may delay the definitive treatment for as long as one to two weeks. Initial treatment should be either traction or external fixation to control pain, restore length, and bring about reduction of some fragments by ligamentotaxis. Great caution must be exercised in using internal fixation on the metaphyseal portion of the injury to prevent breakdown of the wound and sepsis.

Discussions of fractures of the talus contained here show that their treatment must be based on a sound understanding of the biological and biomechanical idiosynchrasies of this bone. The classification of Hawkins, with some slight modifications, is now universally accepted. It was also agreed that very early open reduction and stable screw fixation be used to minimize avascular necrosis. More frequent use of the bilateral or posterolateral approach instead of a standard single medial incision was also suggested. The key to reduction of the multifragmentary fractures of the neck is reduction of the subtalar joint. Titanium screws are preferred for internal fixation since they do not interfere with MRI, which may be desirable in the postoperative period if vascularity of the talus is to be evaluated. Some controversy still persists in the treatment of open complete dislocation of the talus. Treatment must be tailored of the individual, but most surgeons prefer not to sacrifice the talus during the initial stages of treatment. Weight bearing is allowed once the fractures unite, even if partial or total avascular necrosis is anticipated. There is no evidence that avoidance of weight bearing has any beneficial influence on the prevention of collapse of the avascular talus.

The book also makes clear that great progress has been made in the treatment of fractures of the os calcis. Classification of these fractures and the rationale for surgical treatment is based on the CT morphology of the fracture, since this has a direct correlation with the result. Surgical reconstruction of the calcaneal height, length, and width is of fundamental importance in the preservation of the normal biomechanics of the foot and in the preservation of function of the ankle and subtalar joints. The incidence breakdown of wounds has been decreased markedly by the modification of the extended lateral surgical approach recommended by Benirschke. The maneuvers necessary to secure a reduction and stable fixation have been carefully worked out and are very clearly described here, as is the management of the associated severe injuries of the foot which may be present. The functional results have markedly improved since stable internal fixation of the os calcis without transfixation of the adjacent joints has made functional aftercare possible. The seemingly persistent controversy regarding operative and nonoperative treatment will likely be settled when the modern surgical principles so clearly enunciated in this book are incorporated into prospective randomized and blind trials.

The organizing committee worked hard to make the symposium on which this volume is based a reality. We have strived here to make the ideas and concepts discussed there available to a wider audience, which we trust will contribute to an improvement in the care of these difficult injuries.

Joseph Schatzker
Harald Tscherne

Contents

List of Senior Authors

Beck, E., Prof. Dr.
Universitätsklinik für Unfallchirurgie
Anichstrasse 35, 6020 Innsbruck, Austria

Behrens, F., Prof. Dr.
Department of Orthopaedic Surgery
Metro Health Medical Center
Case Western Reserve University
Cleveland, OH, USA

Benirschke, S. K., MD
Harborview Medical Center, University of Washington
325 9th Avenue, Seattle, WA 98104, USA

Bone, L., MD
Department of Orthopaedics, State University of New York
Buffalo, NY, USA

Buckley, R. E., MD
Department of Orthopaedics, University of British Columbia
The Workers Compensation Board of British Columbia,
Vancouver, British Columbia, Canada

Forgon, M., Dr.
Department of Traumatic Surgery, Medical School
University of Pecs, Pecs, Hungary

Gotzen, L., Prof. Dr.
Chirurgische Abteilung, Philipps-Universität Marburg
Baldingerstrasse, W-3550 Marburg, FRG

Hansen, S. T., Jr., MD
Department of Orthopaedics, Harborview Medical Centre
ZS-48 325 9th Avenue, Seattle, WA 981042499, USA

Heim, U., PD Dr.
Chirurgie, FMH
Mattenstrasse 17, 3073 Gümlingen, Switzerland

Kuner, E. H., Prof. Dr.
Department Unfallchirurgie, Albert-Ludwigs-Universität
Hugstetterstrasse 55, W-7800 Freiburg, FRG

Mast, J., MD
Department of Orthopaedic Surgery, Hutzel Hospital
Wayne State University, 4707 St. Antoine Boulevard
Detroit, MI 48201, USA

Muhr, G., Prof. Dr.
Chirurgische Universitätsklinik
Berufsgenossenschaftliche Krankenanstalten "Bergmannsheil"
Hunscheidtstrasse 1, W-4630 Bochum 1, FRG

Poigenfürst, J., Prof. Dr.
Unfallkrankenhaus Lorenz Böhler
Donaueschingerstrasse 13, 1200 Wien 20, Austria

Raaymakers, E. L. F. B., Dr.
Orthopädisch-Traumatologische Universitätsklinik AMC
Meibergdreef 9, 1105 AZ Amsterdam, The Netherlands

Regazzoni, P., Prof.
Departement für Chirurgie, Kantonsspital Basel
4031 Basel, Switzerland

Rüedi, T., Prof. Dr.
Departement für Chirurgie, Kantonsspital
7000 Chur, Switzerland

Sanders, R., MD
Florida Orthopaedic Institute
4175 East Fowler Avenue, Tampa, FL 33617, USA

Schatzker, J., Prof. Dr.
Sunnybrook Medical Centre, University of Toronto
2075 Bayview Avenue, Toronto, Ontario M4N 3MS, Canada

Szyszkowitz, R., Prof. Dr.
Department für Unfallchirurgie, Chirurgische Unversitätsklinik
Auenbruggerplatz, 8036 Graz, Austria

Trentz, O., Prof. Dr.
Departement Chirurgie, Klinik für Unfallchirurgie
Universitätsspital Zürich
Rämistrasse 100, 8091 Zürich, Switzerland

Tscherne, H., Prof. Dr.
Unfallchirurgische Klinik, Medizinische Hochschule Hannover
Konstanty-Gutschow-Strasse 8, W-3000 Hannover 61, FRG

Waddell, J. P., MD
Department of Surgery, University of Toronto
St. Michael's Hospital, Toronto, Ontario, Canada

Zwipp, H., Prof. Dr.
Unfallchirurgische Klinik, Medizinische Hochschule Hannover
Konstanty-Gutschow-Strasse 8, W-3000 Hannover 61, FRG

PART I · PILON FRACTURES

Treatment of Pilon Tibial Fractures: State of the Art

T. Rüedi

Intra-articular fractures of the distal tibia were already observed a century ago, as nicely illustrated in a textbook of that time. At the same time, around the turn of the century, the Belgian surgeon Albin Lambotte even demonstrated how these fractures should be treated by stable internal fixation – with screws and plates – to allow early mobilization. Unfortunately, Lambotte's personal series of highly successful operative fracture management could not be reproduced by others, and most attempts at internal fixation ended with sepsis, fusion, or even amputation.

The choice of treatment for decades thereafter was either prolonged traction through the calcaneus or primary fusion of the ankle. Until the 1960s the results were consistently poor after nonoperative as well as operative treatment (although Sir John Charnley stated that "in the case of intra-articular fractures good results could only be expected after anatomical restoration and freedom of joint movement, both of which required internal fixation").

In the late 1950s the pioneers of the Swiss AO group started to apply their new implants and techniques based on Danis' principle of interfragmentary compression. As demonstrated by Rüedi and Allgöwer as well as Heim and others, open reduction and internal fixation (ORIF), if performed properly, can lead to consistently good functional results in about 75% of cases. Post-traumatic osteoarthritis usually manifests itself early, within 1–2 years after the accident. If after that interval the functional result is still good, it may be expected to remain so for many years to come. This is illustrated by a patient of Dr. Allgöwer, who after ORIF returned to full activity as a skiing instructor. At a recent follow-up some 22 years later the patient showed no signs of osteoarthritis and was still an enthusiastic skier.

Already in the early days, but even more so after a considerable learning curve, four principles of treatment were established and their strict application considered essential in order to obtain a good result:

1. Reconstruction of fibula fracture
2. Restitution of articular surface of tibia
3. Autologous bone graft
4. Medial buttress of tibia

Despite of repeated warnings, the optimistic reports of the Swiss AO group unfortunately encouraged numerous 'knife-happy' surgeons around the world to do the same. The results were often disastrous. It soon became evident, that the importance of the soft tissues and their careful handling of was generally underestimated by most surgeons. Anatomical reconstruction of the joint and stable fixation is only part of the whole operation. Gentle soft tissue handling and careful skin closure are of paramount importance for a good, uneventful postoperative outcome.

Where do we stand today, 25 years after the AO group's first report? Perfect anatomical reconstruction (other than in the diaphysis) is still considered the most important goal in articular fractures, and interfragmentary compression as the basic principle of stable internal fixation remains the only way to maintain reduction and to allow early movement. Bone loss must be replaced by either autologous bone or ceramics.

The four basic principles have remained the same, but a number of tactical changes have been introduced in recognition of the fact that the original Swiss experience and expertise were obtained mainly from a rather homogeneous population of mostly young skiers, who were in the hospital and ready for surgery within a few hours of their accident.

Few other surgeons have had the similar fortune to deal with such an ideal patient population. In most instances patients are admitted some time after their accident when they have already developed problematic soft tissue conditions. This is particularly true of the elderly pedestrian hit by a vehicle or the workman injured at work, who arrives with a full-thickness skin contusion or open injuries.

Under such circumstances surgery has to be minimized or postponed. In order to maintain temporary reduction, several techniques have been advocated:

1. Conventional traction with a calcaneal pin
2. External fixator between talus and tibia
3. ORIF of the fibula and external fixator between talus and tibia
4. Percutaneous adaptation of articular fragments with Kirschner wires or canulated screws in combination with an external fixator
5. Combinations of the above

The aim of all these techniques (except the first) is to immobilize the fracture area while the soft tissues recover, and yet allow movement of the limb. Once edema has subsided, classical ORIF can be accomplished more safely.

Especially in delayed cases it is advisable to apply different techniques of gentle indirect reduction as described in detail by Mast et al. [1].

As far as implants are concerned, most of us have stopped using the bulky 4.5/6.5 mm screws and plates, as similarly good fixation can be obtained with 3.5/4.0 mm implants – especially in combination with a reinforced cloverleaf plate.

In young and cooperative patients with a good quality of bone and large fracture fragments, screw fixation alone may be sufficient. A further possibility for improving the support within the impacted epi- and metaphyseal area is to use a large corticocancellous wedge graft, as has been described for the tibial plateau [2]. The better mechanical properties of this graft allow earlier loading of the injured limb, so that practically no casts are applied any more and in cooperative patients partial weight-bearing can be started as early as 6 weeks postoperatively.

Although today we see considerably more open pilon fractures, and also more in older patients, our overall results have not changed much. Around 75% of cases are considered as having a good or acceptable outcome. We believe, therefore, that these fractures do profit from ORIF, provided it is tactically and technically performed correctly.

References

1. Mast J, Jakob R, Ganz R (1989) Planning and reduction technique in fracture surgery. Springer, Berlin Heidelberg New York
2. Rüedi T (1989) Treatment of displaced metaphyseal fractures with screws and wiring systems. Orthopedics 12:55–59

Pilon Fractures of the Distal Tibia: A Test of Surgical Judgment

J. Mast

Introduction

Intra-articular fractures of the distal tibia are difficult fractures to manage [1, 6–11, 13, 31, 40]. In the 1960s, in the hands of certain members of the AO group, successful surgical treatment of this group of fractures was carried out. By the 1970s, papers on operative management based on the AO principles began to appear in the British orthopedic literature [14, 15, 34–37]. These clinical studies were optimistic about what might be expected to be achieved by the application of the AO group's methods. Until these references appeared British literature on the pilon fracture was, at best, cautionary to pessimistic. Jergesen, of California, typified this thinking when in his article "Fractures of the Ankle", written in 1959 [19], he stated that "explosion fractures of the distal end of the tibia were not amenable to open reduction and internal fixation". Later papers by Leach [23], Sheck [39] and Rouff and Shnider [4] tried to illustrate through limited clinical studies, techniques that had been helpful to the authors in their attempts to salvage ankles in patients with these fractures. These techniques were directed toward internal fixation of the fibula as an isolated event, and preoperative planning with isolated percutaneous fixation of the major articular fragments.

In the 1980s there appeared to be a controversy over the results that could be obtained with this fracture. The AO literature remained quite optimistic, with Rüedi and Allgöwer [35–78], Heim and Naser [15], and Hackenbruch [14] reporting results in the 80% good/excellent range. At the same time other authors such as Kellam and Waddell [20], Maale and Seligson [24], Pierce and Heinrich [33], Ovadia and Beals [31], Bourne et al. [4], and Teeney and Wiss [41] were less optimistic, sharing the view that the pure compression type of fracture (type C Rüedi-Allgöwer) had a relatively dismal complication rate and, frequently, suboptimal end results (Fig. 1).

There is no doubt that many surgeons have had problems achieving success in the operative treatment of these fractures, as anyone involved in a referral type of reconstructive practice knows. How do we interpret these variations of clinical experience in the 1990s? The advances that have been made in internal fixation have allowed us to offer our patients an improved chance of an almost full functional recovery from many fractures that would not have been successfully treated by other means [2]. The problem is that in many areas in the United States the level of sophistication of operative fracture care remains surprisingly low.

Hospitals, for many reasons, do not have the variety of instruments and implants necessary to carry out successful operative interventions on difficult fractures such as the pilon of the tibia. In addition, perhaps due to a low level of interest in fracture surgery, local hospital staff surgeons, taking rotating accident surgery call as a requirement of hospital privileges, often lack the expertise to recognize and treat the problems that accompany this fracture (Fig. 2). Unfortunately the injuries that may present to the Emergency Department can be devastating and even the highly experienced fracture surgeon may do well if the patient escapes only with complications of treatment such as a deformity to be corrected at a later time, or a pseudoarthrosis, or even an arthrodesis (Fig. 3).

Frequently the patient is a young person with a high-energy, open articular fracture with severe fragmentation of the joint surface coupled with a low fibula fracture segmentally comminuted at the syndesmosis. What have we learned in the past decades to be the safest yet most effective way to guide such a patient through the treatment of the injury and subsequent rehabilitation.

Soft Tissue Assessment

Increasing sophistication of methods of documenting associated soft tissue injuries has definitely improved our ability to determine the appropriateness of various treatment alternatives. These schemes have been developed independently by Tscherne and Gotzen [40], and Border et al. [3]. They are presented in the AO manual [29].

More extensive soft tissue involvement requires a modification of usual methods of treatment. In fact, extensive injuries involving muscle–tendon units and neurovascular structures require that treatment is also directed to correction of these deficits along with modification of the standard approaches of fracture care.

Radiographs

Good quality anteroposterior, lateral, and oblique radiographs are mandatory. In addition, preoperative planning requires comparison views of the sound extremity [28]. Additional studies such as tomography, and CT scans with three-dimensional reconstruction may be useful in selected cases. Imaging of this type allows a precise classification of the injury to be made, and is helpful in developing the preoperative plan.

Many classification schemes have been proposed, for fractures of the distal tibial articular surface [1, 9, 20–22, 24, 26, 29, 31, 32, 35–38]. The extended AO morphological classification allows a better appreciation of the fracture problems which need to be overcome. This may influence the surgeon to modify the standard approach that he would use on a type A or B fracture once he realizes that he is dealing with a problem fracture of type C [29]. The preoperative plan should include not only a drawing of "the desired end result", but also the method for achieving the reduction [27] (Fig. 4).

Timing of Surgery and Surgical Approach

It is well known that the optimum time for surgical intervention is during the first 4–8 h after injury. After that time interstitial edema becomes apparent and jeopardizes the safety of the surgical wound over the anteromedial distal tibia (Fig. 5). The classic AO surgical approach to the distal tibia has been a problem in the hands of many surgeons [4, 31, 33, 41]. Marginal necrosis of the medial edge of the wound is not uncommon, and when it occurs with the base of the wound over the anterior tibial tendon, it becomes difficult to manage. This is because the tendon becomes exposed and, with time, desiccated. Ultimately it becomes infected, requiring debridement. In the vast majority of instances this starts a sequence of events leading to an eventual bone or joint infection. For many years the author has been modifying the classic AO anteromedial approach by straightening it out somewhat, and crossing over the front of the leg from medial distally to lateral proximally at the level of the tibialis anterior muscle belly. The deep portion of the incision is made transretinacular distally and is extended at the level of the joint capsule as far laterally as necessary, even to the anterior tibial tubercle of Chaput, deep to the tendons and anterior neurovascular bundle. Care is taken to produce no superficial flaps through undermining the area between the subcutaneous tissue and the fascia, and to leave intact the soft tissue attachments to fragments in the fracture zone.

If the patient presents more than 8 h after the injury, or if there are extenuating circumstances, the patient is placed in calcaneal traction on a Böhler frame with elevation of the leg until the skin wrinkles, which signifies that the inflammatory edema has resolved. This usually takes from 7 to 10 days. During this period helpful information may be obtained from anteroposterior and lateral radiographs in traction. If the fracture is reducing with the pull of the calcaneal pin, it is a good prognostic sign. It indicates that distraction techniques carried out during the surgical procedure may be expected to be helpful in reducing the fracture [28] (Fig. 6). If reduction does not occur during the period of calcaneal traction, the presence of interposition of tendons or other significant structures within the fracture fragments must be suspected, as well as marked impaction.

Internal Fixation

The standard approach to the pilon fracture has been well described by Rüedi and Allgöwer [35–38], and reinforced and restated at countless AO courses. Unfortunately, the full realization of all the steps may not be achievable in every clinical situation or in all fracture types. As has been mentioned above, individual circumstances may call for a modification of the methods employed. Some of these alternative maneuvers are described below.

Reduction and Fixation of the Fibula

Under almost all circumstances (the exception being when the fibula is segmentally fragmented beyond recognition of known landmarks) the fibula can be reduced and stably fixed. Because of the ligamentous attachments of this bone to the fracture fragments of the tibia, an improvement in the articular fragments of the tibia may be expected to occur. As has been noted, several authors have described using only this step as a definitive treatment [23, 34]. In principle the method is unacceptable as a definitive treatment, because it does not fulfill the requirements of stability to allow early return of functional activity to the ankle joint. However, under certain circumstances, such as compromised medial soft tissues or a pulverized tibial articular surface, this method alone or, preferably, in combination with a logically proportioned medially mounted external fixator, may be employed as a temporary step in a staged procedure, or as a definitive treatment [17] (Fig. 7).

Reconstruction of the Articular Surface

Reconstruction of the joint in most cases is significantly easier using the principles of ligamentotaxis [5]. As has been mentioned above, an indication as to the efficacy of this technique can be gained by observing the effect of calcaneal pin traction on the reduction of the displaced articular surface.
The benefit of such an approach is that one is always operating in an environment of relative stability. Each step further stabilizes the fracture until it is fixed. All this is accomplished because of the soft tissue attachments, not in spite of them. Having arrived at a reduction through ligamentotaxis, stabilization on a temporary basis may be achieved by the application of large-diameter clamps, one point being placed against the bony fragment through the wound, the other percutaneously against the bone on the other side of the fracture. Ultimately the clamp points, which contact the fracture fragments and hold the reduction, serve as indicators for the location of lag screws. The lag screws are inserted percutaneously where appropriate, using the sleeve system of the standard external fixation set (Fig. 8).

Cancellous Bone Graft

The addition of a cancellous bone graft to support a reduced articular fragment that has been impacted into the epi-metaphysis may be likened to a true biological buttressing implant.
Because the cancellous bone graft is contributing to the stability of the fixation, it is generally of benefit to use it at the time of the original open reduction. In the case of a contaminated open fracture it is prudent to delay bone grafting until the time of secondary closure. Antibiotic-impregnated methylmethacrylate cement as temporary filling may then be employed to give support to the

reduced articular surface. These fillings may be removed and replaced by autogenous cancellous bone graft at or after the time of definitive wound closure.

Medial Buttress Plate

A medial buttress plate supports the fractured tibial metaphysis and prevents a late varus deformity. In cases associated with medial soft tissue damage the use of such a plate may be too precarious. The buttressing function can be carried out using a mini-external fixator, 4.0-mm Schanz screws being inserted into the anteromedial surface of the tibial diaphysis proximally and into the reconstructed articular block distally. The Schanz screws are then connected by two adjustable clamps and a 4.0-mm connecting rod. Such a montage may be used as the definitive fixation. The external fixator can usually be removed after 6–8 weeks, as bony consolidation precludes the need for buttressing.
When there is no possibility of anchoring the frame directly to the distal fragment, the joint may be spanned and the distal tibia neutralized by a frame mounted from the tibia to the os calcis [5, 44]. Definitive soft tissue reconstruction, bone grafting, and buttress plating can then be carried out as a delayed procedure over the ensuing several weeks [17].

Wound Closure

Frequently the problems begin when the bone work is completed. The problem presents as a loss of elasticity of the wound edges, which will no longer mobilize easily over the anteromedial aspect of the tibia. To leave the wound open means leaving the implant exposed. In such cases it is usually possible to close the wound over the tibia with 4.0 nylon suture. Vertical mattress-type suture with an Allgöwer modification will generally allow a good approximation of the dermis even under these circumstances provided the lateral wound is left open.
The fibular plate is left covered by closing the posterior margin of the anterior fibular wound edge to the anterior margin of the peroneal longus muscle belly. In the distal aspect of the lateral wound it is usually possible to close skin to skin in a similar fashion as with the tibial wound. A delayed or primary split-thickness skin graft based on the exposed peroneal musculature completes the reconstruction of the soft tissue sleeve.
In the worst circumstances the wounds may be left open and an occlusive or biological dressing applied together with a thickly padded compressive dressing and a splint to hold the ankle at 90°. Postoperatively the extremity is elevated and a delayed primary closure carried out at 3–5 days. If needed, a delayed local rotational flap or a remote free vascularized flap may be employed for coverage.

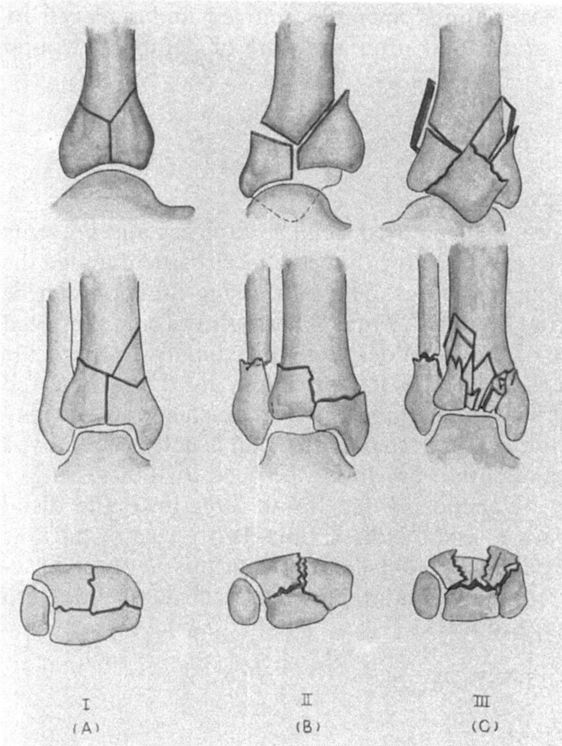

Fig. 1. Classification of pilon fractures according to Rüedi and Allgöwer. Type A, a simple cleavage fracture without intra-articular involvement. Type B, intra-articular displacement with little comminution. Type C, intra-articular displacement with marked comminution

Fig. 2. **a, b** Anteroposterior (AP) and oblique radiographs of a 43-year-old woman with a Grade I open fracture of the distal tibia. There is comminution at the level of the joint and mild displacement. **c, d** Oblique radiographs of the immediate postoperative result. The patient had been taken to surgery where irrigation and debridement had been carried out. The fixation had been obtained by a half tubular plate seen on the fibula and bent threaded Steinmann pins through the medial malleolus into the tibial diaphysis. The articular fracture was fixed by a single lag screw. The choice of implants implied a poor understanding of the principles of internal fixation. The implants were not in harmony with the size of the bone, the screws were haphazardly placed, and the use of an epiphyseal to diaphyseal intramedullary fixation caused a displacement of the epiphysis in the lateral direction. The result of this surgery, not surprisingly, was postoperative wound slough along the medial aspect of the leg, infection, and necrosis of bone in the area of the medial metaphysis. ▶

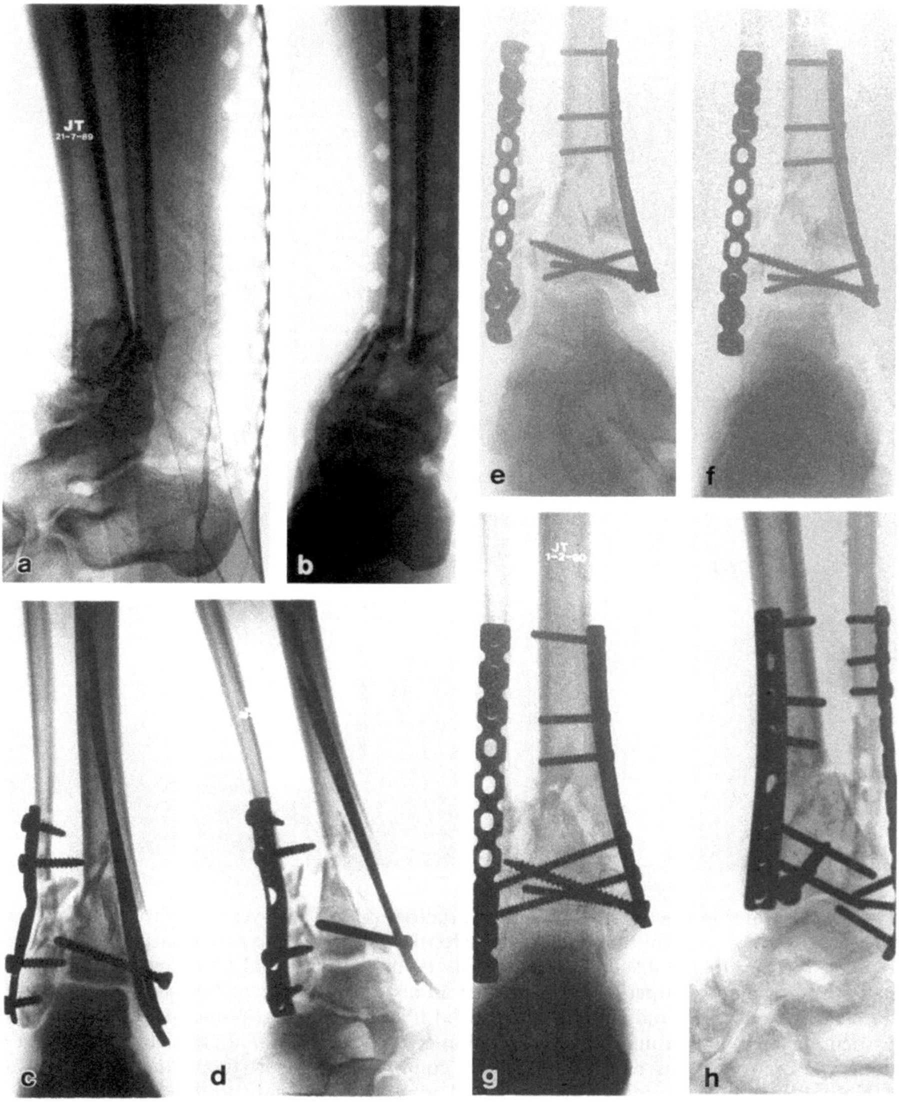

Fig. 2 *(continued)*. **e, f** AP and oblique radiographs of the distal tibia and fibula. Reconstruction of this significant problem consisted of removal of the fibular plate and posterior bridge plating of the fibula at length, the area of necrotic metaphyseal cortex and plugging of the defect with antibiotic-impregnated methylmethacrylate cement, and buttress plating of the medial tibia with a 3.5 DC plate and screws. Coverage was obtained simultaneously with a free flap from the rectus abdominus. **g, h** Six weeks later, with maturing of the free flap, the final surgical procedure was carried out. During this procedure the methylmethacrylate antibiotic spacer was removed and replaced by autogenous cancellous bone graft. Stability was obtained by transyndesmotic screws traversing the distal tibial epiphyseal fragment and finding purchase in the fibula. The patient subsequently went on to heal, and the metal has been removed. The patient's function is excellent with 15° of dorsiflexion, 30° of plantar flexion

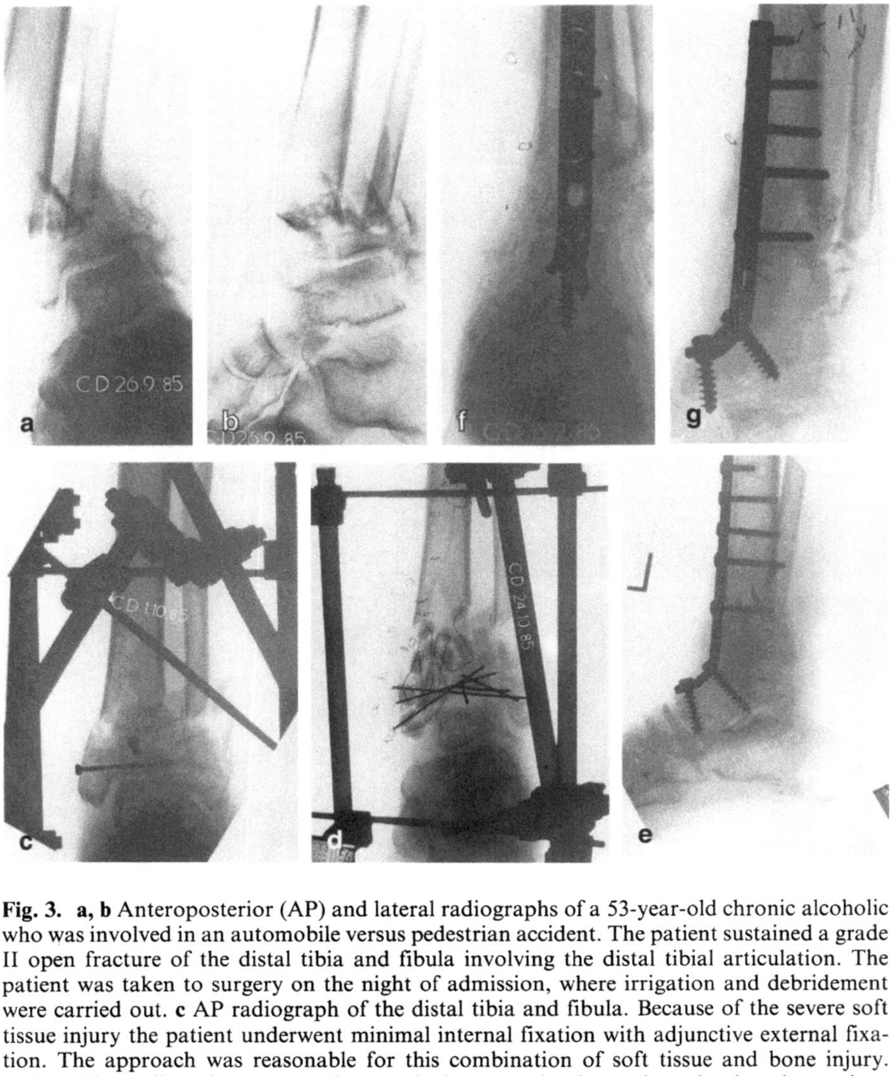

Fig. 3. **a, b** Anteroposterior (AP) and lateral radiographs of a 53-year-old chronic alcoholic who was involved in an automobile versus pedestrian accident. The patient sustained a grade II open fracture of the distal tibia and fibula involving the distal tibial articulation. The patient was taken to surgery on the night of admission, where irrigation and debridement were carried out. **c** AP radiograph of the distal tibia and fibula. Because of the severe soft tissue injury the patient underwent minimal internal fixation with adjunctive external fixation. The approach was reasonable for this combination of soft tissue and bone injury. **d** Notwithstanding the conservative surgical approach, the patient developed a serious postoperative infection requiring debridement, removal of necrotic bone and the use of methylmethacrylate antibiotic beads. The screws were removed, and the thin bony plates remaining were stabilized as well as possible with Kirschner wires. **e** On the third surgical intervention, approximately 3 months after the original injury, the patient's ankle was arthrodesed. The arthrodesis was accomplished by a cancellous bone graft between the talus and the tibia and an anterior plate. Soft tissue coverage was obtained by a free flap. **f, g** The final result after the arthrodesis had healed, 5 months after the original injury. This example illustrates a difficult case which was managed initially by external fixation with limited internal fixation in anticipation of problems. Nevertheless, despite the original good decision-making, a problem developed because of the severe soft tissue injury. In the end this problem was solved by a free tissue transfer and an arthrodesis. The final result was successful, and the patient had a functionally good extremity despite an arthrodesis of the ankle joint

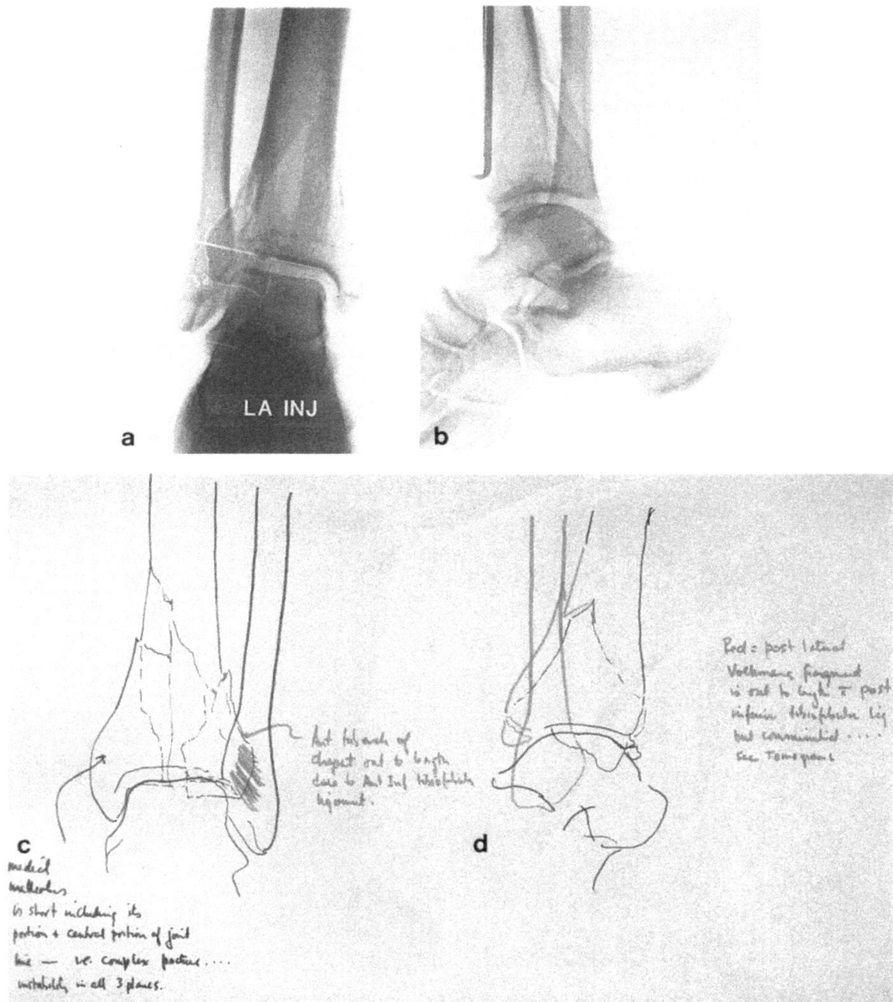

Fig. 4. a, b A closed type B fracture of the pilon in a 38-year-old. On the anteroposterior (AP) view, the radiographic shadow of the anterior tibial tubercle can be seen, which is at length because of the intact syndesmotic ligaments. **c, d** Tracings of the AP and lateral radiographs. The problem was identified on the tracings, and that was that during surgery the medial fragment of the distal tibia had to be brought out to length, reducing the talus underneath the intact portion of the anterolateral joint surface. With this landmark as reference, reduction and fixation of the distal tibial articular surface were correct from the standpoint of length. To accomplish this an AO femoral distractor was used. **e–j** see p. 16

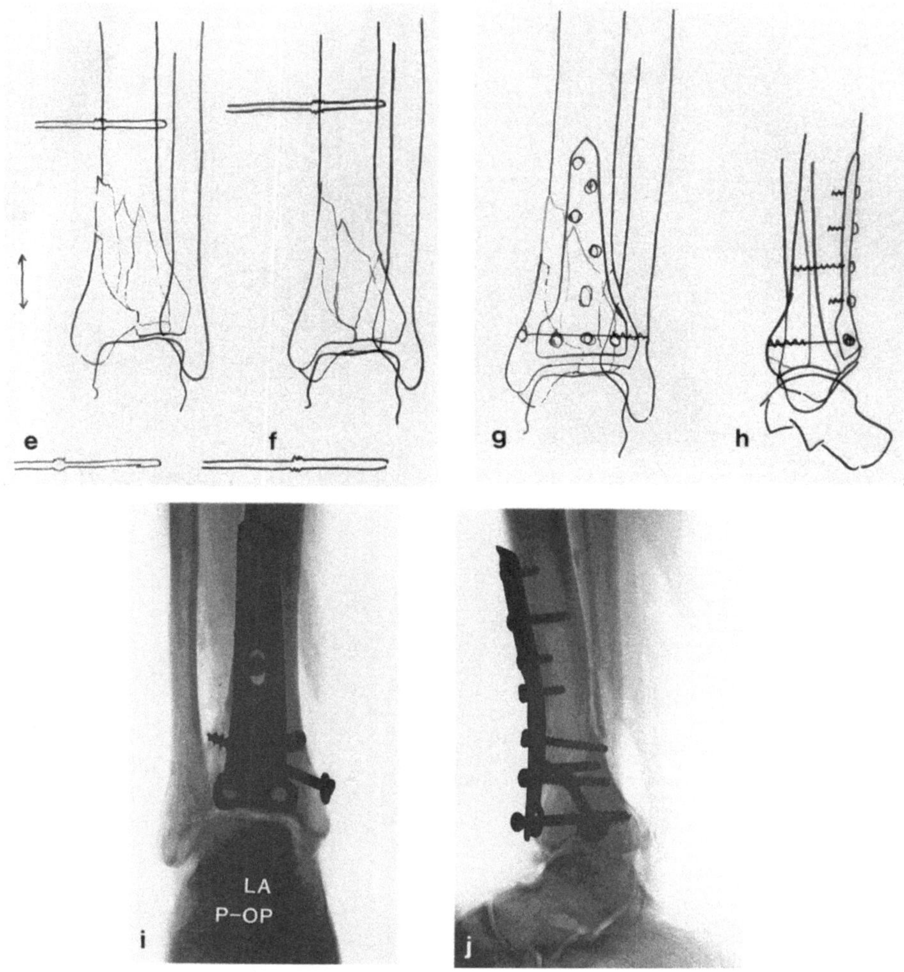

Fig. 4 *(continued)*. **e, f** Schematic drawing of the same fracture with the femoral distractor included. This first regained by distraction. By doing this, the medial fragment is adjusted until the subchondral line reduction is complete and, following this, fixation accomplished. This illustrates the method that will be used to obtain reduction. **g, h** The drawing of the desired end result utilizing an anterior spoon plate and a transverse lag screw from the medial malleolar fragment to Chaput's tubercle. **i, j** The postoperative result, which reveals the execution of the essential steps of the preoperative planning

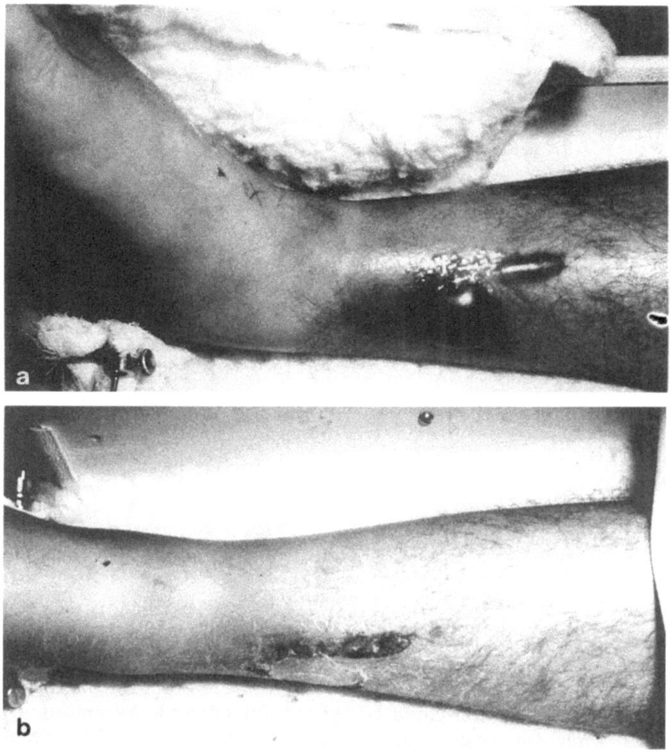

Fig. 5. **a** Clinical photograph of the leg of a patient with a distal intra-articular fracture of the tibia. Two days after the operation the patient has developed edema and secondary fracture blisters. It is obvious that a surgical intervention at this time would not be wise. **b** The same patient viewed after 10 days of calcaneal pin traction in a modified Böhler-Braun frame. The fracture blisters have subsided. The skin has dried and has begun to wrinkle. Although some of the elasticity of the soft tissues has been lost, the leg is now safe for an operative intervention

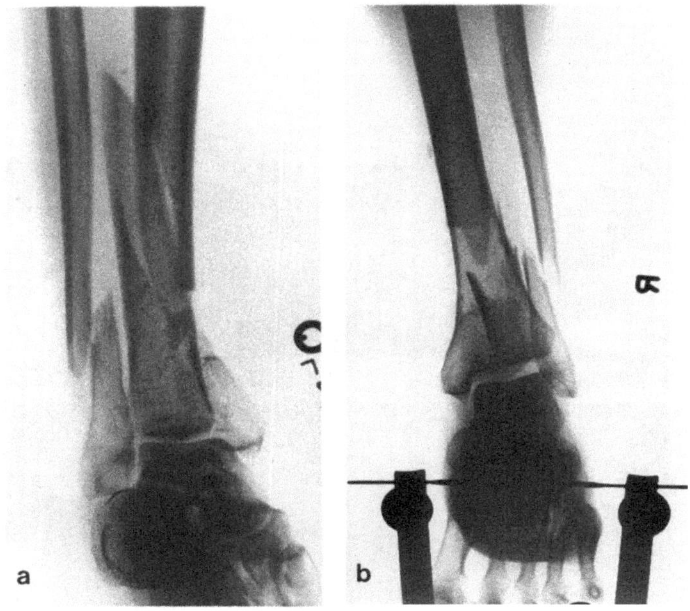

Fig. 6. **a** A type B pilon fracture in the preoperative displaced position. Because of the delay in reaching the emergency room and concomitant soft tissue swelling, the patient was placed in calcaneal traction on a Böhler-Braun frame in order for the swelling to subside so that an operative intervention could be carried out safely. **b** An anteroposterior (AP) radiograph taken while the patient was in calcaneal traction. Note how the fracture has practically anatomically reduced during the holding period. This is a good prognostic sign as it means an indirect reduction technique with distraction should be equally successful in reducing the fracture during surgery

Fig. 7. **a–c** Anteroposterior (AP), oblique, and lateral radiographs of a type B pilon fracture. This fracture was associated with severe soft tissue contusion which contraindicated an immediate operative intervention. **d, e** Calcaneal pin traction was instituted on a Böhler-Braun frame. Note the improvement of the reduction of the joint with distraction. Again, this is a very good prognostic sign. **f–i** see pp. 20/21 ▶

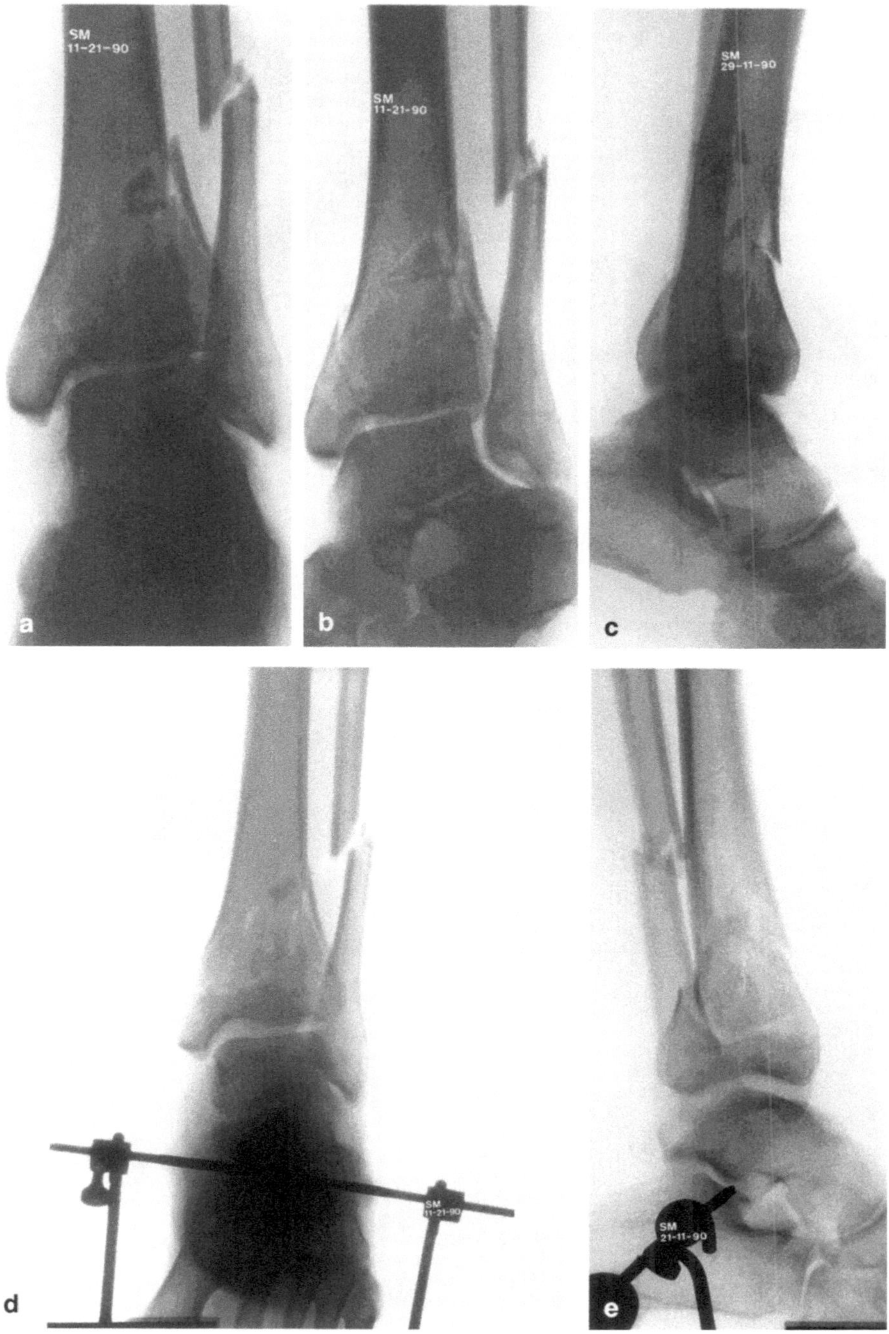
SM
11-21-90
a
SM
11-21-90
b
SM
29-11-90
c
d
SM
11-21-90
SM
21-11-90
e

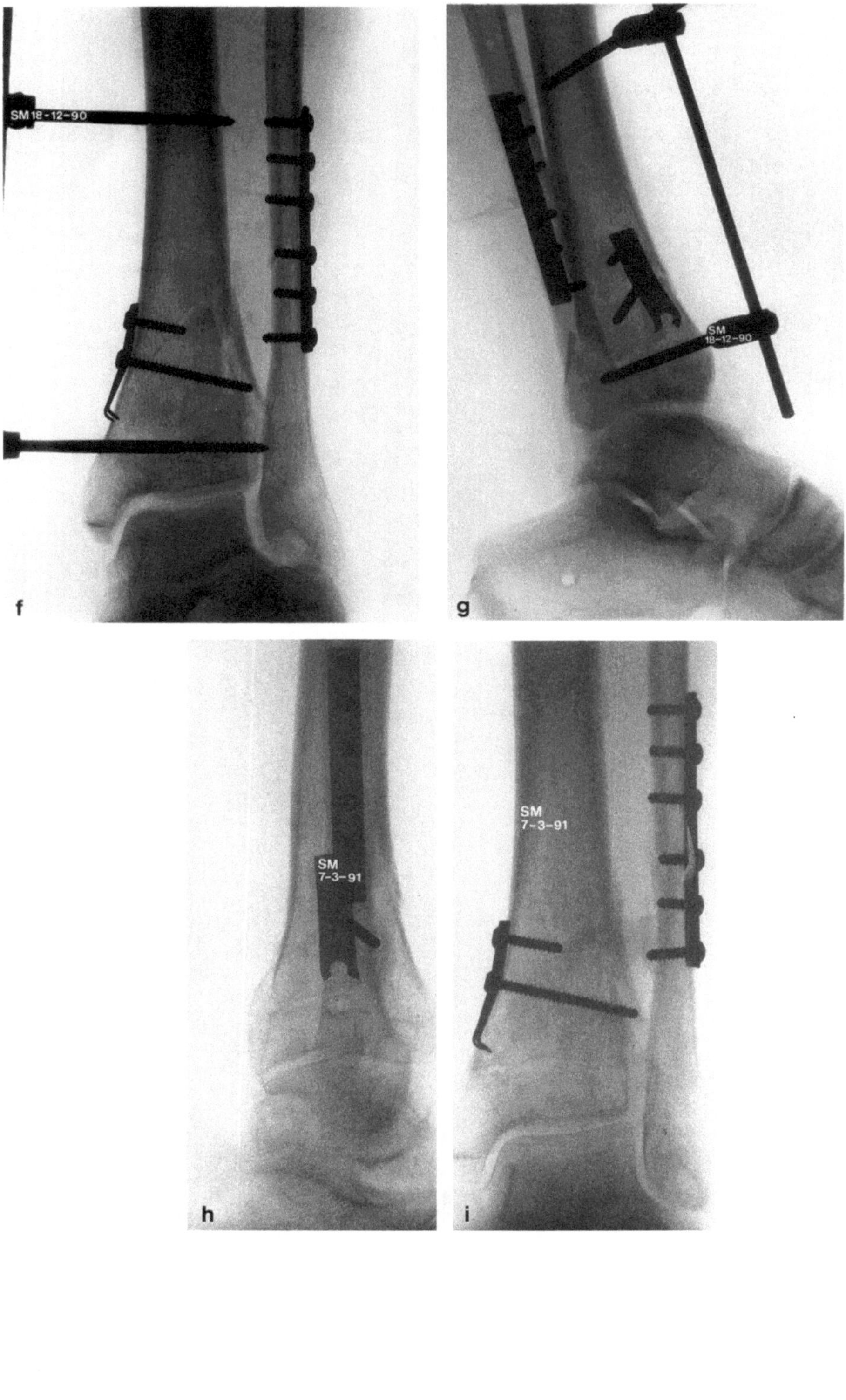
SM 18-12-90
f
SM
18-12-90
g
SM
7-3-91
h
SM
7-3-91
i

◀ **Fig. 7** *(continued)*. **f, g** At 10 days, the patient's leg was felt to be in an optimal condition for an operative intervention. Nevertheless, the soft tissue injury had left a residual full-thickness defect medially at the level of the medial malleolus. Therefore, it was elected to proceed with fixed reduction and fixation of the fibula, minimal internal fixation at the level of the metaphyseal instability, and neutralization with a mini-external fixator. These radiographs show the postoperative results approximately 1 month after the fracture. **h, i** AP and lateral views approximately 3 months after the injury. The fractures have healed. Although the patient is slightly osteoporotic, he has had functional treatment and has an excellent range of motion equal to that on the opposite side. The third-degree defect over the medial malleolus healed by secondary means

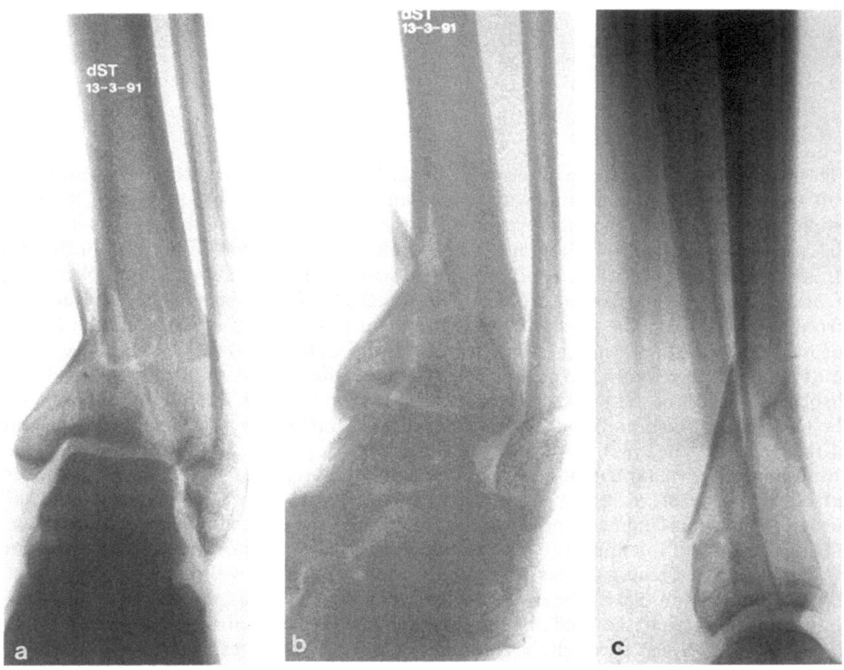

Fig. 8. a–c A type B pilon fracture. This fracture clearly had a supination adduction mechanism. There is a low fibular fracture at the level of the joint. There is a lateral gap of the articular surface along with the supramalleolar fracture with displacement of the medial malleolus upwardly and inwardly. Although the lateral column is fractured, it is relatively nondisplaced. There is a diaphyseal extension. **d–l** see pp. 22–25

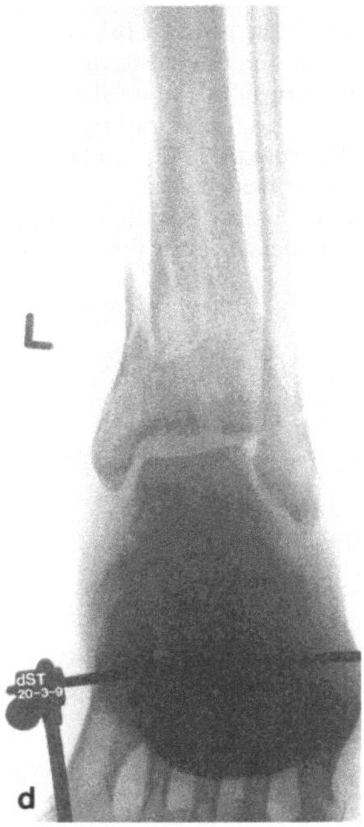

Fig. 8 *(continued)*. **d** Because of the delay in reaching the emergency room, there was enough soft tissue swelling to contraindicate immediate surgery. Therefore, calcaneal traction was employed. Once more, the information as to the ease of reduction during surgery is seen in the anteroposterior (AP) radiograph taken while the patient was in traction in the Böhler-Braun frame. Again, this is a good prognostic sign. **e, f** Preoperative tracings of the original fracture in the AP and lateral projections respectively. The *arrows* in the AP tracing point (from left to right) to the possibility of entrapment of the posterior tibial tendon behind the medial malleolus, the opening in the metaphysis through which autogenous cancellous bone graft may be inserted into the metaphysis to support the epiphysis once it is reduced, and the displaced portion of the joint which must be corrected through the fracture before reducing the metaphyseal comminution. On the lateral view, the *arrows* point to these same features of the fracture. The *lower arrow* posteriorly shows the possibility of posterior tibial tendon entrapment, the metaphyseal comminution, and the area that will be used to reduce the intra-articular fracture and to support it with bone graft. The *arrow inside* on the displaced posterior articular fragment indicates the fracture fragment needing an articular reduction. **g** Diagram illustrating application of the medium-sized distractor that will enable reduction by distraction. **h** Tracing of the desired end result. The fibula will be approached first and fixed with a tension plate. The distractor will then be applied as shown in the diagram, and following distraction the medial buttress plate will be applied to cause reduction of the displaced metaphysis. Through the comminuted metaphyseal area, reduction of the epiphysis may be carried out along with bone grafting. The lag screws in the diagram will be placed percutaneously. ►

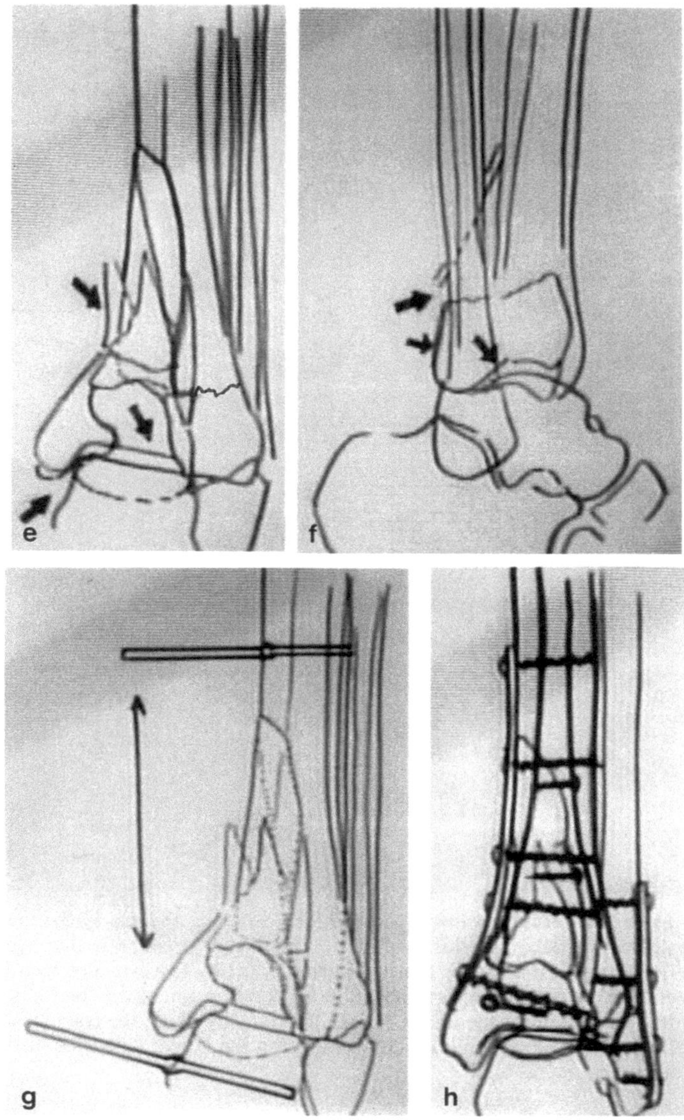
e
f
g
h

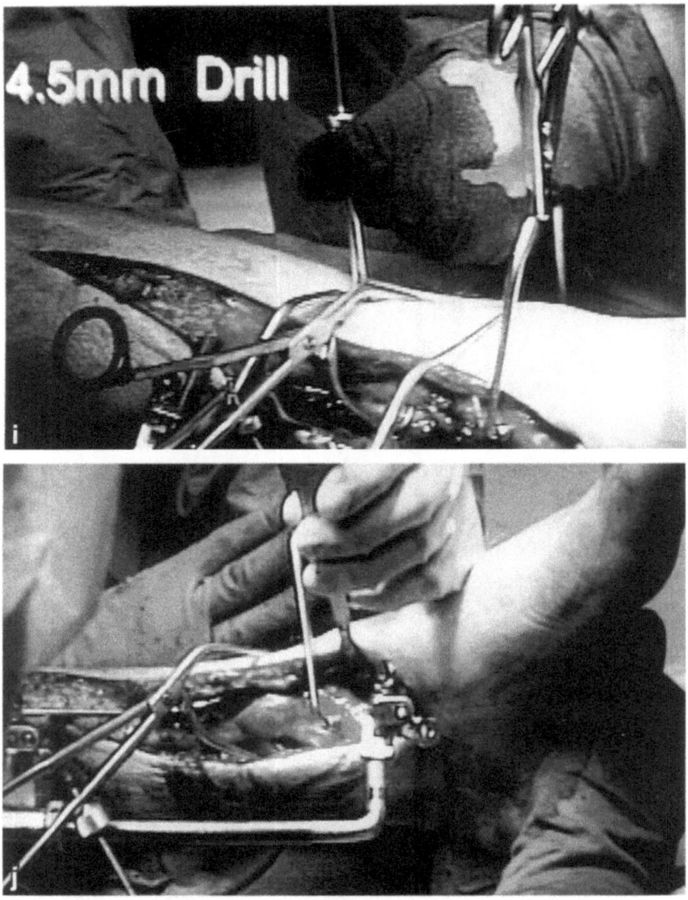

Fig. 8 *(continued)*. **i** Intraoperative view showing the use of Synthes external fixator drill sleeves to place anterior-to-posterior lag screws fixing the diaphyseal component of the fracture percutaneously. Synthes pelvic reduction forceps, also seen here, serve as excellent clamps for percutaneous application for stabilization of the fractures. **j** Another intraoperative view showing the use of clamps temporarily fixing the fracture lines on the medial side through the wound and percutaneously on the lateral side. The medium-sized distractor is also seen in this view.

Conclusion

Successful management of tibial pilon fractures requires significant experience in fracture surgery.

Problems resulting from this fracture can be divided into two categories: those related to the surgeon and his environment, and those related to the severity of the fracture itself. The first group of problems have been and will continue to be addressed by continuing education, but as long as the present arrange-

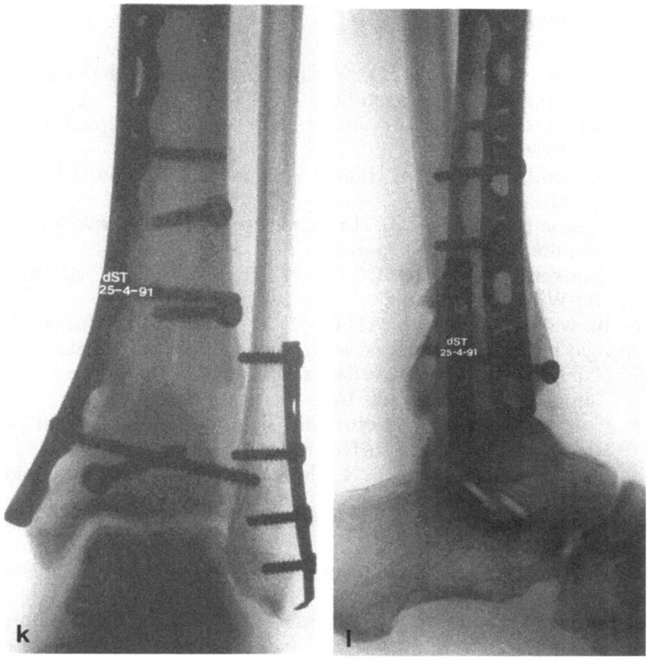

Fig. 8 *(continued)*. **k, l** AP and lateral views of the postoperative result taken 6 weeks after the fracture. With this type of surgical technique the bone remains attached to its soft tissue connection. Bone union is rapid and, frequently, healing is convincingly present in as little as 6 weeks after the injury. The patient's function at this time was excellent

ments in the United States exist for the coverage of accident surgery in community hospitals there will be a wide variation in the standard of care. Difficult fractures with bad prognostic characteristics must be handled with techniques that enable the special circumstances present to be dealt with. In these cases the goal must be to avoid making matters worse by the accumulation of surgical complications. Some techniques to allow individual modification of the basic principles in management of this fracture have been discussed. If complications can be avoided, late surgical reconstruction can frequently yield very satisfactory end results.

References

1. Ashurst A, Bromer R (1922) Classification and mechanisms of fractures of the leg bones involving the ankle. Arch Surg 4:51
2. Bone L (1987) Fractures of the tibial plafond. The pilon fractures. Orthop Clin North Am 18:95–104
3. Border J, Allgöwer M, Hansen S, Rüedi T. Blunt multiple trauma. Dekker, New York, pp 441–448
4. Bourne RB, Rorabeck CH, Nacnab J (1983) Intraarticular fractures of the distal tibia; the pilon fracture. J Trauma 23:591–596
5. Brooker AG, Edwards CC (1979) External fixation – current state of the art. Williams and Wilkins, Baltimore
6. Burwell HN, Charnley AD (1965) The treatment of displaced fractures at the ankle by rigid internal fixation and early joint movement. J Bone Joint Surg 47:634
7. Childress HM (1976) Vertical transarticular pin fixation for unstable ankle fractures. Clin Orthop Rel Res 120:164
8. Coonrad RW (1970) Fracture-dislocations of the ankle joint with impaction injury of the lateral weight bearing surface of the tibia. J Bone Joint Surg 52:1337
9. Dabezies E, D'Ambrosia R, Shoji H (1978) Classification and treatment of ankle fractures. Orthopedics 1:365
10. Decoulx P, Razemon JP, Rousdelle Y (1961) Fractures du pilon tibial. Rev Chir Orthop 47:563
11. Destot E (1911) Traumatismes de pied et rayons X malléoles, astragale, calcaneum, avant pied. Masson, Paris
12. Franklin JL, Johnson KD, Hansen ST (1984) Immediate internal fixation of open ankle fractures; report of thirty-eight cases treated with a standard protocol. J Bone Joint Surg [Am] 66:1349–1356
13. Gay R, Evard J (1961) Les fractures récentes du pilon chez l'adulte. Rev Chir Orthop 49:397
14. Hackenbruch W (1977) Die Pilon-Fraktur des Skifahrers. Fortschr Med 95:219 (English abstr)
15. Heim V, Naser M (1876) Die operative Behandlung der Pilon-Tibial-Fraktur. Technik der Osteosynthese und die Resultate bei 128 Patienten. Arch Orthop Unfallchirurg 86:341 (English abstr)
16. Heim V, Pfeiffer KM (1974) Small fragment set manual. Springer, Berlin Heidelberg New York
17. Montzsch D, Karnatz N, Jansen T (1990) One- or two-step management (with external fixator) of severe pilon-tibial fractures. Aktuel Traumatol 20:199–204
18. Jahna H, Wittich H, Hartenstein H (1980) Der distale Stauchungsbruch der Tibia. Unfallheilkunde [Suppl] 137:1
19. Jergesen F (1959) Fractures of the ankle. Am J Surg 98:136
20. Kellam JG, Waddell JP (1979) Fractures of the distal tibial metaphysis with intra-articular extension: the distal tibial explosion fracture. J Trauma 19:593
21. Lauge-Hansen N (1952) Fractures of the ankle: IV. Clinical use of genetic Roentgen diagnosis and genetic reduction. Arch Surg 64:488
22. Lauge-Hansen N (1953) Fractures of the ankle: V. Pronation-dorsiflexion fracture. Arch Surg 67:813
23. Leach IRE (1964) A means of stabilizing comminuted distal tibial fractures. J Trauma 4:722
24. Maale G, Seligson D (1980) Fractures through the weightbearing surface of the distal tibia. Orthopedics 3:517
25. Mast JW, Spiegel PG (1984) Complex ankle fractures. In: Meyers MH (ed) The multiply injured patient with complex fractures. Lea and Febiger, Philadelphia
26. Mast J, Spiegel PG, Pappas J (1988) Fractures of the tibial pilon. Clin Orthop 230:68–82

27. Mast JW (1987) Reduction techniques in fractures of the distal tibial articular surface. Techniques Orthop Surg 2/3:29–36
28. Mast JW, Jakob R, Ganz R (1989) Planning and reduction techniques in fracture surgery. Springer, Berlin Heidelberg New York
29. Müller ME, Allgöwer M, Schneider R, Willenegger H (1990) Manual of internal fixation, 3rd edn. Springer, Berlin Heidelberg New York
30. Nelson MC, Jensen NK (1940) The treatment of trimalleolar fractures of the ankle. Surg Gynecol, Obstet 71:509
31. Ovadia DN, Beals RK (1986) Fractures of the tibial plafond. J Bone Joint Surg [Am] 68:543–551
32. Pankovich MM (1979) Adult ankle fractures. J Cont Med Educat Orthop 3:17
33. Pierce RO Jr, Heinrich JH (1979) Comminuted intra-articular fractures of the distal tibia. J Trauma 19:828
34. Rouff AC III, Snider RK (1971) Explosion fractures of the distal tibia with major articular involvement. J Trauma 11:866
35. Rüedi T, Allgöwer M (1979) The operative treatment of intra-articular fractures of the lower end of the tibia. Clin Orthop Rel Res 138:105
36. Rüedi T, Allgöwer M (1969) Fractures of the lower end of the tibia into the ankle joint. Injury 1:92
37. Rüedi T, Allgöwer M (1978) Spätresultate nach operativer Behandlung der Gelenkbrüche am distalen Tibiaende. Sog. Pilon-Frakturen. Unfallheilkunde 81:319 (English abstr)
38. Rüedi T (1973) Fractures of the lower end of the tibia into the ankle joint, results nine years after open reduction and internal fixation. Injury 5:130
39. Scheck M (1965) Treatment of comminuted distal tibial fractures by combined dual pin fixation and limited open reduction. J Bone Joint Surg [Am] 47:1537
40. Tscherne H, Gotzen L (1984) Fractures with soft tissue injuries. Springer, Berlin Heidelberg New York
41. Teeny SM, Wiss DA (1991) Open reduction and internal fixation of tibial plafond fractures: variables contributing to poor results and complications. Presented at annual meeting of American Academy of Orthopedic Surgeons
42. Trojan E, Jahna H, Wittich H, Hartstein H (1980) Der distale Stauchungsbruch der Tibia. Unfallheilkunde [Suppl] 137:1
43. Weber BG (1972) Die Verletzungen des oberen Sprunggelenkes. Han Huber, Stuttgart
44. Weber BG, Brunner CF (1982) Special techniques in internal fixation. Springer, Berlin Heidelberg New York, pp 115–132, 176–179

Morphological Features for Evaluation and Classification of Pilon Tibial Fractures*

U. Heim

Introduction

The term "pilon tibial fractures" must be strictly limited to fractures of the weight-bearing surface of the tibial plafond, as defined by the radiologist Destot [4] in 1911. These lesions are rare and appear in such a diversity that it has always been extremely difficult to classify them.

In 1955, Lorenz Böhler [2] tried to explain the different split fractures according to the position of the foot during the impact (Fig. 1). His drawings show mostly partial fractures. In 1963 Gay and Evrard [5] classified complete fractures, calling them "bicondylar fractures", looking only at the concavity of the plafond (Fig. 2). The typical ski pilon fracture was analyzed in 1970 by Bandi [1], who explained why a sudden deceleration leads to a metaphyseal comminution.

The newly emphasized distinction between "low" and "high" velocity impact is difficult to apply to these lesions: Is a fall from scaffolding high velocity? Is the sudden stop of the foot of a fast skier high velocity? The energy released is certainly sometimes comparable to that resulting from a traffic accident.

Classification Principles

The new principles of classification are based on an analysis of the severity of the injury. This in turn depends on the soft tissue damage and on the morphology of the fracture itself, as visualized by radiographs [10].

Articular fractures are in general divided into two main types:

1. *Type B*. In these a part of the articular surface is not damaged and remains in anatomical contact with the diaphysis.
2. *Type C*. These are complete fractures, which means that there is no anatomical connection between the articulation and the diaphysis. Type C fractures are more unstable and often badly vascularized. The treatment will therefore be more difficult and the prognosis usually worse.

---

* This analysis is based on data at the AO documentation centre in Berne, covering the years 1979 to 1985. It consists of 1077 fractures of the distal tibia segment, 397 being extra-articular type A fractures, 289 being partial articular type B fractures, and 391 being complete articular type C fractures.

Anatomical Aspects

The articular surface of the tibial plafond represents an irregular rectangle, slightly concave in the sagittal plane (Fig. 3a). The modest tibiotalar mobility is practically limited to this plane. There exist neither condylar nor pillar-like structures. The opponent bone, the talus, is a very hard bone with sharp edges. The situation is therefore different from that in the radiocarpal joint, where all articular elements are curved and allow a lot of movement in all planes, and where the radial styloid process participates fully in the transmission of axial forces (Fig. 3b).
For these reasons the schemes of Gay and Evrard [5], which consider only the radiograph in the sagittal plane, and the scheme of Vivès [14], who analyzed the injury only from the frontal plane, do not properly represent reality. As Gay himself stated and showed in his drawings, fracture lines in the tibial plafond are irregular and often oblique or concave.

Morphological Elements

In all articular fractures we first have to consider the basic morphology. The first morphological form is the *split*. Except in cases of extreme displacement the fragments remain in contact with the periosteum or the articular capsule and are thus not devitalized. A proper reduction may be possible by external traction. The split leaves the cartilage nearly intact. Reduced fractures therefore do not lead to posttraumatic arthritis.
The second form is *depression*, caused by the blow of an opposing bony edge (Fig. 4). It is usually combined with a split. This fracture morphology does not exist in all articular fractures. It is most common in the tibial plateau and surprisingly also in articular fractures of the hand and forefoot. A depressed area cannot be reduced by external or indirect means. If reduced by an open reduction, it leaves a defect in the subchondral bone.
When the articular fracture pattern is more complicated, the term *multi-fragmentary* has been introduced [10] to characterize the morphology.

Fracture Patterns in the Tibial Plafond

We will now look at the occurrence of these fracture patterns in the weight-bearing parts of the articular surface of the tibia.
Split fractures are very common (Fig. 5). They cross the articulation in all planes, are often oblique and include the medial malleolus. They may be angulated and very often it is impossible to distinguish clearly between simple or T-shaped fracture lines even with convential radiographs.
In partial articular fractures (type B) the plane of a fracture line can be more or less distinguished because the intact part of the articulation acts as a guide. If the fracture line is not concave or angulated it may be better visualized in

the radiograph of one plane. It can then be assigned to the frontal or sagittal plane, even if there is some obliquity. In complete articular fractures (type C) such a distinction is not realistic.

The *depressions* of pilon fractures are of many types [8, 13]. It is quite understandable that they are more frequent in partial B fractures (57 of 289), but we found them also in many of the complete C fractures (50 of 391). When they occur in C fractures, they are then not so deep due to the fact that the main fracture gives way.

The most common feature of depressions can be compared to a wing or an open door. It may be triangular or rectangular. It is mainly found in the border areas – medially, laterally, anteriorly, or posteriorly – and is always preceded by a small split fragment acting as a vanguard (Fig. 6). Pistil-like depressions, where all contact with the surrounding cartilage is disrupted, are not so frequent (Fig. 7). Their blood supply is more commonly compromised than in a wing depression, especially if they are in central areas. In order to be certain that it is really a pistil morphology, the depression has to be clearly seen in the radiograph of both planes or proved by tomography. If the depression is at the border of the articulation, the vascularized capsule may remain attached. Its attachment to the fragment should be carefully preserved during reduction. It is necessary to emphasize, that the depression can only be recognized if it is adjacent to an intact area or a really large fragment that was able to resist the sudden pressure of the injury.

The third important, but much less common morphology of the articular surface is *disintegration* (in French and German better called "dissociation") of the surface. Usually this morphology is considered as characteristic of a "typical pilon fracture" [7, 12]. But it is not so common. In our case material disintegration occurred in 16 of 289 B fractures and 45 of 391 C fractures, a total of 61 (or 9%) of 680 pilon fractures. In these cases the multiplicity of splite and depressions are such that a proper distinction of the morphological elements is no longer possible (Fig. 8). This pattern of course must be confirmed by oblique radiographs or tomography to distinguish it from the effect of overlapping larger fragments.

It is clear that disintegrations (B3 and C3 fractures) have the worst prognosis since reconstruction of the articular surface by internal fixation is almost always unsatisfactory or even impossible. Surprisingly traction alone may sometimes lead to acceptable results in such cases [9].

Disintegrations exist also in other articulations, but they are then not combined with specific metaphyseal patterns.

Combination with Metaphyseal Lesions

For a suitable evaluation of the severity of these fractures we have to consider their appearance in the metaphysis. For a proper judgement, reference is needed to the morphology of the extra-articular (A) fractures of the distal tibial segment. As in other metaphyseal segments, the features seen are the

simple fracture line, the metaphyseal *wedge* and the *complex* [10]. They appear also in pilon fractures.
A specific morphological type found in the distal tibia is *impaction* (Figs. 9, 10), the destruction of bone caused by a crushing mechanism. Impactions are well known in fractures of the distal radius, but there, due to the short cancellous area and the large difference in cross-section between articular surface and diaphysis (trumpet shape), the impaction is cortico-spongious (Fig. 3). In the distal tibia, the spongious area is wider and the difference between the weight-bearing surface and the diaphysis is much smaller. The impactions are cortico-spongious or spongio-spongious and are often combined with splits prolonged into the articulation [6]. The reduction of an impaction leads to a metaphyseal defect which has to be filled in with a graft to avoid a later repetition of the initial malpositioning. Impacted fractures are almost always closed, but the deep soft tissue damage can be significant and of major clinical importance.
Axial deviations can also originate in this area. Surprisingly, our analysis showed that in pilon fractures valgus (Fig. 10) is much more frequent than varus and that antecurvation and recurvation are only of very limited importance [8].

Classification of Pilon Fractures

If we now combine these metaphyseal patterns with those of the articular surface, we get a realistic classification of the various pilon tibial fractures.
In partial (B) fractures multiple fracture lines in the metaphysis indicate a higher degree of severity. Such fractures are classified as subgroup 3.
In C fractures combination of the different extra-articular patterns with a simple articular split is very common.
Specific to pilon fractures is the combination of an articular split with metaphyseal impaction or complex elements. This gives us group C2, the largest group in our case material (220 cases). Impacted fractures are usually closed except when there is a valgus deviation. If there is complex metaphyseal morphology, open fractures are very common (39 of 86 cases = 45%). The same applies to the extra-articular fractures A2 and A3.
B3 and C3 fractures with disintegration of the articular surface can be subdivided according to their extension into the metaphysis.
Finally, extension of the fracture into the diaphysis has to be considered (Fig. 8). This does not only produce increasing instability and additional difficulties for reduction, but also impairment of the diaphyseal circulatory system. For this reason fractures extending into the diaphysis are classified as being of a higher degree of severity (subgroup .3) [10].

Surrounding Lesions

When analyzing the surrounding lesions we found some surprising facts [8]:

1. The *internal malleolus* is very often fractured. There certainly seems to be some pressure on the internal malleolus too, but it must be excluded from the classification because, in contrast to the distal radius, it takes no part in supporting axial body weight. Surprisingly, ruptures of the *deltoid ligament* are not seen, a fact that distinguishes pilon fractures from malleolar fractures.
2. The most important but old observation [11] is, that (with a few exceptions) *the tibiofibular ligaments remain intact.* Again this is a clear distinction between pilon and malleolar fractures. It also explains why traction methods may be effective in achieving reduction of pilon fractures [9].
3. On the other hand, ruptures of the *fibulotalar* and *fibulocalcanear ligaments* are not uncommon. The talus is then dislocated medially or proximally. In such cases of lateral instability traction is ineffective.
4. *Fibula fractures* are very common. Being connected with the main tibial displacement, they show some peculiarities (e.g. cortico-spongious impactions) which again help to distinguish them from malleolar fractures.
5. If the *fibula* remains *intact,* there is always at least one tibial fragment attached via a ligament to the fibula. True ruptures of the tibiofibular ligaments that can be detected on radiographs, are extremely rare. In the literature some are mentioned as intraoperative findings [3].

Conclusion

The articular split, articular depression, and even disintegration of the articular surface are not specific to pilon fractures. But combinations of these with the metaphyseal pattern are characteristic of the so-called typical pilon fracture. The morphological combinations seen are split plus impaction and split plus complex metaphyseal fractures. Lesions of the surrounding structures (fibula, medial malleolus and ligaments) are also frequent and may be sometimes specific, but must not be included in the classification.
Our purpose here is to focus attention on these distinguishing features which allow a proper classification of pilon fractures into the classical nine groups and 27 subgroups [8] (Fig. 11).

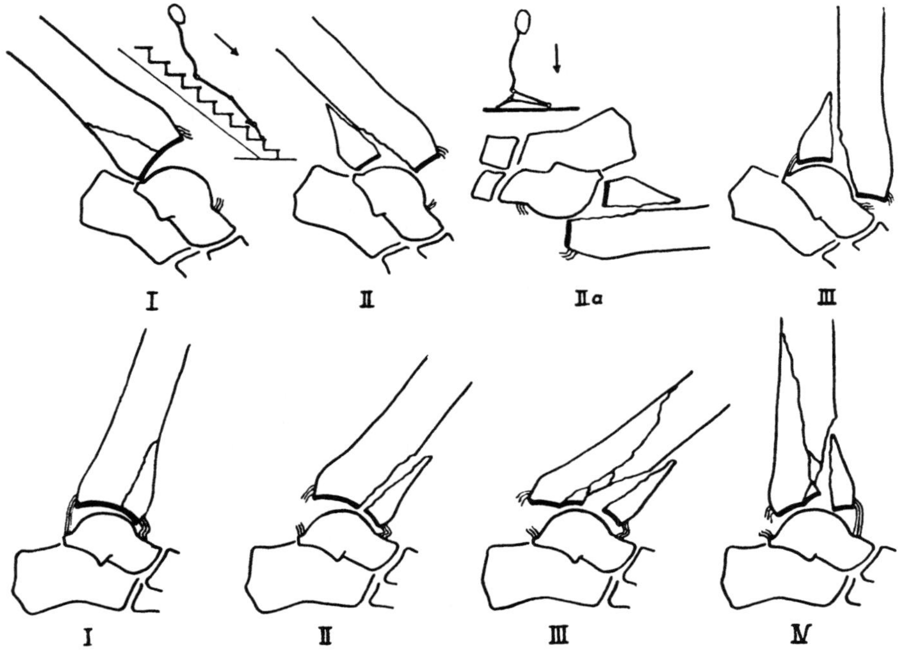

Fig. 1. Partial fractures as illustrated by Böhler in 1955, explaining how the morphology of the fracture depends on the position of the foot during impact [8]

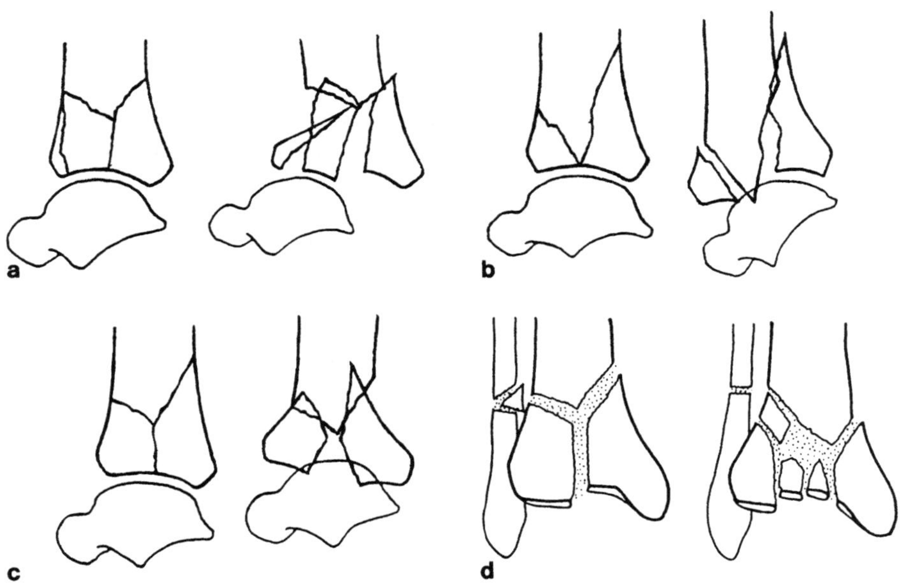

Fig. 2 a–d. Complete fractures. **a–c** Drawings by Gay and Evrard [5] illustrating "fractures bimarginales" (sagittal aspect). **d** Scheme proposed by Vivès [14] for simple and complex fractures (frontal aspect) [8]

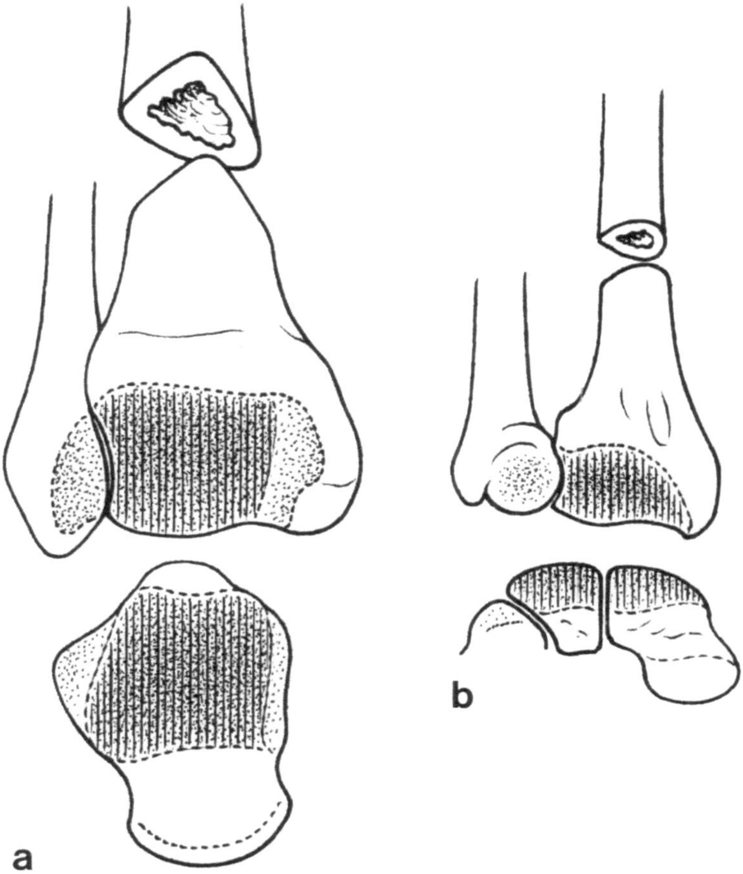
a b

Fig. 3 a, b. Comparison of the weight-bearing articular surfaces and of the cross section of the diaphysis. **a** Distal tibia. **b** Distal radius. The difference in cross-sections in the radius (trumpet-like shape) is much more marked than in the tibia

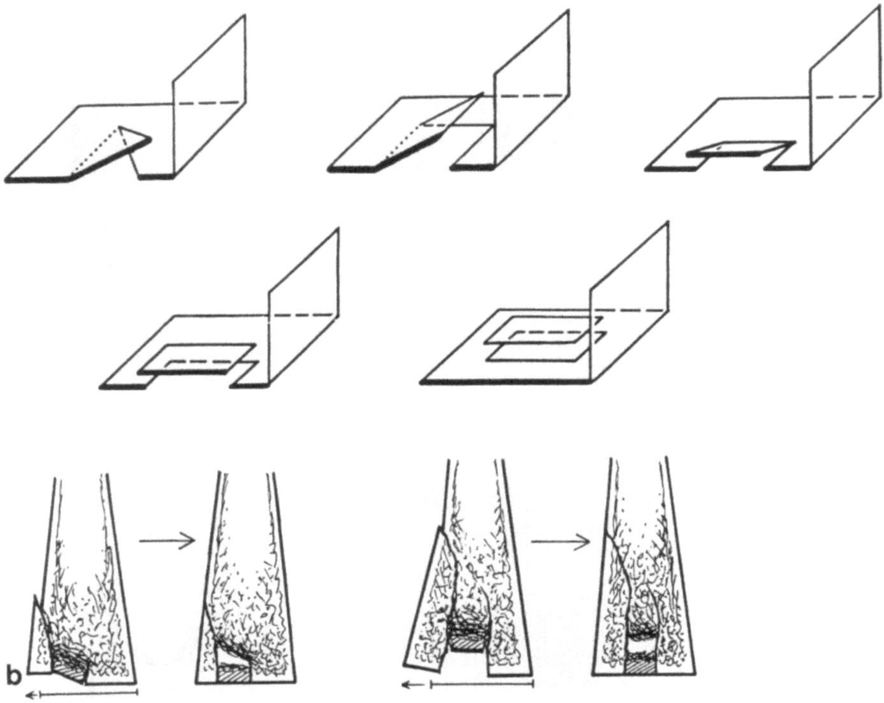

Fig. 4a, b. Types of articular depressions. **a** Triangular, "open door" and pistil-like (marginal or central) depressions. **b** Marginal and central (pistil-like) depressions enlarging the epiphysis lead to a spongious defect after reduction

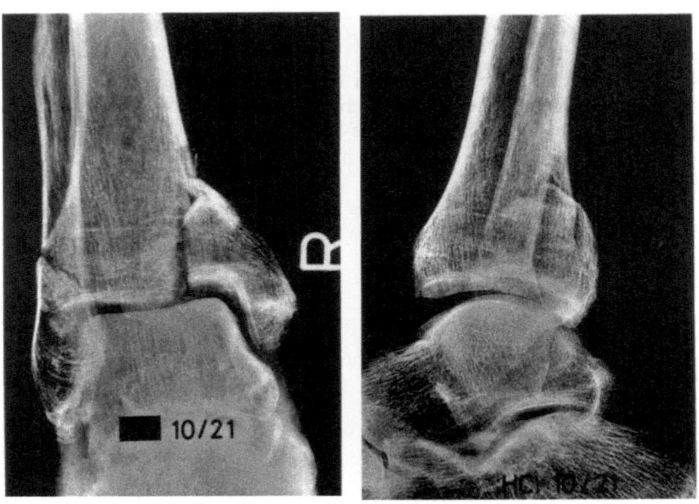

Fig. 5. Radiograph showing split fracture in the sagittal plane; partial fracture; varus position with a typical oblique fibula fracture

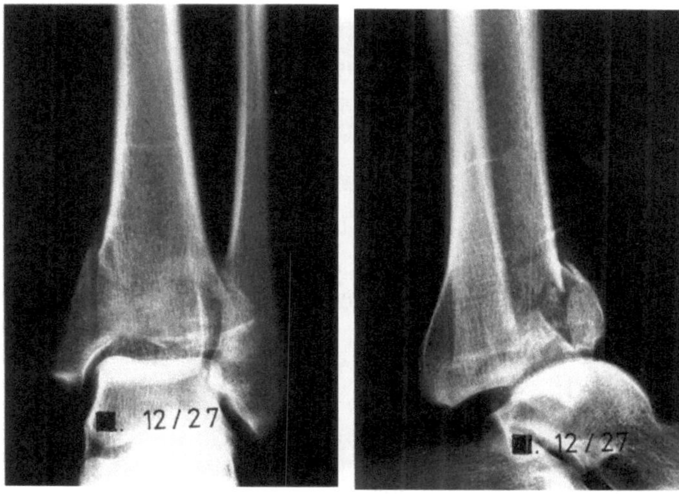

Fig. 6. Radiograph showing anteromedial marginal depression with a vanguard split fragment; partial tibia fracture; oblique distal fibula fracture; vertical fracture of the medial malleolus

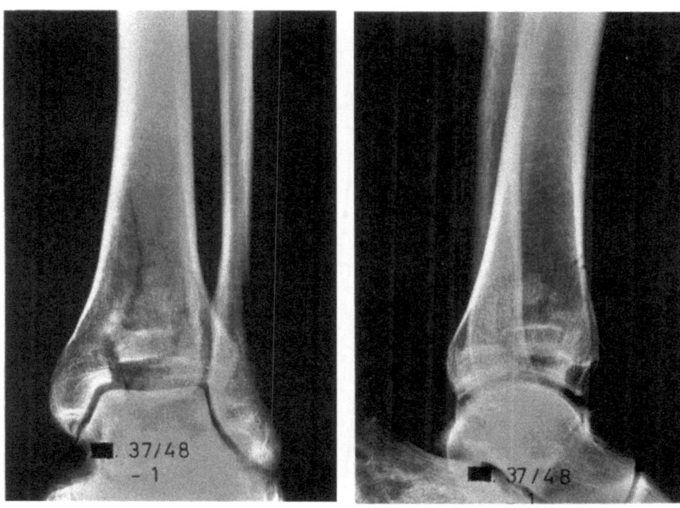

Fig. 7. Radiograph showing pistil-like anterior depression, better visualized in the anteroposterior view; partial fracture, intact fibula

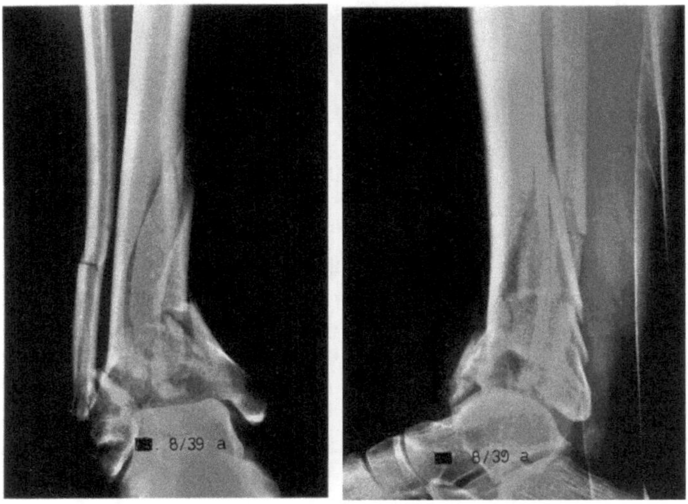

Fig. 8. Radiograph showing disintegration of the articular surface; extension into the diaphysis, varus position; segmental fracture of the fibula

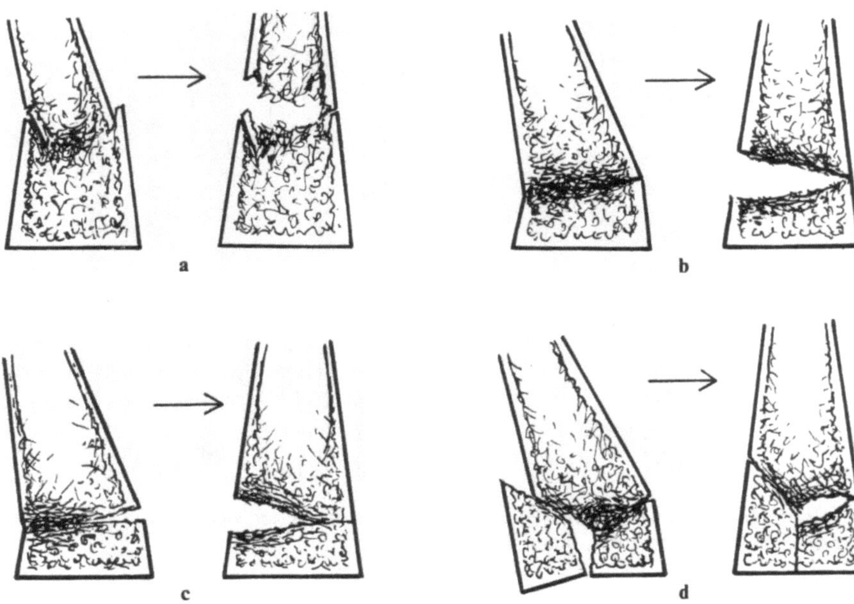

Fig. 9 a–d. Types of impaction, and the resulting defect after reduction: **a** cortico-spongious; **b** complete spongio-spongious; **c** partial spongio-spongious; **d** partial spongious with split fragment

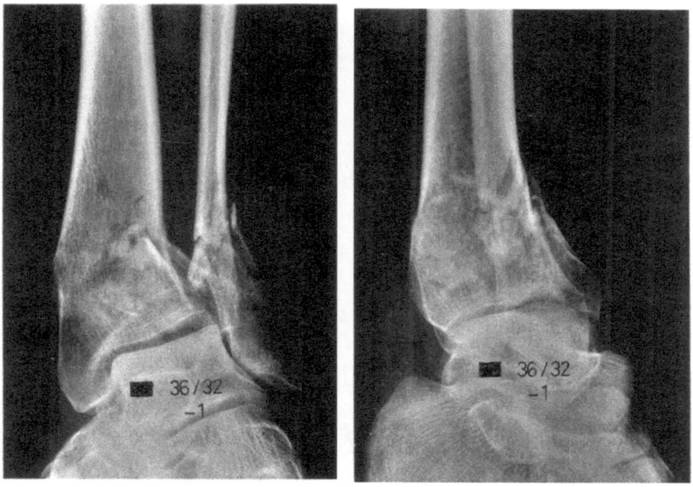

Fig. 10. Radiograph showing impaction plus lateral articular split; valgus position; supramalleolar impacted fibula fracture

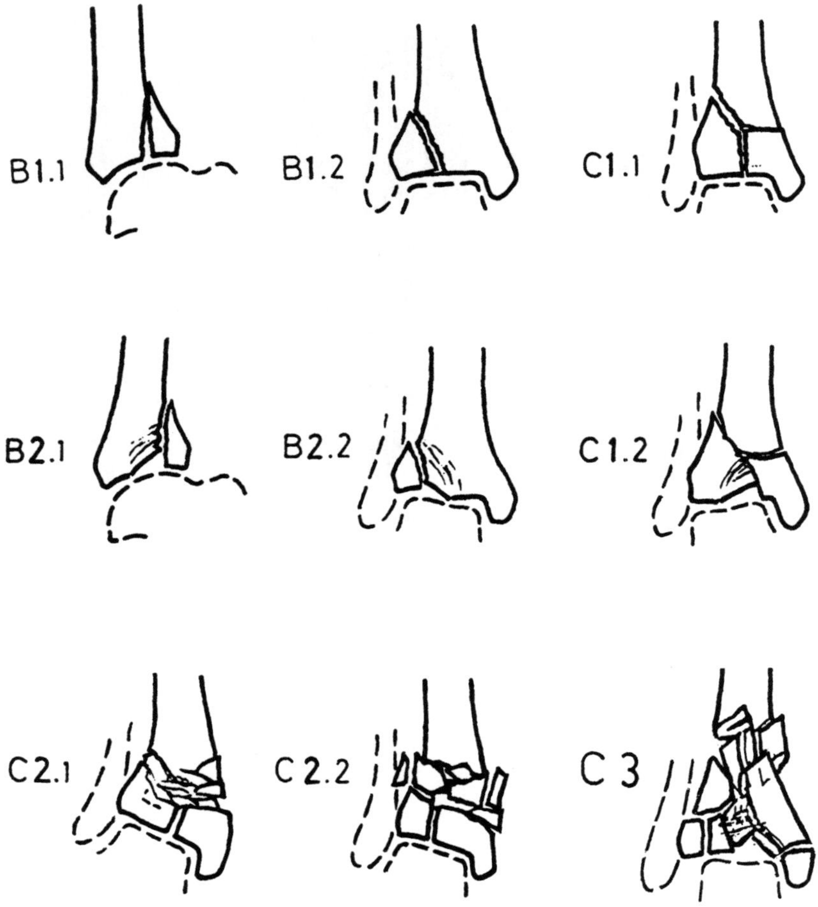

Fig. 11. Typical pilon fractures. *B1*, partial split fractures in both planes. The split may also be posterior, central or nearer to the medial malleolus. *C1.1*, complete articular split fracture plus simple metaphyseal fracture. *B2*, partial depression fractures in the same location as in B1. The depression may also be posterior, central or medial. *C1.2*, complete fracture with articular depression, plus simple metaphyseal fracture. *C2.1*, complete fracture: articular split plus metaphyseal impaction. Valgus position. The split may also be located in the sagittal plane. *C2.2*, complete articular split fracture plus complex metaphyseal fracture. *C3*, disintegrated (multi-fragmentary) articular surface plus extension into the proximal metaphysis.

References

1. Bandi W (1970) Zur Mechanik der supramalleolären intraartikulären Schienbeinbrüche des Skifahrers. Proceedings, congress of Société Internationale de Traumatologie et Medecine des Sports d'Hiver (SITEMSH). Nebel-Verlag, Garmisch-Partenkirchen
2. Böhler L (1951) Die Technik der Knochenbruchbehandlung, 12–13 edn. Maudrich, Vienna (reprint 1977)
3. Börner M (1982) Einteilung, Behandlung und Ergebnisse der Frakturen des Pilon tibial. Unfallchirurgie 8:230–235
4. Destot E (1911) Traumatisme du pied et rayons X. Masson, Paris
5. Gay R, Evrard J (1963) Les fractures récentes du pilon tibial chez l'adulte. Rev Chir Orthop 49:397–512
6. Heim U (1972) Le traitement chirurgical des fractures du pilon tibial. J Chir (Paris) 104:307–322
7. Heim U, Pfeiffer KM (1987) Small fragment set manual, 3rd edn. Internal fixation of small fractures. Springer, Berlin Heidelberg New York
8. Heim U (1991) Die Pilon-tibial-Fraktur: Klassifikation, Operationstechnik, Ergebnisse. Springer, Berlin Heidelberg New York
9. Lechevallier J, Thomine JM, Biga N (1989) Le fixateur externe tibiocalcanéen dans le traitement des fractures du pilon tibial. Rev Chir Orthop 74:52–60
10. Müller ME, Nazarian S, Koch P, Schatzker J (1990) The comprehensive classification of fractures of long bones. Springer, Berlin Heidelberg New York
11. Rieunau G, Gay R (1956) Enclouage du péroné dans les fractures supramalléolaires. Lyon Chir 51:594–600
12. Rüedi T, Allgöwer M (1979) The operative treatment of intraarticular fractures of the lower end of the tibia. Clin Orthop 138:105–110
13. Stampfel O, Mähring M (1977) Komplikationen und Ergebnisse 40 operierter Pilon-tibial-Stauchungsfrakturen. In: Kraft-Kinz K, Kronberger L (eds) Proceedings, Congress of Oesterreichische Gesellschaft für Chirurgie, Graz, May 19–21, pp 639–642
14. Vivès P, Hourlier H, De Lestang M, Dorde T, Letot P, Senlecq F (1984) Etude de 84 fractures du pilon tibial de l'adulte. Rev Chir Orthop 70:129–139

Tibial Plafond Fractures

J. P. Waddell

Fractures of the distal articular surface of the tibia have a reputation for uncertain outcome regardless of the method of treatment [1, 3, 9]. A combination of fracture configuration [4, 6, 11], metaphyseal crush with instability [2, 8], primary articular cartilage damage [4], and persisting joint surface incongruity [7] all contribute to this reputation (Fig. 1).
Recognizing the problems inherent in this fracture type it was hoped that results could be improved by addressing the problems in a planned fashion which would allow anatomic reconstruction of the articular surface, stabilization of supporting metaphyseal bone, and early joint motion [6]. To achieve these goals plate fixation was chosen as the preferable method of treatment [10] (Fig. 2).

Materials and Methods

Based on our previous experience with this particular fracture type, a protocol for treatment was developed. This includes:

a) Restoration of fibular length
b) Anterior ankle arthrotomy
c) External fixator to apply distraction to the ankle joint
d) Restoration of lateral articular and metaphyseal fragment
e) Restoration of central fragment
f) Supporting bone graft
g) Restoration of medial pillar
h) Anterior or medial buttress plating (Fig. 3)
i) Early motion
j) Delayed weight bearing

Thirty-eight patients treated according to this protocol have been followed up to the conclusion of treatment: 29 males and nine females aged 19 to 62 years with a mean of 41.2 years. The duration of follow-up ranged from 1 to 11 years with a mean of 4.9 years. Thirty patients were injured in falls from a height, six in motor vehicle accidents, and two as a result of crushing injuries. Thirty-one fractures were closed, six were grade I open injuries, and one was a grade II open fracture. The time to surgery varied from 3 to 96 h with a mean of 20 h.

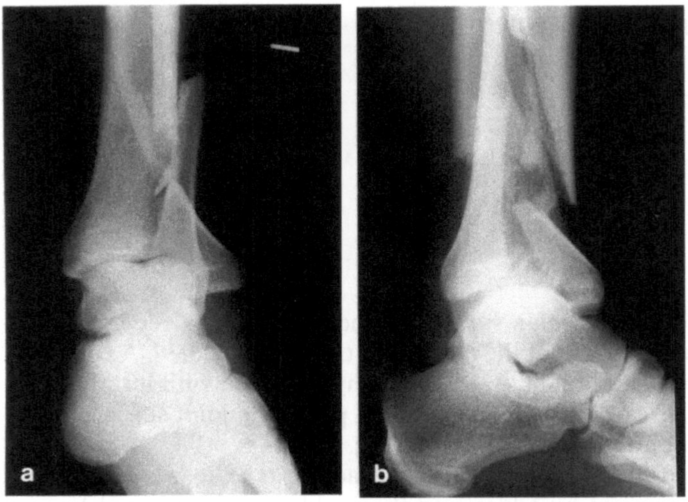

Fig. 1. **a** AP and **b** lateral radiographs showing fibular fracture, metaphyseal crush, articular surface incongruity, and joint subluxation

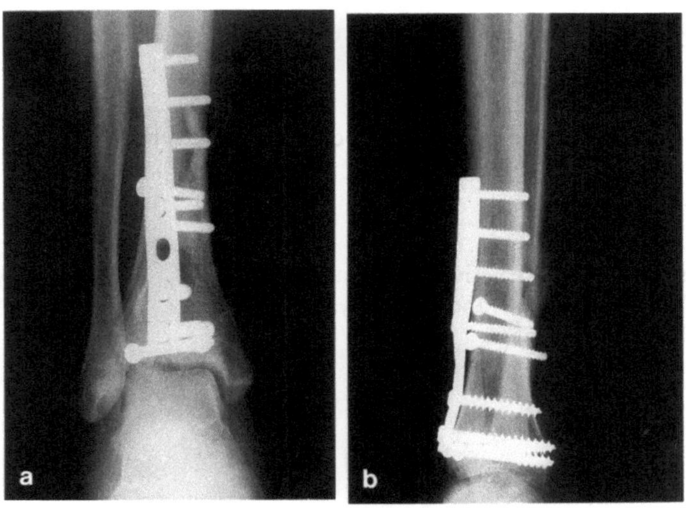

Fig. 2. **a** AP and **b** lateral radiographs demonstrating anatomic articular surface maintained with anterior buttress plate

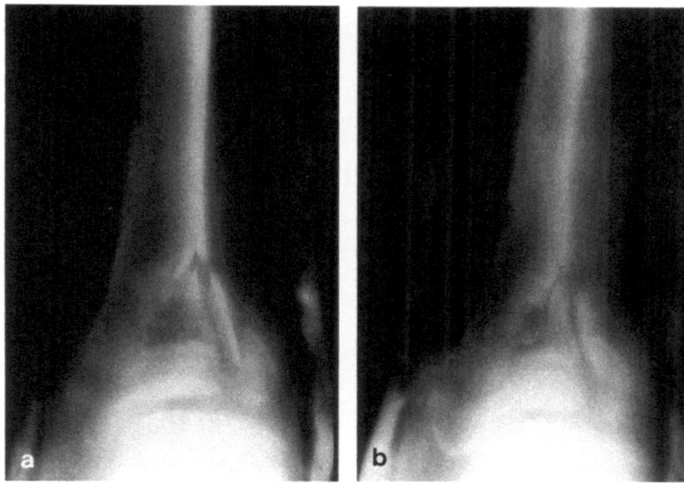

Fig. 3a, b. AP tomograms demonstrating separate medial and lateral pillar fragments, lateral metaphyseal crush, and separate central fragment. All of these fragments must be reduced and maintained for a satisfactory outcome

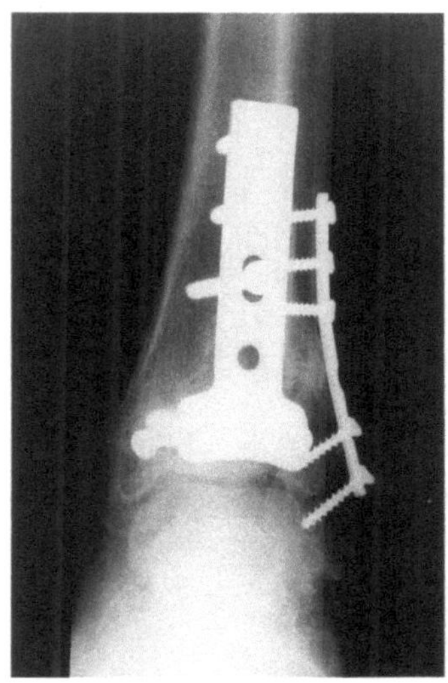

Fig. 4. AP radiograph showing <2 mm discrepancy between central and lateral fragment: anatomic reduction between central and medial fragment

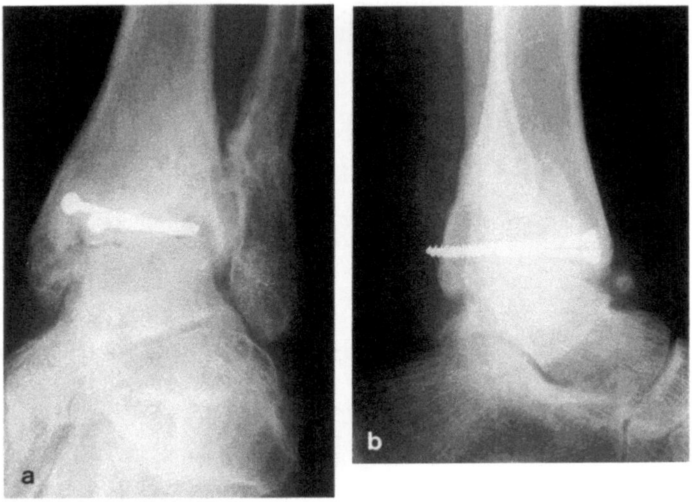

Fig. 5. a AP and **b** lateral radiographs showing severe degenerative arthritis secondary to failed fracture reduction

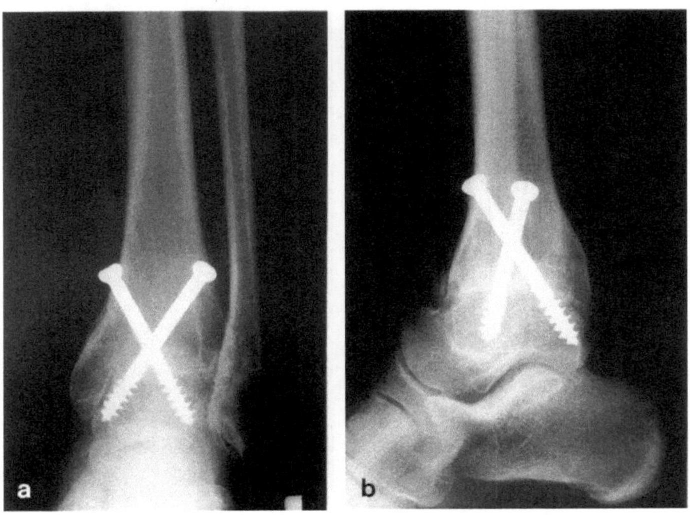

Fig. 6. a AP and **b** lateral radiographs demonstrating successful arthrodesis using crossed screws

Results

Thirty-three patients achieved primary wound healing. Of the five patients with delayed wound healing, two healed spontaneously, two required split-thickness skin grafting, and one required a local flap [5].
There were four documented wound infections, three superficial and one deep. All responded to antibiotic treatment; debridement and repeat closure was used for the deep infection under antibiotic coverage.
Eight patients demonstrated evidence of persistent fracture line on radiographs, pain on stressing, or local tenderness at 16 weeks from the date of surgery. A diagnosis of delayed union was made. At 26 weeks five of these delayed unions had resolved, leaving three patients in whom a diagnosis of non-union was made. These three patients required cancellous bone grafting and all had a satisfactory outcome. None of the eight patients with delayed union required further additional immobilization for this reason.
At review, 31 patients had an anatomic articular surface as demonstrated by radiography. Five patients demonstrated less than 2 mm of articular surface discrepancy (Fig. 4) and two demonstrated greater than 2 mm of articular surface discrepancy.
Range of motion was measured as a combination of ankle and subtalar motion compared with the opposite foot and ankle. No patient had normal motion. Twenty-eight patients had a greater than 75% aggregate range of motion, four had 50%–75% of the motion of the opposite leg, and six had less than 50% of motion.
On direct questioning 26 patients stated that they had no or inconsequential pain. Eight patients had pain which required some modification of activity, while four reported severe disabling pain (Fig. 5).
Fourteen patients underwent secondary surgery. Three required skin closure procedures, one had debridement for control of infection, six underwent hardware removal, and four had ankle arthrodesis to control pain (Fig. 6).

Discussion

The results of surgical treatment of fractures of the tibial plafond continue to be somewhat disappointing. A high proportion of our patients required subsequent surgery; many had pain sufficient to modify daily activities. Some restriction of ankle/subtalar motion is almost certain following this injury and the treatment as described; however, the proportion of patients with significant disability is small.
Review of our cases in which the outcome was unsatisfactory suggests a high correlation between persistent pain and the following:

a) Severe articular damage at the time of initial injury
b) Deep infection as a consequence of surgical intervention or original compounding wound

c) Significant (greater than 2 mm) articular surface incongruity
d) Reflex sympathetic dystrophy.

While obviously not all of these can be overcome with techniques available to us today, the review of our satisfactory results suggests that early surgery accomplished with atraumatic dissection, resulting in anatomic reduction secured by rigid fixation and followed by early active motion and delayed weight bearing, gives the best chance of successful outcome in these most difficult fractures.

References

1. Ayeni JP (1988) Pilon fractures of the tibia: a study based on 19 cases. Injury 19(2):109–114
2. Bone LB (1987) Fractures of the tibial plafond. The pilon fracture. Orthop Clin North Am 18(1):95–104
3. Bourne RB, Rorabeck CH, Macnab J (1983) Intra-articular fractures of the distal tibia: the pilon fracture. J Trauma 23(7):591–596
4. Brennan MJ (1990) Tibial pilon fractures (review). Instr Course Lect 39:167–170
5. Dillin L, Slabaugh P (1986) Delayed wound healing, infection, and nonunion following open reduction and internal fixation of tibial plafond fractures. J Trauma 26(12):1116–1119
6. Kellam JF, Waddell JP (1979) Fractures of the distal tibia. J Trauma 19(8):593
7. Mainwaring BL, Daffner RH, Riemer BL (1988) Pylon fractures of the ankle: a distinct clinical and radiologic entity. Radiology 168(1):215–218
8. Mast JW, Spiegel PG, Pappas JN (1988) Fractures of the tibial pilon. Clin Orthop Rel Res (230):68–82
9. Miller BN, Krebs B (1982) Intra-articular fractures of the distal tibia. Acta Orthop Scand 53(6):991–996
10. Ovadia DN, Beals RK (1986) Fractures of the tibial plafond. J Bone Joint Surg (Am) 68(4):543–551
11. Rüedi TP, Allgöwer M (1979) The operative treatment of intra-articular fractures of the lower end of the tibia. Clin Orthop Rel Res 138:105–110

Results of Operative Treatment of Pilon Fractures

E. Beck

Patients and Methods

Between 1972 and 1985, a total of 380 tibial pilon fractures were managed by open reduction at the accident hospital in Feldkirch and the university clinic in Innsbruck, Austria. In Feldkirch almost all of these fractures were managed by open reduction whilst in Innsbruck about one half were managed closed [6]. A total of 256 patients (68%) were followed for at least 2 and 15 years after surgery, with a mean follow-up time of 7.5 years [2, 5]. The right side was slightly more frequently involved than the left (53% vs 45%) and there was bilateral involvement in 2% of cases. The average age of the patients was 34 years (range 15–74 years) and there were more male patients (123) than females (71). Three hundred and forty-two fractures (90%) were closed and 38 (10%) open. The most common cause of the fractures was a skiing injury, which would be anticipated as both the hospitals are in the centre of popular skiing areas (Table 1). Using Heim's classification there were 89 (22%) cleavage-type fractures, 177 (44%) fracture dislocations and 114 (34%) distal tibial fractures with extension into the ankle joint [3, 4].

We used screws and a plate for fixation in 75% of cases. Generally a cloverleaf plate was used, but sometimes a T plate or DC plate. In the remaining 25% of cases, mainly cleavage fractures, fixation with screws alone provided sufficient stability. We never used an external fixator, even in open fractures [1]. Even in the most severely comminuted cases we always attempted reconstruction of the articular surface rather than primary arthrodesis. The usual postoperative management was functional, although weight bearing was generally not permitted until 12 weeks.

Table 1. Etiology of 380 pilon tibial fractures

Skiing accident	214 (56%)
Fall from a great height	92 (24%)
Fall from a lesser height	38 (10%)
Traffic accident	31 (8%)
Soccer	5 (2%)

Results

In the 256 patients that we were able to follow up, we used a scoring system based on pain, range of movement, gait disturbance, and radiological appearance (Table 2) [9–11]. Overall, the results were classified as excellent in 58%, good in 24%, fair in 15% and poor in 3% of patients (Table 3). When these figures were analyzed in accordance with Heim's classification, we achieved the best results in cleavage-type fractures and in distal tibial fractures which extended into the articular surface. There were not so many good results from fracture dislocations of the joint (Fig. 1).

Table 2. Scoring system used for the follow-up results of pilon tibial fractures

Excellent	No pain, normal range of movement, normal gait, normal radiograph
Good	Slight pain, loss of movement less than 10°, slight restriction of gait, normal radiograph
Fair	Some pain, loss of movement more than 10°, some restriction of gait, slight osteoarthritis
Poor	Severe pain, marked restriction of movement, marked restriction of gait, severe osteoarthritis

Table 3. Follow-up results of 256 operated pilon tibial fractures

Excellent	147 (58%)	(82%)
Good	62 (24%)	
Fair	38 (15%)	
Poor	9 (3%)	

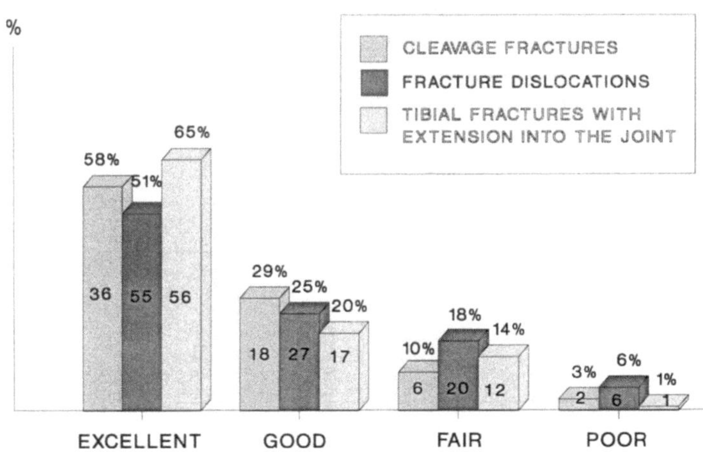

Fig. 1. Long-term operative results for different types of pilon fractures

There were 8 nonseptic complications (2%): One necrosis of a bony wedge, 4 supramalleolar non-unions requiring re-osteosynthesis, 2 refractures following removal of implants, and 1 late arthrodesis. There were also 9 cases of infection (2.5%): 5 were primary infections, 4 of which healed without further complications, while 1 patient with an infection related to a secondary external fixator died of cardiac arrest. There were also 2 secondary infections and 2 others following removal of implants. These cases healed without further complications.

Conclusion

Good results can be achieved with open reduction and internal fixation of tibial pilon fractures, if the surgeon is experienced and accurate reduction of the articular surface is obtained [7]. If there is any incongruency of the articular surface, poor results can be expected. Our infection rate was low, probably because of the high proportion of skiing accidents without marked disruption of soft tissues.

Acknowledgment. The author wishes to thank Drs. Häfele and Lippay in Feldkirch and Doz. Dr. Resch, Prof. Dr. Benedetto, and Dr. Pechlaner in Innsbruck for their assistance with follow-up of patients.

References

1. Beck E (1990) Verletzungen des distalen Schienbeinendes und des Sprunggelenkes. In: Beck E (ed) Traumatologie: 4. Untere Extremität. Urban and Schwarzenberg, Baltimore (Breitner, chirurgische Operationslehre, vol 11)
2. Häfele H, Lippay S (1976) Komplikationen und Schwierigkeiten bei der operativen Behandlung distaler intraartikulärer Schienbeinstauchungsbrüche. Acta Chir Austriaca [Suppl]: 534–535
3. Heim U, Mäser M (1976) Die operative Behandlung der Pilon-tibial-Fraktur. Technik der Osteosynthese und Resultate bei 128 Patienten. Arch Orthop Unfallchir 86: 341–356
4. Heim U (1990) Die Pilon-tibial-Fraktur. Springer, Berlin Heidelberg New York
5. Lippay S (1977) Frühergebnisse operierter distaler Stauchungsbrüche des Unterschenkels. In: Kraft-Kinz J, Kronberger L (eds) Kongreßbericht der Österreichischen Gesellschaft für Chirurgie. Dorrong, Graz, pp 659–661
6. Resch H, Pechlaner S, Benedetto KP (1986) Spätergebnisse nach konservativer und operativer Behandlung von Pilon Tibial-Frakturen. Aktuel Traumatol 16: 117–123
7. Resch H, Benedetto KP, Pechlaner S (1986) Die Entwicklung der posttraumatischen Arthrose nach Pilon-Tibialfrakturen. Unfallchirurg 89: 8–15
8. Rüedi T, Matter P, Allgöwer M (1968) Die intraartikulären Frakturen des distalen Unterschenkelendes. Helv Chir Acta 35: 556–582
9. Rüedi T (1973) Frakturen des Pilon tibial: Ergebnisse nach 9 Jahren. Arch Orthop Unfall Chir 76: 248–254
10. Rüedi T (1973) Fractures of the lower end of the tibia into the ankle-joint. Injury 5: 130–134
11. Rüedi T, Allgöwer M (1978) Spätresultate nach operativer Behandlung der Gelenksbrüche am distalen Tibiaende (sog. Pilon-Frakturen). Unfallheilkunde 81: 319–323

External Fixation of Severely Comminuted and Open Pilon Fractures

L. Bone, P. Stegemann, K. McNamara, and R. Seibel

Introduction

We are indebted to Rüedi and Allgöwer for their early work and recommendations for the management of intra-articular distal tibia fractures (pilon fracture). Their classification and guidelines for stable internal fixation with early mobilization have improved the outcome of these severe injuries. It is important to appreciate, though, their particular patient population and type of injury: The majority of their patients had fairly low-energy skiing injuries. Their articular reconstructions and final outcome were excellent [5–7]. Similar results have not been obtained, however, in injuries from high-energy falls or road traffic accidents that involve severe comminution of the intra-articular plafond and distal tibia, especially when these injuries were open [3]. Because of this, an alternative method of stabilization of severely comminuted and/or open pilon fractures has been used at the Erie County Medical Center of the State University of New York at Buffalo over the past 2½ years. This consists of reduction and stabilization of the intra-articular component with screws or small plate fixation and the use of an external fixator across the ankle joint as an external neutralization device.

Patients and Methods

Twenty patients (13 male and 7 female) with severely comminuted and/or open pilon fractures were managed with the use of an external fixator with limited internal fixation of the intra-articular component.

Patient ages ranged from 19 to 69 years (average 44 years). In all cases they had suffered significant high-energy injury: 10 in falls from a height, 8 from road traffic accidents, 1 from a gunshot injury and 1 from a motor vehicle-pedestrian injury.

Eighteen of the injuries were classified as pure pilon fractures. There were 2 additional injuries: one an intra-articular distal tibia, from a fracture from a gunshot injury, and the other a severe fracture dislocation of the ankle. There were 12 open fractures (10 of the pilon fractures): with 1 of grade I, 2 of grade II, 3 of grade III A, and 4 of grade III B plus the grade III fracture dislocation of the ankle and the grade I gunshot injury.

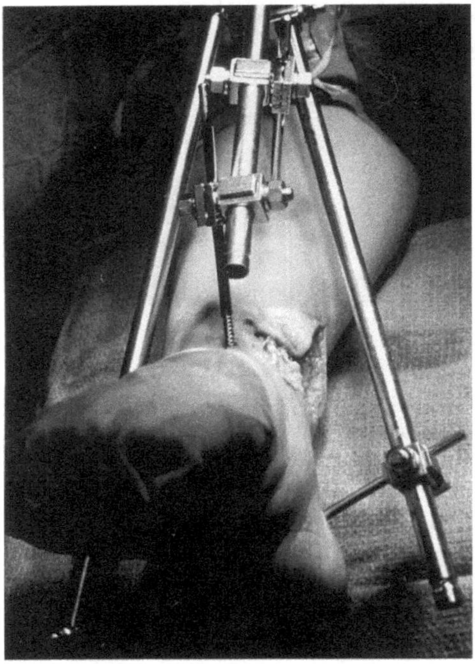

Fig. 1. Open pilon fracture treated with external fixator from tibia to calcaneus

All open fractures were managed acutely with debridement of the wound, application of an external fixator across the ankle joint with pins in the calcaneus, talus and the tibia (Fig. 1), reconstruction of the ankle mortis, and stabilization of the fracture with screws (Fig. 2d, e) and/or small plate fixation with a modified cloverleaf plate. All but 1 patient had open reduction and internal fixation (ORIF) of the fibula to obtain length and stabilization prior to joint reconstruction (Fig. 2c). The 8 closed injuries consisted of severely comminuted pilon fractures. Four had severe comminution of the metaphysis of the distal tibia and 3 had a combination of diaphyseal and metaphyseal fractures (Fig. 2a, b). The closed injuries were operated on an average of 5 days after the injury (range 3–7 days) when the swelling had subsided. Preoperative management consisted of either calcaneal skeletal traction or plaster immobilization.

Results

All 20 patients were followed prospectively with an average follow-up time of 18 months (range 12–36 months). The external fixator was in place for an average of 2.5 months (range from 6–12 weeks). Union of the fracture oc-

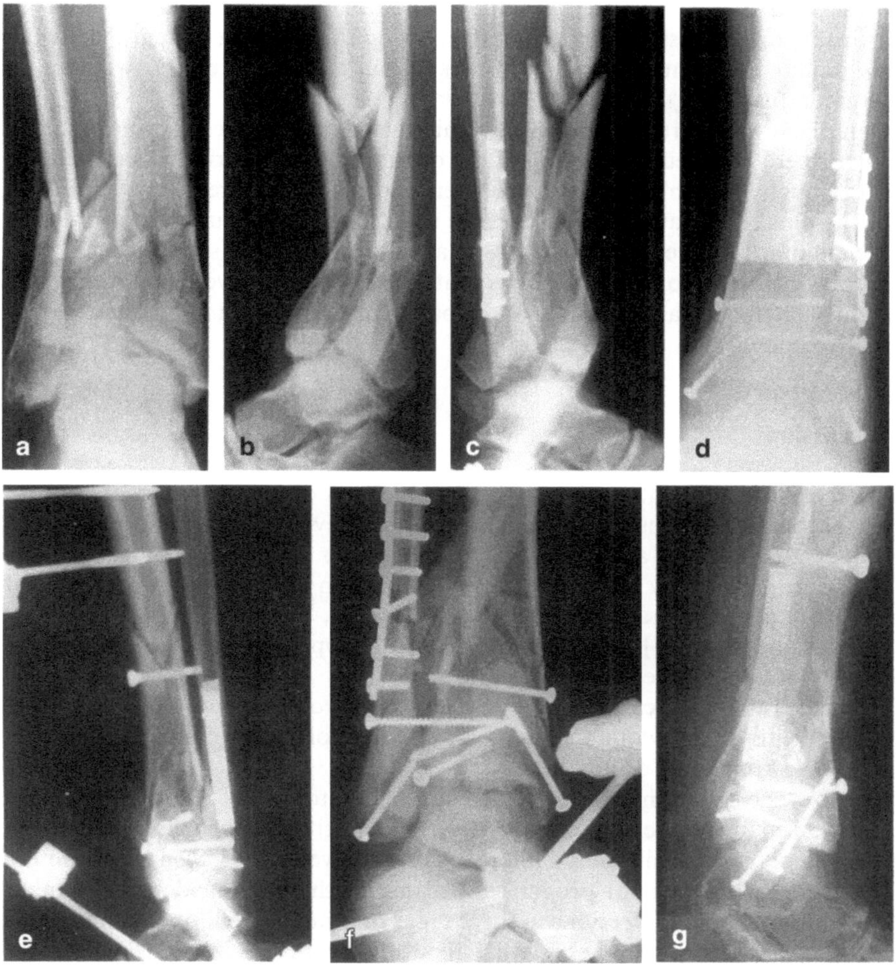

Fig. 2a–g. Distal tibia fracture with extension into the ankle, treated with limited internal fixation and external frame as the neutralization device

curred at an average of 4.5 months. There were 3 delayed or non-unions that required bone grafting. Two required additional plate stabilization. The range of motion of the affected ankle at the last follow-up was excellent in 6 patients, with at least 10° of dorsiflexion and 30° of plantar flexion; good in 9 patients, with at least 5°–10° of dorsiflexion and 25° of plantar flexion; fair in 3 patients, with 0°–5° of dorsiflexion and 20° of plantar flexion; and poor in 2 patients who required fusion. Overall results were graded as "good" in those patients who had no pain, no deformity, an anatomically restored articular surface and no stiffness. "Fair" were those who had pain with sports or intense activity, no deformity, minimal radiographic changes, and minimal stiffness. "Poor" were those who had pain with walking, radiographic deformity, post-traumatic arthritis, or stiffness greater than 50%. Using this grading system there were six good to excellent results, nine fair results, and five poor results, two because of ankle fusions.

Complications were minimal using this technique on these severe injuries. There were no infections in any of the open or closed injuries. There were no skin sloughs and only 2 pin-tract problems, which were corrected with removal of the pins. One patient's fracture was not adequately reduced and healed in a malunion. Three patient's had delayed or non-unions requiring repeat surgery before union occurred. Two patients developed severe post-traumatic arthritis requiring ankle fusion, and 4 patients had mild pain with mild degenerative changes on their radiographs.

Discussion

There is little in the literature on the management of open pilon fractures and few recommendations for management of the severely comminuted fracture that cannot be either anatomically reduced and/or stably fixed after reduction [4]. There is similarly little about the combination of diaphyseal-metaphyseal and intra-articular fractures of the tibia (Fig. 2a, b).

Ovadia and Beals [3] had 25 grade II and III open pilon fractures in their review, of which 9 became infected.

Their overall complication rate consisted of 10 wound infections, 10 cases of osteomyelitis and 5 wound sloughs. Twenty-one of their total of 145 patients required arthrodesis or amputation.

The low-energy pilon fracture which can be anatomically reconstructed and stably fixed with plate and screw fixation has a fairly good prognosis. The open pilon or severely comminuted pilon fracture, however, has been shown in the literature to have a poor prognosis. Because of the high incidence of wound sloughs and wound infections in these types of injuries we adopted a modified form of fixation using the external fixator as a neutralization device after reconstruction of the articular surface and screw or small plate fixation of the fracture in 20 severely comminuted or open pilon fractures.

The advantages of the external fixator during the surgical procedure for obtaining length and helping to stabilize the limb for reconstruction of the intra-articular component were first proposed by Kellam and Waddell [1] and by Mast and Spiegel [2]. Placement of the external fixator with a calcaneal pin and a half pin in the tibia, with traction on the calcaneal pin, will allow ligamentotaxis to occur. This will help in reduction of the fracture and allow easier access to the ankle joint for joint reconstruction (Fig. 2c). When the external fixator is used as a neutralization device there is no need for large plates with their increased risk of skin slough (Fig. 2f, g). The greatest advantage of the external fixator, though, is in open fractures in which wounds are left open: since no plate is used none has to be left exposed. In addition it is an excellent device in those severely comminuted fractures in which stable fixation cannot be achieved with the use of a plate, and in those fractures with proximal metaphyseal and diaphyseal extension in which stable fixation could only be obtained with extremely long plates and thus additional extensive soft tissue dissection. While the final outcome of these 20 patients cannot be stated because of the short follow-up, the early complications have been minimal considering the severity of the injuries. An infection rate of zero in 12 open fractures, seven of which were grade III, is a decided improvement over the 30% infection rate in the grade II and III open fractures reported by Ovadia and Beals [3]. This may in part be due to the decreased soft tissue dissection required the external fixator and emphasis is placed on maintaining viability of the bony fragments. The overall results in these 20 patients, while not excellent, appear to be an improvement considering the severity of their injuries. The 2 patients who required ankle arthrodesis developed severe post-traumatic arthritis secondary to articular cartilage damage/sustained at the time of their injury. The second surgical procedures required by 3 patients to obtain union could perhaps have been avoided if bone grafting of the most proximal fracture lines on the lateral aspect of the tibia had been performed at the time of delayed closure of the open wounds or at the time of the initial surgery. Their non-union site was at the most proximal fracture line and the problem did not occur when this area was bone grafted primarily. In general these patients obtained a very adequate range of motion despite having their ankle joints immobilized for an average of 2.5 months. The reason for this may be that the ankle joint was maintained in slight distraction, which kept the soft tissues stretched during the immobilization and not compressed and shortened as occurs with plaster immobilization.

While this series is small and the follow-up relatively short, the use of the external fixator to stabilize severely comminuted and/or open pilon fractures appears to be an improvement over plate fixation. The lowered complication rate of infection, skin sloughs, and arthrodeses appears to prove that point. These injuries were of the high-energy type which may have produced irreversible joint damage. Reconstruction of the intra-articular component, in combination with the use of the external fixator to obtain and maintain proper metaphyseal or diaphyseal fracture reduction and stabilization, may be the better alternative in these severe injuries to formal open reduction and plate fixation.

References

1. Kellam JF, Waddell JP (1979) Fractures of the distal tibial metaphysis with intra-articular extension: the distal tibial explosion fracture. J Trauma 19:593–601
2. Mast JW, Spiegel PG (1984) Complex ankle fractures. In: Meyers MH (ed) The multiply injured patient with complex fractures. Lea and Febiger, Philadelphia, p 304
3. Ovadia DN, Beals RK (1986) Fractures of the tibial plafond. J Bone Joint Surg [Am] 68:543–551
4. Pierce R, Heinrich J (1979) Comminuted intraarticular fractures of the distal tibia. J Bone Joint Surg 19:828–832

5. Rüedi T (1973) Fractures of the lower end of the tibia into the ankle joint: results nine years after open reduction and internal fixation. Injury 5:130–134
6. Rüedi TP, Allgöwer M (1969) Fractures of the lower end of the tibia into the ankle joint. Injury 1:92–99
7. Rüedi TP, Allgöwer M (1979) The operative treatment of intra-articular fractures of the lower end of the tibia. Clin Orthop 138:105–110

Critical Soft Tissue Conditions and Pilon Fractures

O. Trentz and H. P. Friedl

Introduction

The microcirculation of the distal part of the lower leg is very precarious and notoriously poor soft tissue healing and inadequate venous drainage (leading frequently to unstable scar conditions, chronic edema, and stasis ulceration) are common around the distal tibia [3, 5, 8]. In addition to this the distal tibia and ankle are predisposed to high-energy trauma, as a result of combination of compressive and shearing forces. In pilon fractures three different mechanisms have been recognized to be responsible for major soft tissue injuries: direct high-energy impact, shearing injuries, and axial compression with explosion-like injuries of the bone stock.

Any high-energy injury may traumatize the skin and subcutaneous tissues from within by means of fracture fragments. The resultant massive swelling may lead to the early formation of post-traumatic bullae, and skin necrosis may ensue if the soft tissues are further traumatized by ill-advised or poorly timed surgical procedures. Since the state of the skin and subcutaneous tissues is of major importance in pilon fractures we strongly recommend that surgeons modify the established standard procedures (as recommended by the AO/ASIF group) and individualize treatment according to the nature of the injury, and the state of the bone and the soft tissues.

This paper deals specifically with the appropriate modifications of the recommended standard procedures in cases where there are critical, severely critical, and extremely critical soft tissue conditions.

General Principles

The operative strategy used in dealing with pilon fractures is frequently much influenced by precarious soft tissue conditions. Therefore, timing of surgery, appropriate operative strategies, and delicate, atraumatic handling of the soft tissues are of vital importance in the management of these fractures.

Any additional tension, and distraction or "ligamentotaxis" should be strictly avoided, if critical soft tissue conditions exist in a primary closed injury (without an open wound being present) or where the soft tissues have been closed artificially by suture.

Furthermore, preoperative planning should include the optimal timing of surgery, consider further impairment of critical soft tissues during the post-traumatic course, and focus on two "windows" (Fig. 1):
(1) primary surgery as soon as possible and preferably within the first 6 h after trauma, or (2) delayed surgery following recuperation of the soft tissues approximately between the sixth and 12th day after trauma. Surgery performed beyond the 12th day after trauma appears to be less advantageous due to the fact that anatomical reconstruction of the articular surface becomes increasingly difficult.
Since the microcirculation of injured tissues is so precarious, any rough handling, kinking of skin flaps or inadvertent distraction of damaged tissues – especially with a tourniquet in place – will definitely amplify the initial insult and interfere with wound healing. Delicate handling of the soft tissues is thus of major importance in the management of these complex injuries. The general principles are outlined in Table 1.

Critical, Severely Critical, and Extremely Critical Soft Tissue Conditions: Modifications of the Standard Procedure

With critical soft tissue conditions we prefer gradually to modify the established standard procedure [4] (Table 2) according to our protocol (Fig. 2).

Critical Soft Tissue Conditions (IC2-IO1)

With critical soft tissue conditions (Table 3), graded IC2-IO1 according to the AO/ASIF classification [6] or grade I according to Oestern and Tscherne [7], internal buttressing may be modified by placing the buttress plate in either an anterior or a posterior position.
Soft tissue defects should be covered temporarily with skin substitutes. Free tissue transfer should be used frequently.

Table 1. General principles and tissue handling of pilon fractures with critical soft tissue conditions

1. *Internal buttressing intended:*
Skin bridges > 7 cm
Extended straight incisions
Fasciocutaneous dissection
"Holding sutures"
2. *Distant buttressing intended* (see text):
Stab incisions for percutaneous reconstruction of the articular surface

Table 2. Standard procedures in the absence of critical soft tissue conditions

1. Fibular reconstruction
2. Articular reconstruction
3. Bone grafting
4. Internal buttressing
Medial buttress plate
(Anterior buttress plate)

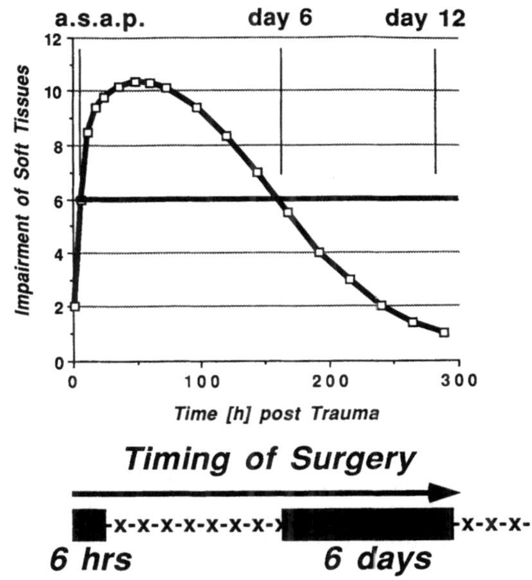

Fig. 1. Optimal timing of surgery should consider additional impairment of critical soft tissues after trauma and focus on two "windows": (1) primary surgery as soon as possible and preferably within the first 6 h after trauma, (2) or delayed surgery following recuperation of the soft tissues between the 6th and 12th days after trauma

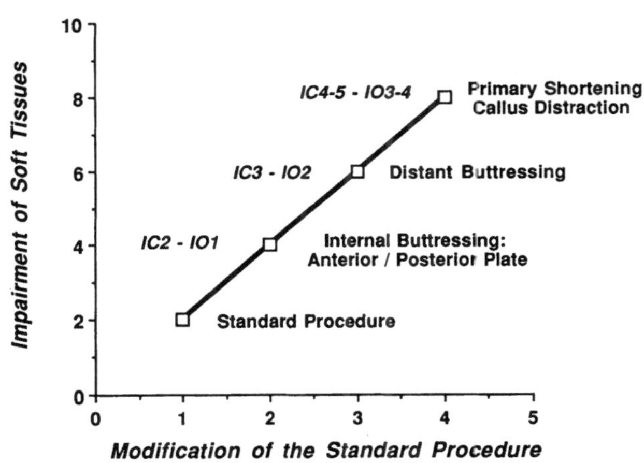

Fig. 2. Gradual modification of the standard procedure according to the severety of soft tissue injuries. For further details refer to Tables 2 (standard procedure), 3 (modified internal buttressing), 4 (distant buttressing), and 5 (primary shortening/callus distraction)

Severely Critical Soft Tissue Conditions (IC3-IO2)

With severely critical soft tissue conditions (Table 4) a distant buttressing technique may be used to give adequate support and to prevent secondary deformity. In these cases reconstruction of the articular surface is performed percutaneously through stab incisions (Table 1). Following this a triangular unilateral external fixator may be used for temporary or auxiliary medial buttressing, particularly if critical soft tissue conditions (graded IC3-IO2 [6], or grade II according to [7]) do not permit primary internal (plate) buttressing of the tibia. Alternatively the "comb" ("en peigne") technique of Judet et al. [4] may be considered.
Soft tissue defects should be covered temporarily with skin substitutes (e.g. Epigard) and definitively by a free tissue transfer (preferably musculocutaneous flaps) as soon as is feasible. Following restoration of the soft tissues external fixators should be replaced as soon as possible (to preserve the articular function of the ankle joint) by a scheduled re-osteosynthesis employing an internal buttressing technique. With the availability of titanium plates we prefer to use LC-DC plates (3.5 or 4.5 mm) for this purpose. Free tissue transfer should be resorted to frequently since unstable scar conditions usually limit scheduled re-osteosynthesis or reconstructive surgical procedures.

Table 3. Procedures in the presence of critical soft tissue conditions

1. Fibular reconstruction
2. Articular reconstruction
3. Bone grafting
4. *Modified internal buttressing*
   Anterior internal buttressing
   (Posterior buttress plate)
5. *Free tissue transfer*

Italic type denotes differences from the standard procedure detailed in Table 2.

Table 4. Procedures in the presence of severely critical soft tissue conditions

1. Fibular reconstruction
2. Articular reconstruction
3. Bone grafting
4. *Distant buttressing*
   External fixator
   ("Comb" technique)
5. *Free tissue transfer*
6. *Scheduled re-osteosynthesis*
   Internal buttressing

Italic type denotes differences from the standard procedure detailed in Table 2.

Table 5. Procedures in the presence of extremely critical soft tissue conditions

1. Fibular reconstruction/*shortening*
2. Articular reconstruction
3. *Shortening/impaction*
4. *Internal or distant buttressing and* (if required)
5. *Free tissue transfer*
   and
6. *Scheduled re-osteosynthesis* (if required)
7. *Reconstitution of the original length by callus distraction*

Italic type denotes differences from the standard procedure detailed in Table 2.

Extremely Critical Soft Tissue Conditions (IC4-5-IO3-4)

In cases with extremely critical soft tissue conditions (graded IC4-5-IO3-4, or grade III) combined with comminuted fibula fractures we recommend primary impaction of the fracture fragments and shortening to obtain contact of vital soft tissues aside from the primary impact (Table 5). Fixation depends on the conditions of the soft tissues and can be achieved by using either technique of internal or distant buttressing.
Remaining soft tissue defects may be covered first with skin substitutes and then by a free tissue transfer (preferably musculocutaneous flaps) as soon as is feasible. Scheduled re-osteosynthesis is only required if a distant buttressing technique was chosen for fixation.
Compensatory reconstitution of the original length can be achieved by employing callus distraction techniques at the earliest convenient time, preferably after restoration of the soft tissues [1, 2].

Salvage Procedures with Osteitis, Malunions, and Non-unions

Secondary complications following operative treatment are frequently accompanied by poor soft tissue conditions. Debridement of bony structures, soft tissues, and unstable scars is therefore followed by the reconstruction of a vital and stable soft tissue envelope. As a rule definitive bony reconstruction should be achieved secondary to the restoration of the soft tissues.

Conclusion

The operative strategy in dealing with pilon fractures with critical soft tissue conditions should involve appropriate modifications of the standard procedures. In summary, where the condition of the soft tissues is extremely critical consider: (1) preliminary dressing of tissue defects with skin substitutes; (2) delayed internal buttressing; (3) frequent use of free tissue transfer; and (4) primary shortening and compensatory callus distraction.
Since delicate, atraumatic handling of the soft tissues is of vital importance in the management of these fractures the operative strategy should strictly avoid any additional tension, distraction, or "ligamentotaxis", if critical soft tissue conditions exist in a primary closed injury (without an open wound being present) or where the soft tissues have been closed artificially by suture.
Timing of surgery should focus preferably on two "windows" involving either immediate surgery within the first 6 h after trauma or delayed surgery within the period between the sixth and 12th days after trauma. Free tissue transfer should be used frequently. Following restoration of the soft tissues distant buttressing techniques should be replaced by a scheduled re-osteosynthesis employing an internal buttressing technique.

References

1. Giebel G (1987) Extremitätenverlängerung und die Behandlung von Segmentdefekten durch Kallus-Distraktion. Chirurg 58:601–606
2. Giebel G (1991) Resektions-Débridement am Unterschenkel mit kompensatorischer Kallus-Distraktion. Unfallchirurg 94(8):401–408
3. Heim U (1991) Taktik und Technik beim Weichteilschaden. In: Heim U (ed) Die Pilon-tibial-Fraktur. Springer, Berlin Heidelberg New York, pp 204–208
4. Judet J, Judet R, Letournel E (1967) Un procédé d'osteosynthèse pour fracture multifragmentaire du pilon tibial. Mem Acad Chir 17–18:547–549
5. Mast J, Spiegel PG, Pappas JN (1988) Fractures of the tibial pilon. Clin Orthop 230: 68–82
6. Müller ME, Allgöwer M, Schneider R, Willenegger H (1991) Manual of internal fixation. Springer, Berlin Heidelberg New York
7. Oestern HJ, Tscherne H (1983) Pathophysiologie und Klassifikation des Weichteilschadens. Hefte Unfallheilkd 162:1–9
8. Tile M (1987) Fractures of the distal tibial metaphysis Involving the ankle joint: the pilon fracture. In: Schatzker J, Tile M (eds) The rationale of operative fracture care. Springer, Berlin Heidelberg New York, pp 343–369

Complications After Pilon Fractures

G. Muhr and H. Breitfuß

Introduction

Complications after pilon fractures either result from lesions of the narrow soft tissue layer and the very congruent ankle joint or are brought about by treatment (e.g. infection and malalignment) [2]. To elucidate the complication rate we undertook a retrospective study of 229 patients with pilon fractures treated in the Trauma Department of the Bergmannsheil Hospital, Bochum, between 1969 and 1989.

Patients

Until 1984 our therapeutic approach followed the AO group's recommendations [3]: open reduction, internal plate fixation (ORIF), and early functional rehabilitation. Patients treated in this way ($n = 182$) comprised group 1 in our study. Since 1985 this approach has been used only in cases of simple fractures without soft tissue lesions. In all other fractures, reduction has been by closed means employing traction. The ankle joint is then stabilized with external fixator clamps and a reconstruction of only the joint surface carried out with a minimum of implants (screws, Kirschner wires). If necessary, after soft tissue healing, an internal fixation is done. Patients treated by this modified procedure ($n = 47$) comprised group 2 in our study. Follow-up for patients of group 1 was at 5 years postoperatively, and for group 2 at 2 years on average. The average age of the patients was 46 years.

Fractures and Treatment

Open fractures occurred in 28% of patients in group 1 and in 17% of those in group 2. Only 9% in group 1 and 4% in group 2 sustained their fracture as the result of indirect trauma (e.g. skiing injury); in all other patients a direct blow (e.g. traffic accident, fall) was the cause of the fracture.
Seventy percent of patients in group 1 were treated by open reduction and rigid internal fixation. In group 2 70% of patients had closed reduction, external transfixation of the fracture and, in some cases, primary minimal internal fixation. Only in 30% of group 2 patients was ORIF done.

Complications

In 10% of group 1 and 11% of group 2 patients a compartment syndrome was diagnosed. Since the origin of the problem was the original injury, there was no difference in the rate between groups. Treatment consisted of wide decompression incisions of the skin fascia.

In group 1 the overall infection rate was 13% (10% after closed and 20% after open fractures). In group 2 there were no cases of infection after closed fractures treated by closed reduction and external fixation. Postoperative osteitis occurred in 4.8% of patients who had open reduction and plate fixation. The overall infection rate in group 2 was therefore 4.8%.

Three patients in group 2 had malalignment, with an axial deformity of up to 8°. In each case fixation of the tibia and of the fibula was done according to different biomechanical methods (static-dynamic).

The results for function in the uninfected cases were as follows. Sixteen percent of patients in group 1 had unlimited function of the ankle joint, as did 26% of those in group 2. Loss of up to 20° of dorsiflexion was noted in 57% of group 1 and 67% of group 2 patients. Severe functional restrictions were present in 7% of patients in group 1 and 4% in group 2.

Narrowing or irregularities of the ankle joint space were found in radiographic controls in 28% of group 1 patients and 33% of those in group 2. Twenty-eight percent of group 1 and 4% of group 2 had symptomatic osteoarthritis.

Two years after trauma on average, 18% of group 1 patients required an ankle; fusion 75% of these had had previous septic complications. The fusion rate in group 2 was 6%; all of these patients had had a postoperative infection after fracture treatment.

Discussion

The study shows the problem of the fracture, but also the risks in treatment. Compartment syndromes were evident in the two groups to the same extent (10% and 11% for groups 1 and 2, respectively). This is an expression of the severity of the trauma and therefore unrelated to treatment. The rate of bone infections in the two groups is mainly the result of the high incidence of direct trauma with soft tissue lesions. Bourne [1] in his study of pilon fractures had 22% open fractures and a 13% infection rate, while Raymond and Pierce [4] had 33% open fractures and a 19% infection rate. Only Rüedi [5] had no infections in his patients after skiing injuries. In the present series a significant decrease in osteitis was evident in group 2 (17% open fractures, 4.8% infection rate) compared to group 1 (28% open fractures, 13% infection rate). This was related to the change in therapeutic approach, to closed reduction and external fixation as the norm and ORIF as the exception. All infections in group 2 were seen after primary plate fixation, so this technique seems to be the most likely cause of complications in the treatment of severe pilon fractures with soft tissue injury.

The study also showed the close correlation between bone infection and rate of ankle fusion: 75% of patients in group 1 who required a fusion, and 100% of those in group 2, had had osteitis after fracture treatment.
The overall fusion rate of 18% in group 1 was reduced to 6% in group 2. The difference in the timing of follow-up between the two groups (5 years for group 1 and 2 years for group 2) is less important, because all fusions were performed within a maximum of 2 years after trauma. It is obvious that osteoarthritis and osteitis are an unhappy combination which strongly indicate the need for fusion. Reduction of infection rate therefore reduces the fusion rate.
There was only a small number of axial deviations below 8° (valgus/varus position). They were seen in those cases where the fibula and tibia were stabilized according to different biomechanical principles. A static plate fixing the fibular fracture and a dynamic external fixator on the tibia lead of course to a varus deformity. The best way to avoid axial deviations is to use either a static-rigid or a dynamic fixation on each of the bones.
The similar functional result of the ankle joint in the non-infected cases in both groups gives strong support to the idea that ankle function in these severe comminuted fractures is not improved by ORIF and that similar results can be obtained by external transfixation (external fixation).

Conclusion

The complicated osseous situation of a pilon fracture is exacerbated by the soft tissue lesion. Some complications are induced by the trauma itself (compartment syndrome, osteoarthritis, functional restriction). Others are the result of the treatment (osteitis, fusion rate, axial deviation). Knowledge of these problems should lead to a decrease in the complication rate.

References

1. Bourne RB (1989) Pilon fractures of the distal tibia. Clin Orthop 240:42–45
2. Breitfuß H, Muhr G, Neumann K (1988) Prognose und Therapie des geschlossenen distalen intraartikulären Unterschenkelbruches. Unfallchirurg 91:557–564
3. Heim U (1991) Die Pilon-tibial-Fraktur. Springer, Berlin Heidelberg New York
4. Raymond O, Pierce JHH Jr (1979) Comminuted intraarticular fractures of the distal tibia. J Trauma 19/11:828–832
5. Rüedi T (1983) Die Fraktur des Pilon tibial. Unfallheilkunde 86:259–261

PART II · TALUS FRACTURES

Talus Fractures

E. H. Kuner, H. L. Lindenmaier, and P. Münst

Historical Review

One of the first reports of an injury of the talus is by Herodot (490–420 B.C.) (cited in [8]). King Darius I (522–486 B.C.) is said to have fallen from his horse while hunting a lion, sustaining an open fracture-dislocation. The most important phrase in the original Greek is "the talus dislocated out of the joint". The treatment by an Egyptian surgeon was successful and the king was able to walk without difficulty. In another report in 1608 Fabricius Hildanus [7] mentions a surgeon who, in 1582, successfully treated an open talar dislocation by talectomy. This method, rather than primary amputation, was also suggested by Cooper in 1818 [5]. James Syme in the mid-nineteenth century on the other hand, preferred primary amputation for the treatment of open fracture-dislocations of the talus [24]. He based his suggestion on the known mortality of 84% following such an injury at that time.

In 1892, Ernest von Bergmann in Berlin was the first to try open reduction of a dislocated talus [27]. He reported that at operation the talocalcaneal interosseous ligament was ruptured. This led subsequent authors to believe that the injury represented a subtalar dislocation of the foot with a fracture of the body or neck of the talus, as in a complete dislocation of the body this ligament would not be injured. At that time the general opinion was that the talus was supplied by just one blood vessel located in the talocalcaneal ligament. However, in 1894 Schlatter [22] demonstrated on a post-mortem specimen that a large number of blood vessels nurture the talus, both anteriorly and from the medial and lateral sides.

This brief historical review serves to highlight a number of problems unique to this fracture, which even today causes significant clinical difficulties.

Literature Review

In search of a rational method of treatment, we first made a detailed study of the literature [15]. We then reviewed cases treated in AO clinics, and in 1983 reported the initial results [13]; we will refer to these later in the paper. In our study of the literature, 1204 publications relevant to talus fractures from 37 countries were examined. This review of 2712 fractures in total highlighted several aspects of presentation and management.

The rarity of talus fractures makes them more difficult to manage. They comprise only 0.32% of all fractures and only 3.4% of foot fractures. Injuries most commonly associated with talar fractures are malleolar fractures (in 44%), calcaneal fractures (in 18%), and metatarsal fractures (in 18%). Thirteen percent of talus fractures are open fractures.
One of the central issues in talus fractures is the incidence of avascular necrosis. Rates reported in the literature from 1940 to 1975 vary between 18% and 58%. For example: Bonnin [3], 35%; Watson-Jones [29], 50%; Decoulx and Razemon [6], 45%; Schlag [21], 58%; Herwig [10], 18%; Schulitz [23], 42%. It is important to note that in most of these reports neither the degree of injury nor disruption of the bone fragments was mentioned. From the cases with more detailed data, the risk of necrosis can be calculated:

Comminuted fracture	1: 1.8
Neck fracture with dislocation	1: 2
Body fracture with dislocation	1: 4
Neck fracture without dislocation	1: 8
Body fracture without disolocation	1:10.5
Head fracture	1:20

These findings form the basis of a number of similar classifications of talus fractures which have been suggested by various authors [2, 9, 26, 30].
The avascular necrosis caused by injury to the talar blood vessels is similar to that seen in subcapital fractures of the femoral neck. However, the vascular supply to the talus is perhaps not as vulnerable, as all of the three main arteries of the lower limb – the anterior tibial, the posterior tibial, and the peroneal – provide a contribution (Fig. 1). The most important is the posterior tibial artery from which arises the tarsal canal artery, which in turn supplies almost the entire talar body [16, 29]. The tarsal canal artery anastomoses with the artery of the tarsal sinus, which takes its origin from the anterior tibial artery and also supplies the periosteal network. Kelly and Sullivan [12] demonstrated the ample range of variations of the blood supply.
In an experimental study Peterson [17] demonstrated that with a fracture of the talar neck the tarsal canal artery as well as the artery of the tarsal sinus can be injured, depending on the degree of fracture-dislocation. Unfortunately it is difficult to define the severity of dislocation of the fragments necessary to compromise circulation to the talus and subsequently cause avascular necrosis. This is because the initial radiograph shows only the result of the forces applied not the initial displacement that may have occurred. Thus, our information will always be deficient in this area.
About half of all talar fractures are located within the neck of the talus. A number of publications have shown that this is due to both anatomical factors and the pathomechanics of the injury. The centre of both the ankle and subtalar joints is formed by the irregularly shaped talus. About 60% of its surface is covered by cartilage and this forms the articulations of the ankle and subtalar joints as well as the talonavicular joint (Fig. 2). No muscles insert into the talus so it has no active motion. Rather it acts to transfer the force of the

body weight on to the skeleton of the foot. Its shape, ligamentous constraints, and trabecular development are all designed to assist in this function.

Lindenmaier [14] demonstrated the trabecular pattern on the basis of radiographs of 9 mm-thick saw cuts of the talus, one group coming from young persons (average age 16) and one group from elderly persons (average age 75 years). He found a reduced density of trabeculae going from the body to the neck, with trabeculae in the region of the body being very dense and, due to the force transmitted, almost perpendicular to the joint surface. In the region of the talar neck and head the trabeculae were positioned horizontally and were less dense (Fig. 3).

In force-pressure studies on the surface of the talus Lindenmaier [14] found that at the transition from the neck to the body there is a weak spot which, especially in dorsiflexion, breaks with pressure. Coltart [4], in his studies on British Air Force personnel stressed the importance of force applied to the dorsiflexed foot. This led to the phrase "aviator's astragalus." All of the other main injuries of the talus result from multidirectional force, either direct or indirect. Rotation and compression is the most common mechanism of injury as a rule. These forces also lead to the commonly seen associated injuries in the foot.

In earlier times the cause of the injury was a fall from a height in more than half of cases (52%). Road traffic accidents (18%) played a minor role [15]. In Germany today the main cause is automobile and motorbike accidents, which account for 48% of injuries.

Classification

To develop a consistent method of management a reliable classification of the injury is needed. This classification must be simple, requiring only a few clinical and radiological details to evaluate the treatment necessary and the prognosis. It should also differentiate between central and peripheral talar fractures. In central talar fractures the degree of dislocation is the decisive factor to predict the risk of avascular necrosis. Peripheral talar fractures include fractures of the processes (posterior and lateral) and flake fractures. Fractures of the body, neck, trochlea, and head are included in central fractures. Fractures of the talar neck can be further classified into three groups [9]:

Type I Undisplaced talar neck fracture with no subluxation. The circulation is patent and there is no risk of avascular necrosis.

Type II Talar neck fracture with subluxation or dislocation of the subtalar joint. There is a risk of necrosis because the circulation is impaired and only the auxiliary circulation is intact.

Type III Fracture of the talar neck with dislocation of the body out of the subtalar joint. In these cases all of the three main vessels are damaged, so that even the auxiliary circulation is impaired. There is a high incidence of avascular necrosis.

Necrosis is also a risk in comminuted fractures of the body of the talus.
The prognosis is influenced not only by the topographic and anatomical location of the fracture but also by the damage to the surrounding tissues. This is true for closed as well as open fractures.

Diagnosis

The diagnosis of a talar fracture is relatively simple. After taking the history of the trauma and doing a complete clinical examination, very detailed local examination of the foot is necessary. The degree of tissue swelling, the deformity, the peripheral circulation, and the motor power and sensation of the toes are all important. Standard radiographic views include the ankle joint and the subtalar joint, as well as two oblique views designed to demonstrate even better the subtalar situation. It is of great importance to detect the entire injury. In some cases tomograms or CT scans are necessary.

Treatment

The aim of treatment is an immediate reduction, as close as possible to an anatomical reduction, with avoidance of secondary tissue damage.
Apart from direct damage to cartilage, an important factor causing secondary arthrosis is incongruity due to residual subluxation. On the basis of these considerations we have formulated guidelines for treatment. Central fractures which are not subluxated (type I) can be treated conservatively.
We are now extending our indications to operative treatment because stable fixation has many advantages, as has been previously seen in fixation of intra-articular fractures. The surgical technique will therefore be described in some detail.

Surgical Technique

The incision is anteromedial and should not be too small. It starts at the level of the ankle joint in the medial third and continues in an arc distally to the tuberosity of the navicular [25] (Fig. 4). If necessary it can be extended proximally and distally. The dissection through the subcutaneous tissue preserves the saphenous vein and nerve. The fascia is incised in the line of the incision and the capsule opened first at the level of the ankle joint and then distally. A good view of the anterior trochlea, the medial ankle joint, and the neck and head of the talus is obtained. The joint capsule of the transverse tarsal articulation (Chopart's joint) is opened if necessary.
With this exposure, all talar neck fractures can be reduced exactly and stabilized. Fixation is obtained with either 4.0 mm cancellous screws or one screw together with a 1.8 mm Kirschner wire (Fig. 5). Sometimes a 6.5 mm cancel-

lous screw can be used. Small peripheral fragments or fresh osteochondral fragments can be held with absorbable pins (i.e. Ethipins or Biofix) or possibly with fibrinous glue. The screw is inserted from the head of the talus, its head being countersunk beneath the articular surface. Zones of osteochondral indentation are elevated and the defects filled with cancellous bone.
Dislocated trochlear fragments of type III can be very difficult to reduce. In these cases various reduction aids have to be used. If there is no ankle fracture then an osteotomy of the medial malleolus can be performed. Using an image intensifier the exact position of the osteotomy is determined and holes drilled for subsequent insertion of cancellous screws to fix the medial malleolus. Only then is the osteotomy done, which should be perpendicular to the screw holes (Fig. 6).
In very difficult cases a temporary external fixator is applied to gain length. With two pins in the calcaneus the distraction can be increased either anteriorly (volarly) or dorsally as needed, so that room is made for the reduction of a dislocated body or trochlear fragment (Figs. 7 and 8). Rarely Schanz screws have to be used to reduce a dislocated fragment of the talar body.
Only rarely a second lateral exposure is necessary. Postoperatively a lower limb plaster slab is applied immediately to prevent equinus.

Subsequent Management

The following questions need to be answered clearly:

1. What is the state of the soft tissues?
2. What is the fracture type?
3. Can the fracture be treated conservatively?
4. Has an operation been performed?
   a) Stable internal fixation with screw?
   b) Co-aption of fragments with fixation used as a buttress?
   c) Cast necessary for protection?

The non-subluxated central talus fracture, with no displacement, wherever located, can be treated conservatively with good results. This is also true for the subluxated talar neck fracture (type II) if it can be reduced exactly. Immobilization with a split cast in an elevated position is carried out until the tissue swelling is reduced. After 8–10 days the patient is put into a walking cast, which is left on for 5–6 weeks in the case of a non-subluxated fracture. With an initially subluxated fracture the cast is left on for a period of 8–10 weeks, depending on the radiographic findings. After that, physiotherapy is best performed in the thermal pool.
In the case of a stable screw osteosynthesis in type II talar neck fractures we use a split cast postoperatively to prevent equinus. On the second postoperative day active movement is carried out under the supervision of a physiotherapist. Later passive motion using the continuous passive movement (CPM) machine is carried out (Fig. 9a–l).

If wound healing is satisfactory the patient is mobilized and after 10–12 days is discharged. For the first 10–12 weeks loading of 10–15 kg on the affected side is permitted. After this time, depending on the case, gradual increase to full weight-bearing is permitted. This usually takes 4–6 weeks.

If the comminuted fragments have been co-apted without complete stable fixation, then management is the same as for conservative fractures except with prolonged immobilization.

Fractures with severe comminution or open fractures in association with a dislocation are treated primarily by operation. The reduction is as close as possible to anatomical. In most cases, unfortunately, co-aption only of the fragments is possible and prolonged immobilization is required. A primary astragalectomy has yet never been performed.

Prolonged non-weight-bearing has been advised to reduce the risk of avascular necrosis and promote revascularization in type III fractures; however, this is now debatable. In the literature, more and more single case reports can be found where revascularization has taken place with a prolonged period of non-weight-bearing [11, 19]. Other pathophysiological and morphological reports point to the fact that prolonged non-weight-bearing produces secondary damage rather than being a positive factor. For talar neck fractures of type III one has to assume that the talar body is devoid of all blood supply. Anatomical reduction with stable fixation is an important prerequisite for undisturbed bone healing, but an intact blood supply is also important for healing and maintenance of anatomical shape.

In weight-bearing areas, indentations and irregularities are subsequently seen which lead to radiological opacities in the cancellous bone. The surrounding bone tissue attempts to heal with a spread of new blood vessels ("creeping substitution") which leads to re-ossification [18]. However, these healing processes stop early, especially in loaded areas, and secondary bone infarctions with demarcation occur. The radiograph shows an osteolytic area around a separated fragment. Further consequences are the destruction and partial removal of necrotic material through the new blood vessels so that small cavities result [1].

Because of the low chance of revascularization, even after the restitution of normal anatomical form and structure, prolonged non-weight-bearing cannot be advised. Hyaline cartilage is nurtured through diffusion and thus depends on movement and pressure though normal weight-bearing, so long-term immobilization can lead to a secondary arthrosis [23]. These pathophysiological considerations form the basis of our general approach to operative management.

It is important in our view to find a method which enables assessment of the viability of the talus at an early stage. The above changes on the plain radiograph (changes in shape, density and cysts) are late signs. Riess [20] carried out an osseous venogram in three cases and demonstrated that injecting 3–4 ml of contrast medium into the talus leads to immediate filling of the lower limb veins if the circulation is patent. If the contrast medium remains in the talar body and no venous filling is observed, avascular necrosis is likely (Fig. 10).

Today magnetic resonance imaging (MRI) provides a noninvasive technique for assessing avascular necrosis. Stainless steel implants have to be removed first, but the titanium screws that we use now do not impair the MRI scan at all.

The AO Multicenter Study

Finally we would like to present some data from the AO multicenter study. It has to be pointed out that the experience with talus fractures varied significantly from one hospital to another. Thus the indication for conservative or operative treatment was not always based on the same indications. Furthermore, follow-up was carried out after only 34 months, so that the question of delayed damage could not be answered completely. Thirteen percent of the talus fractures were open, with an infection rate of over 30%. Seventy-seven percent of patients had additional injuries, of which subtalar subluxation/luxation (63%) and tibiotalar joint injuries (20%) were the most prominent and had a significant influence on the final result. In most cases a ventromedial incision was performed; a dorsal approach was chosen in only 7 cases (Table 1). An additional osteotomy was necessary in 30 cases. Most implants were screws or Kirschner wires, either separately or in combination. Compared with previously reported rates in the literature [3, 6, 10, 21, 29] the rate of postoperative necrosis in this study was relatively low (20%); after conservative treatment it was only 11% (Table 2). The conservatively managed and operative groups cannot be compared, however, because only simple, minimally dislocated fractures were managed conservatively while all severely dislocated fractures were managed operatively.

The rate of post-traumatic arthrosis was 45% and 53% in the conservative and postoperative groups respectively. Presumably in some cases the differentiation between partial necrosis and an exclusively post-traumatic arthrosis is difficult, because in both cases a fairly severe deformation is observed.

Table 1. AO multicenter study: operative approaches and implants used

Operative approach ($n = 137$)	
Medial incision	94 cases
Lateral or ventral incision	27 cases
Associated medial malleolar osteotomy	30 cases
Dorsal incision	7 cases
Implants	
Screws	54.7%
Kirschner wire	45.2%
Plate	0.7%
External fixator	0.7%
None	6.6%

Table 2. AO multicenter study: incidence of avascular necrosis[a]

Operative management ($n = 137$)	
Neck fracture	20.3%
Body/trochlea	21.1%
Conservative management ($n = 125$)	
Neck fracture	11.1%
Body/trochlea	18.8%

[a] Avascular necrosis was not seen in peripheral fractures

Table 3. AO multicenter study: functional results following central talus fractures

Functional result	Treatment group	
	Conservative ($n = 125$)	Operative ($n = 137$)
Excellent	10%	25%
Good	37%	26%
Poor	53%	49%

Functional results were evaluated according to the criteria used by Weber [31] for the ankle joint (Table 3). Results in one half of the cases were unsatisfactory. It has to be pointed out that symptoms were often less than would have been expected from the radiographs.

Conclusion

From our experience with talus fractures the following conclusions can be drawn:

1. Central dislocated fractures of the talus have to be treated as an emergency. At least the reduction must be carried out as an emergency in an effort to preserve the blood supply.
2. The reduction has to be anatomical irrespective of whether management is conservative or operative.
3. A stable osteosynthesis with screws enables early motion to be started after 2 weeks, combined with early partial weight-bearing of 15–20 kg.
4. After approximately 3 months an MRI scan should be performed to examine the viability of the talus. This necessitates using titanium screws as stainless steel implants interfere with the scan.

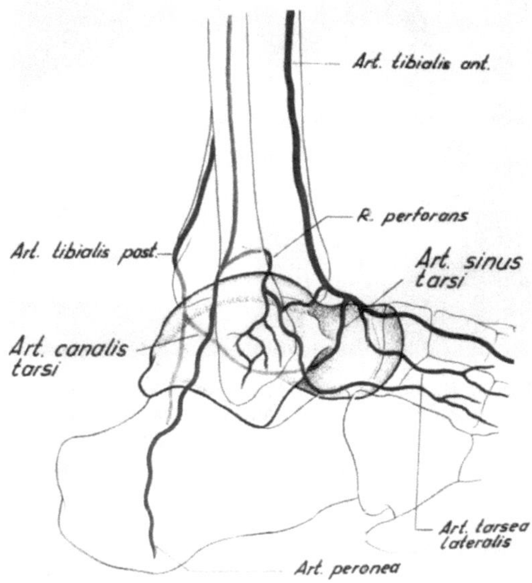

Fig. 1. All three arteries of the lower limb contribute to the vascularization of the talus. The most important, however, is the dorsalis pedis artery with its branch, the tarsal canal artery, which anastomoses with the tarsal sinus artery

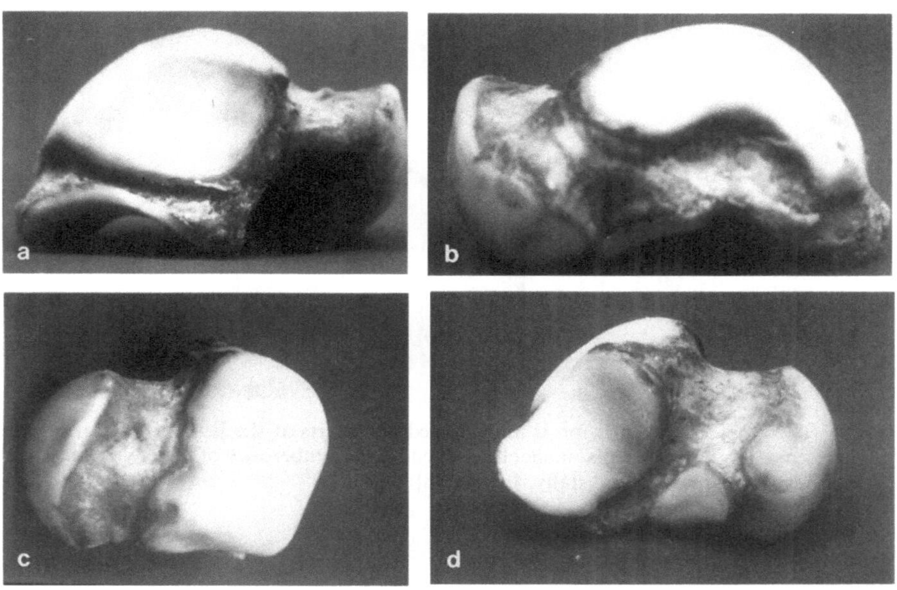

Fig. 2 a–d. About 60% of the talar surface is joint surface. Here the talus is shown in: **a** lateral aspect; **b** medial aspect; **c** from above; **d** from below

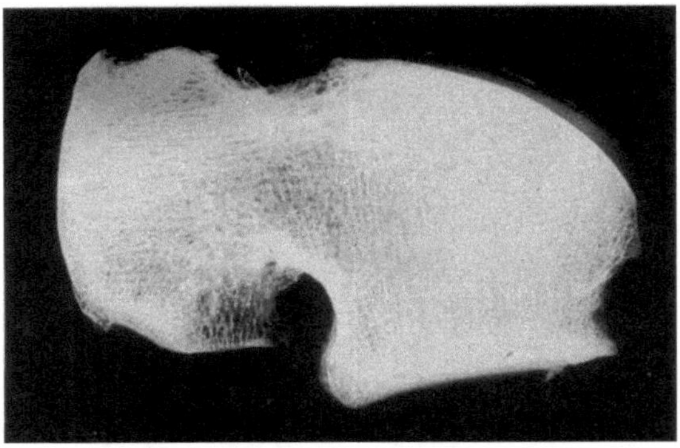

Fig. 3. Radiograph of a 9-mm-thick saw cut of the talus. The reduced density of the cancellous bone between body and neck can be seen clearly. The trabeculae in the region of the body are very dense and almost perpendicular to the subtalar joint, while in the region of the neck they are positioned horizontally but again perpendicular to the articulation

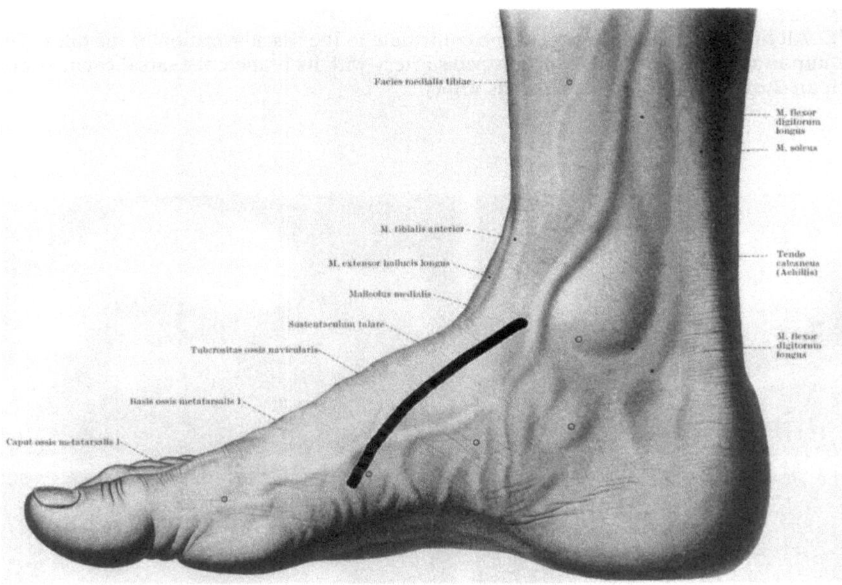

Fig. 4. The anteromedial incision is arch-shaped and starts at the level of the ankle joint about 1 cm lateral of the medial malleolus and ends at the tuberosity of the navicular. It can be extended proximally and distally. (From [28])

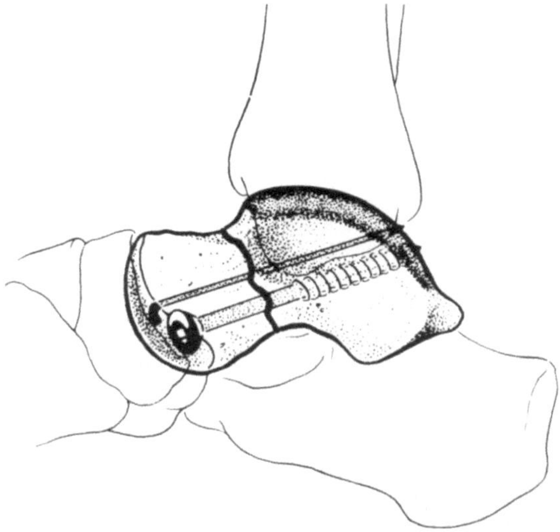

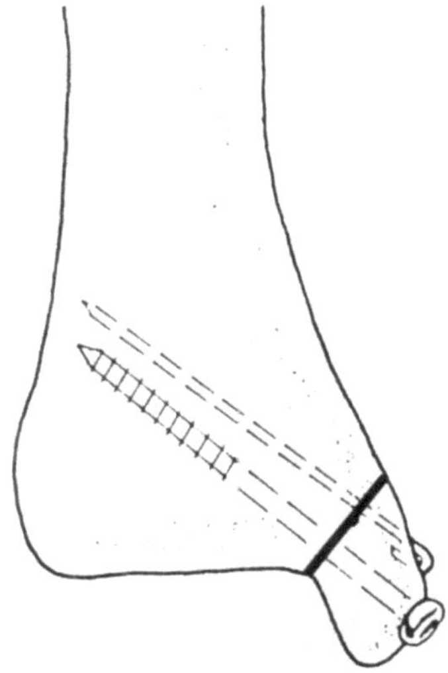

Fig. 5 *(left)*. An exact anatomical reduction of a talar neck fracture stabilized with a malleolar screw and a 1.8 mm Kirschner wire. Alternatively two 4.0 mm cancellous screws can be used

Fig. 6 *(right)*. With a difficult reduction (e.g. type III) an oblique osteotomy of the medial malleolus can be helpful. The dorsal structures have to be protected carefully

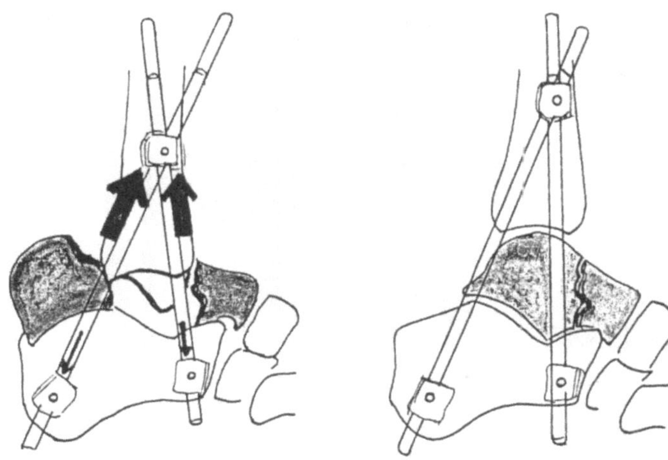

Fig. 7. In the case of a very difficult reduction a temporary external fixator can be applied. Two pins have to be positioned in the calcaneus to control the posterior and anterior distraction

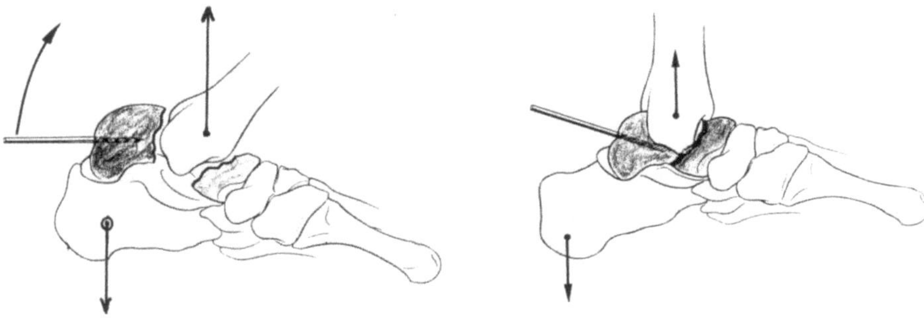

Fig. 8. Occasionally Schanz screws can be helpful in reducing a luxated body fragment

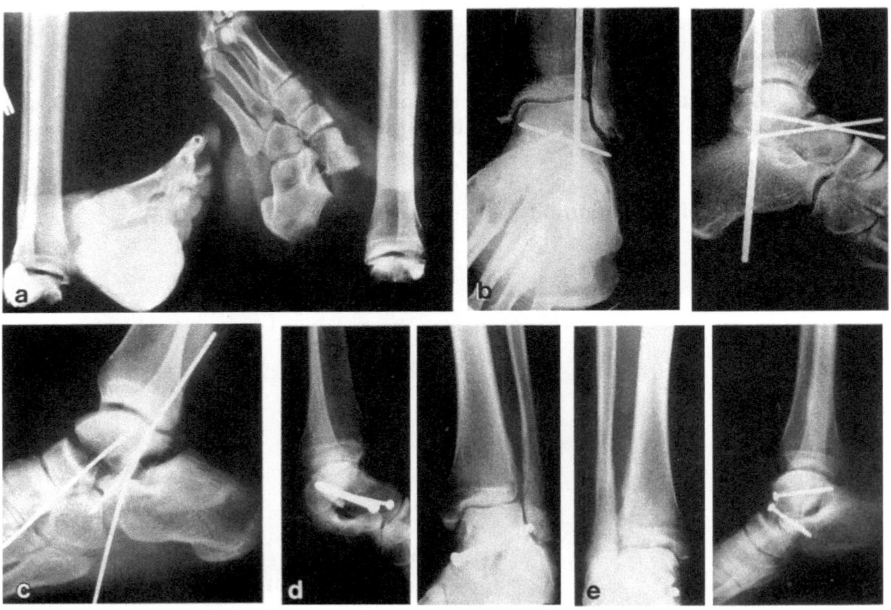

Fig. 9. a Radiograph of a 40-year-old man who fell while hill-climbing, sustaining widely open fractures of the talar neck on both limbs. Rescue and transport were very dramatic. **b, c** Primary treatment: reduction, debridement, temporary fixation with Kirschner wires. On the left side, the head-neck fragment is missing. **d, e** Radiographs taken 4 weeks after ORIF was carried out 2 weeks after the injury. On the right side compression in anatomical position has been achieved using lag screws. On the left, bridging of the defect with a bone graft and primary arthrodesis of the talocalcaneal and talonavicular joint are seen. **f, g** One year later. On both right and left side note the decreased joint space. On the left there is osseous bridging of the arthrodesis. **h, i** Pictures of motion 1 year after trauma: the patient still had good function and few symptoms. **j, k** Five years after trauma there is severe arthrosis with still-endurable symptoms, so that for the moment no special treatment is necessary ►

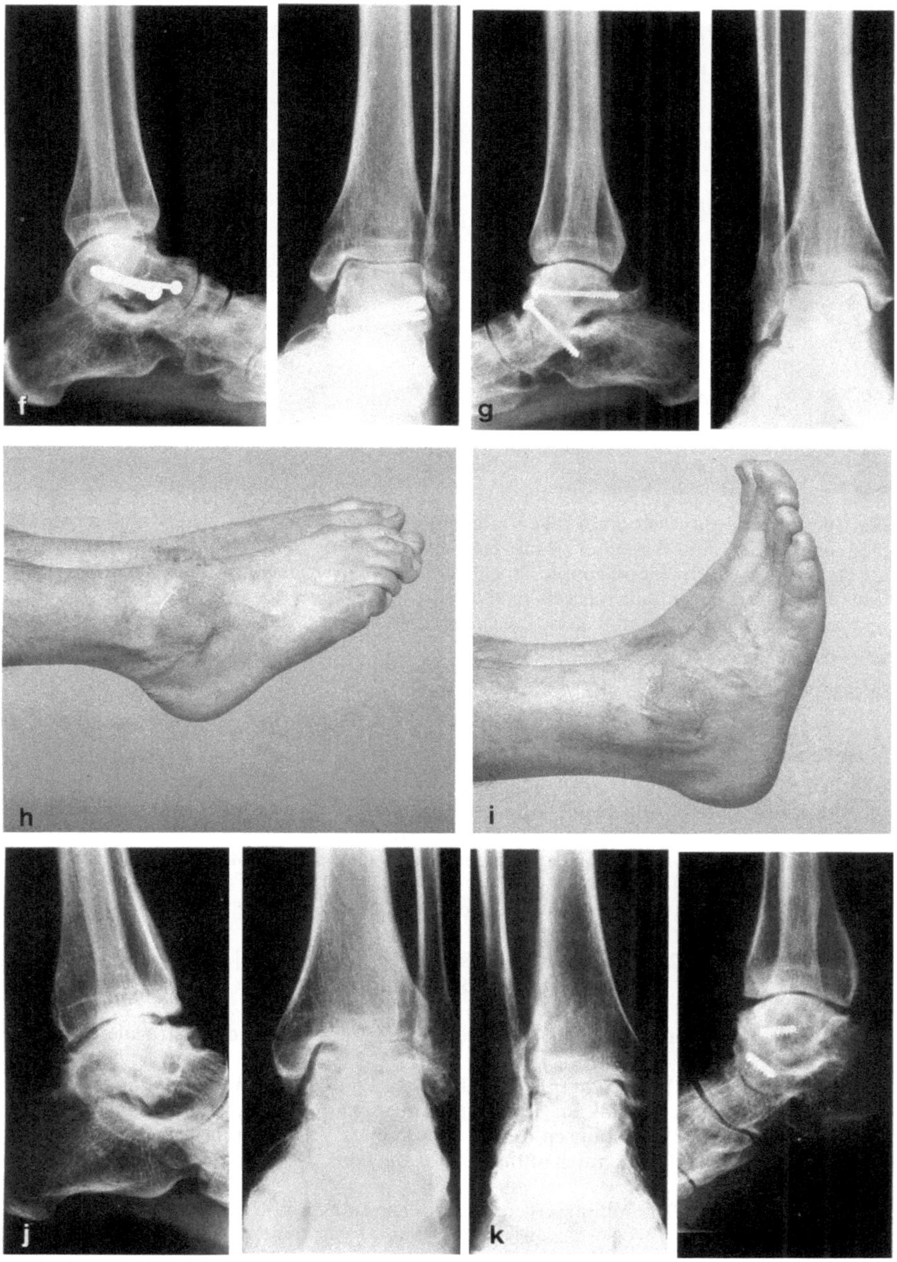
f
g
h
i
j
k

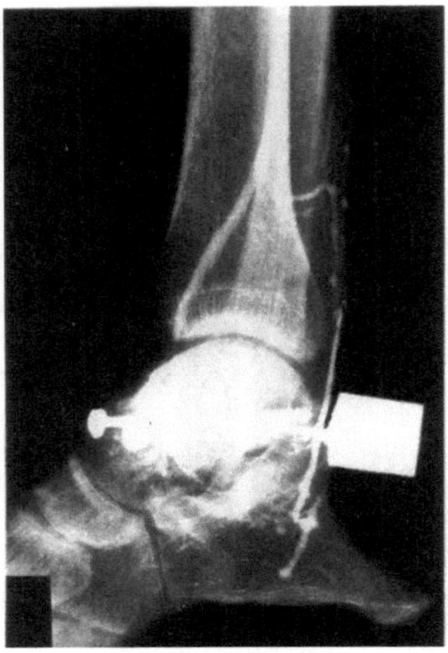

Fig. 10. Intraosseous venogram taken after injection of 3.0 ml of a water-soluble contrast medium into the talus. Already 1–2 min later a visible filling of the veins occurs, demonstrating the viability of the blood supply. In cases of severe arterial compromise (necrosis of the talus) the contrast medium remains in the talus for a longer time. In this venogram after operative treatment of a talar neck fracture (Hawkins II) 6 months after trauma no talar necrosis is seen

References

1. Bessler W (1989) Allgemeine Röntgensymptomatik des pathologischen Skeletts. In: Schinz's radiologische Diagnostik. Thieme, Stuttgart
2. Böhler L (1957) Die Technik der Knochenbruchbehandlung, 13th edn. Maudrich, Vienna
3. Bonnin JG (1940) Dislocations and fracture dislocations of the talus. Br J Surg 28:88–100
4. Coltart WD (1952) Aviator's astragalus. J Bone Joint Surg [B] 34:545–566
5. Cooper A (1818) Treatise on dislocations and fractures of the joints. Wells and Lilly, Boston
6. Decoulx P, Razemon JP (1960) La nécrose posttraumatique de l'astragale. Am Chir 14:771
7. Fabricius H (1608) Observatio LXVII (Letter to Philibertus) Observationum et curationum chirurgicum centurial. In: (1946) Opera quae extant omnia, vol 67. Frankfurt, p 140
8. Crond JTH (1947) Fractuur en luxatie van de talus. Dissertation, Amsterdam
9. Hawkins LG (1970) Fractures of the neck of the talus. J Bone Joint Surg [Am] 52:991–1002
10. Herwig K (1967) Behandlungsergebnisse frischer Talusfrakturen. Z Unfallmed Berufskr 60/2:91–106
11. Jenny F (1952) Über aseptische Nekrosen im Sprungbein. Chirurg 23:300–304
12. Kelly PJ, Sullivan C (1963) Blood supply of the talus. Clin Orthop 30:221–227
13. Kuner EH, Lindenmaier HL (1983) Zur Behandlung der Talusfraktur. Kontrollstudie von 262 Behandlungsfällen. Unfallchirurgie 9:35–40
14. Lindenmaier HL (1985) Experimentelle Untersuchungen zur Biomechanik des Talus. Habilitationsschrift, Faculty of Medicine, University of Freiburg

15. Mueller T (1980) Zur Problematik der Talusfraktur. Inauguraldissertation, Faculty of Medicine, University of Freiburg
16. Mulfinger GL, Trueta J (1970) The blood supply of the talus. J Bone Joint Surg [B] 52:160–167
17. Peterson L (1975) The arterial supply of the talus. Acta Orthop Scand 46:1026–1034
18. Phemister D (1931) Aseptische Knochennekrose bei Frakturen, Transplantationen und Gefäßverschlüssen. Z Orthop Chir 55:161–186
19. Riedl K, Reichelt A (1975) Komplikationen der Talusfrakturen. Z Orthop 113:696–701
20. Riess J (1967) Die ossale Venographie des Sprungbeines. Chirurg 38:72–73
21. Schlag G (1966) Die Talusfrakturen. Aktuel Chir 6:403
22. Schlatter C (1894) Zur Kasuistik der Talusluxationen. Bruns Beitr 11:80
23. Schulitz KP (1975) Die Bedeutung der Vaskularisation für die Talusnekrose nach Frakturen. Z Orthop 113:699–701
24. Syme J (1848) Contribution to the pathology and practice of surgery. Sutherland and Knox, Edinburgh
25. Szyszkowitz R, Reschauer R, Seggl W (1985) Eighty-five fractures treated by ORIF with five to eight years of follow-up: study of 69 patients. Clin Orthop 199:97–107
26. Tile M (1987) Fractures of the talus. In: Schatzker J, Tile M (eds) The rationale of operative fracture care. Springer, Berlin Heidelberg New York
27. von Bergmann (1892) Reposition des luxierten Talus von einem Schnitt aus. Langenbecks Arch Chir XLIII:1–12
28. von Lanz T, Wachsmuth W (1972) Bein und Statik. Springer, Berlin Heidelberg New York (Praktische Anatomie I/4)
29. Watson-Jones R (1956) Dislocation and fracture-dislocation of the talus. In: Fractures and joint injuries, vol 2, 4th edn. Livingstone, Edinburgh, pp 878–900
30. Weber BG (1974) Verrenkungen und Frakturen des Talus. In: Zenker, Deucher, Schink (eds) Chirurgie der Gegenwart. Urban and Schwarzenberg, Munich
31. Weber BG (1966) Die Verletzungen des oberen Sprunggelenkes. Huber, Bern

The Management of Fractures and Dislocations of the Talus

J. Schatzker and M. Tile

Introduction

Fractures of the talus, although rare injuries, can lead to serious disability, which may arise either as a result of the injury itself or its management. Disability as a result of the fracture itself is either due to the serious complication of avascular necrosis and secondary collapse of the body of the talus or due to malunion. Malunion results from malreduction of the fracture. This leads to incongruity and secondary osteoarthritis of the subtalar joint and to altered biomechanics of the foot due to altered alignment of the subtalar joint. Because fractures of the talus are often the result of a high-energy injury, even when closed they are very frequently associated with severe soft-tissue injury, which may not be immediately apparent. Injudicious surgery in combination with such a soft-tissue injury may lead to devastating sepsis with severe disability or even amputation the eventual outcome.

In 1832 Sir Astley Cooper provided the first detailed description of the natural history of dislocation of the talus [3]. In 1919 Anderson collected 18 cases of talar injuries occurring in flyers and coined the term "aviator's astralagus" [1]. The definitive publication on this subject, however, did not come until the publication of Coltart in 1952 [2]. He collected 228 cases, of which 106 were fractures or fracture dislocations of the talar neck. He described the natural history of fractures of the talar neck with no displacement, with subtalar dislocation, and with complete dislocation of the body of the talus, and indicated the prognosis for each. Most of the publications on fractures of the talus since then have embodied the principles expounded by Coltart.

The correct management of fractures of the talus depends on a sound integration of the principles of management of intra-articular fractures with the biological and biomechanical idiosynchrasies of the talus. Because the talus plays such an important part in the ankle and the subtalar joint and because the blood supply to the body of the talus is so precarious, before embarking on treatment the surgeon must have a sound knowledge of the anatomy of the talus and of its blood supply.

Anatomy

The talus is unique: 60% of its surface is covered by articular cartilage, and it has no muscular or tendinous attachments. It possess a head, a neck, and a body. The *head* is directed distally and slightly downward and medially. The *neck* of the talus is the slightly constricted part which connects the head to the body. It is set obliquely on the body and extends farther proximally on the medial side than on the lateral side. The medial part of its plantar surface has a deep groove called the *sulcus tali*. When the talus and the calcaneus are articulated together this groove forms the roof of a bony canal called the *sinus tarsi*.

The *body* of the talus is cuboidal in shape. Its dorsal surface is covered by the trochlear articular surface. It is widest anteriorly and convex from front to back and slightly concave from side to side. The lateral side is triangular in outline and covered by articular cartilage for articulation with the lateral malleolus. It is also concave from above downwards. Of note is the fact that the medial border of the trochlea is straight whereas the lateral border inclines medially at its posterior part. The medial surface is not all cartilaginous. Only its upper part is covered by a comma-shaped articular facet which is broader in front. It articulates with the medial malleolus. Below this facet the surface is pitted by numerous vascular foramina which receive the very important branches of the deltoid artery and branches of the artery of the tarsal canal (Fig. 1).

Vascular Anatomy

Because of the association of certain fractures and dislocations with avascular necrosis of the body of the talus, the extraosseous and intraosseous vascular

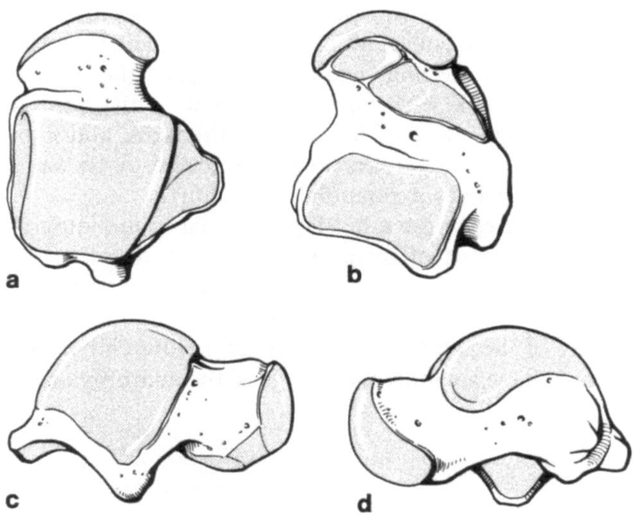

Fig. 1 a–d. Anatomic features of the talus: **a** Superior surface; **b** inferior surface; **c** lateral aspect; **d** medial aspect

anatomy must be appreciated in all its detail. It has been the subject of considerable investigation. Lexor et al. [12], Sneed [18], Phemister [17], McKeever [13], Watson-Jones [19], Kleiger [10], and Wildenauer [20] were the most important early investigators. Wildenauer described fully the blood supply of the talus in 1950, and is credited with being the first to describe the important artery arising from the posterior tibial, the *artery of the tarsal canal*, which runs through the tarsal canal and is responsible for most of the blood supply to the body of the talus. He also pointed out the distinction between the tarsal sinus and the tarsal canal. The tarsal canal lies obliquely from a posterior-medial to an anterior-lateral position and opens into the tarsal sinus. In the canal one finds the interosseous talocalcaneal ligament and the artery of the tarsal canal. Further work by Coltart [2], Lauro and Purpura [11], Haliburton et al. [7], and Montis and Ridola [14] confirmed the work of Wildenauer and especially the importance of the medial blood supply. The most elegant work on the blood supply of the talus is that of Mulfinger and Trueta [15], who used a special injection technique which ensured that only the arterial part of the vascular tree was injected. This work reaffirmed the work of Wildenauer and others and put to rest any remaining controversy regarding the blood supply of the talus.

Extraosseous Blood Supply

The extraosseous blood supply of the talus arises from the posterior tibial, from the anterior tibial, and from the dorsalis pedis arteries.

From the Posterior Tibial Artery

Artery of the Tarsal Canal. This important arterial branch, named by Wildenauer the artery of the tarsal canal, usually arises from the posterior tibial artery 1 cm proximal to the origin of the medial and lateral plantar arteries (see Fig. 2). It then passes anteriorly between the sheath of the flexor digitorum longus tendon to enter the tarsal canal, in which it lies close to the talus. It gives rise to many branches which enter the body of the talus on the medial side as well as branches which enter the body of the talus on its inferior surface from the tarsal canal. The vessel continues through the canal into the tarsal sinus where it anastomoses with vessels in the tarsal sinus which have originated from the peroneal and dorsalis pedis vessels. Thus there is a very rich vascular network under the neck of the talus.

Deltoid Branch. This vessel arises most commonly from the artery of the tarsal canal but may arise directly from the posterior tibial artery. It lies close to the inner aspect of the deltoid ligament and sends many branches which enter directly through the medial surface of the body of the talus. It is responsible for the major portion of the blood supply to the medial half of the body of the talus (see Fig. 3). The surgical significance of this vessel is obvious. First, since

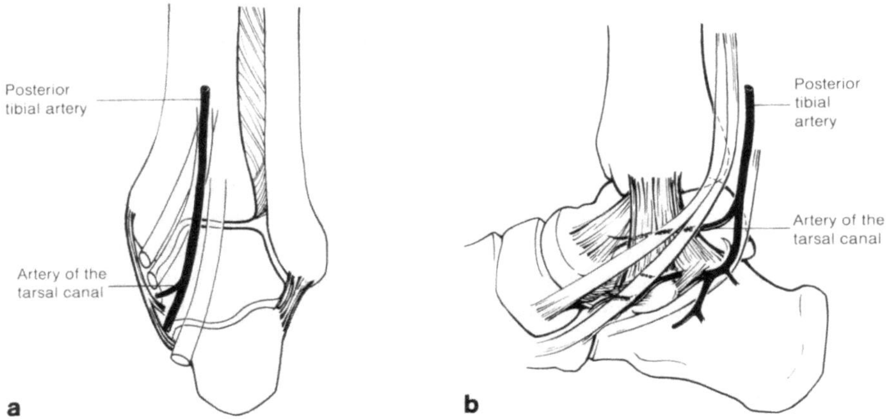

Fig. 2a, b. Extraosseous blood supply to the talus. **a** The artery of the tarsal canal arising from the posterior tibial artery. Note its position along the interior surface of the deltoid ligament. From there, it can be seen entering the tarsal canal (**b**)

most of the injuries occur as a result of forced dorsiflexion and inversion, even in cases of fractures of the neck with significant displacement, the medial vessels may be spared and in this way the blood supply to the body of the talus. Secondly, since these medial vessels may be the only remaining blood supply to the talus, surgeons who choose to approach the talus from the medial side must exercise the greatest caution not to damage the only remaining blood supply to the body of the talus. This applies to any manipulation either of the talus on its medial surface, posterior to the medial malleolus, or deep to the deltoid ligament. Extreme caution must also be exercised whenever an osteotomy of the medial malleolus is performed to gain access to the body of the talus.

From the Anterior Tibial Artery

Superior Neck Branches. The dorsalis pedis artery, the continuation of the anterior tibial artery, sends branches to the superior surface of neck of the talus (see Fig. 3a).

Artery of the Sinus Tarsi. It is formed by the anastomosis of a branch of the dorsalis pedis with a branch of the perforating peroneal artery. It is large and always present, ensuring a very rich lateral blood supply which gains entry into the bone through many vascular perforations (see Fig. 3b).

From the Peroneal Artery

Small branches from the peroneal artery anastomose with some branches from the posterior tibial artery to form the posterior plexus around the talus. As

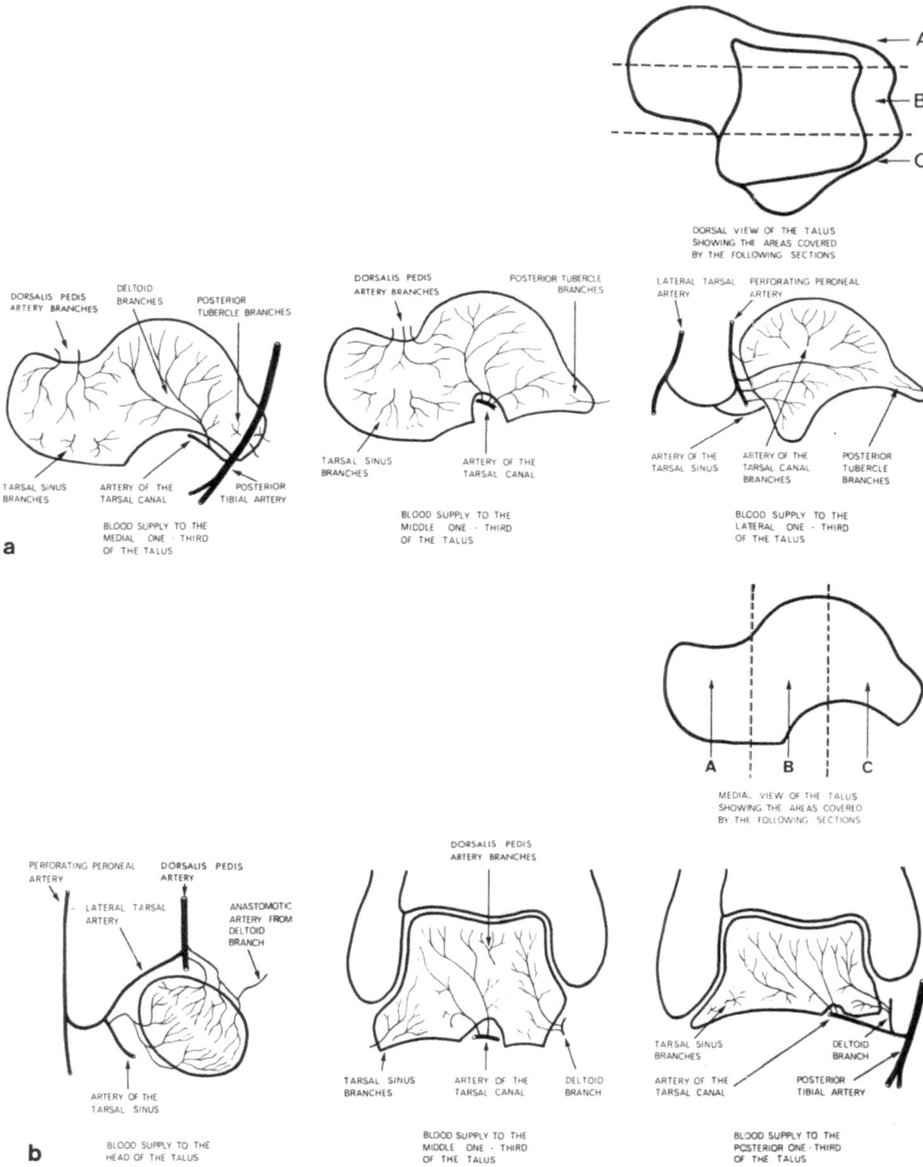

Fig. 3a, b. The deltoid branch. **a** Blood supply to the talus in sagittal sections. The artery of the tarsal canal is shown with the deltoid artery branch arising from it, lying close to the inner surface of the deltoid ligament and entering the body of the talus. **b** Blood supply to the talus in coronal sections. The deltoid branch arising from the artery of the tarsal canal is clearly seen with its relationship to the deltoid ligament and medial malleolus. The other arterial supply, including the perforating peroneal artery, the lateral tarsal artery, the artery of the tarsal sinus, and the dorsalis pedis artery, is also clearly indicated. (From Mulfinger and Trueta 1970)

already stated, the perforating peroneal artery contributes to the artery of the tarsal sinus. The contribution of the peroneal artery to the blood supply of the talus is not important (see Fig. 3b).

Intraosseous Blood Supply

Head of Talus

The head receives vessels medially from branches of the dorsalis pedis artery and laterally from branches of the arterial anastomosis in the tarsal sinus (see Fig. 3b).

Body of Talus

The anastomosis in the tarsal canal between the artery of the tarsal canal and the vessels cursing through the tarsal sinus (*the anastomotic artery*) give rise to four or five vessels on the medial side which supply most of the talar body, that is almost all of the middle third except for the extreme superior aspect, and all of the lateral third except for the posterior aspect. The medial third of the body is supplied by the *deltoid artery* (see Fig. 3b).

Summary

The major blood supply enters posterior to the neck of the talus. Thus, isolated fractures of the neck, unless they are very posterior and are through the body, rarely interfere with the blood supply to the body of the talus. The deltoid artery which lies on the inner aspect of the deltoid ligament may be the only vessel providing a blood supply to the body of the talus. This occurs in most cases of fracture dislocations except where there is total dislocation of the body of the talus with posterior extrusion. The deltoid artery is therefore most important and must be avoided in all surgical approaches.

Mechanism of Injury

Most fractures of the talar neck are caused by a forced dorsiflexion of the foot. The aviator's astragalus described by Coltart was a fracture of the neck of the talus caused by a violent dorsiflexion of the foot resting on the rudder bar of the plane. Most present fractures are the result of high-energy forces occurring in motor vehicle accidents.

At the extreme of dorsiflexion the neck fractures as it impinges on the anteroinferior surface of the tibia and the talus locks in the mortice. If the force continues as medial rotation, the talar head together with the remainder of

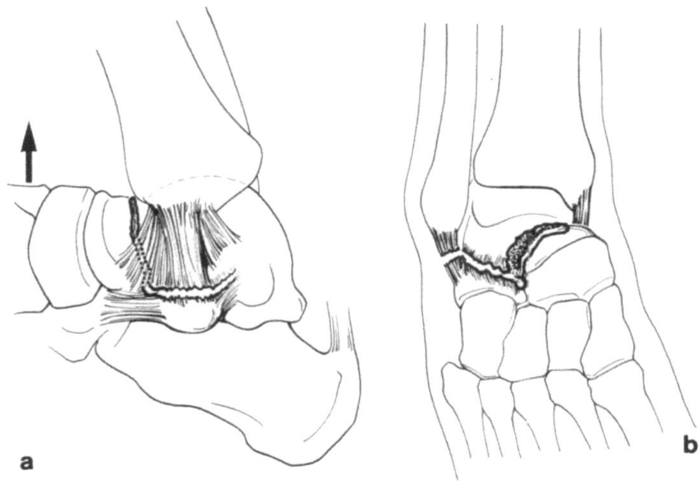

Fig. 4 a, b. Talar neck fractures. Most talar neck fractures are caused by a severe dorsiflexion force. The talar neck abuts the anterior portion of the tibia and the continuing force fractures the talar neck (**a**). A continuing inversion force (**b**) ruptures the lateral subtalar ligaments and often the lateral ligament of the ankle, or causes an avulsion of the lateral malleolus

the foot displaces medially through the subtalar joint causing a subtalar subluxation or dislocation. If the dorsiflexion and medial rotation force is extreme it will also cause a rupture of the interosseous ligament between the talus and the os calcis as well as a rupture of the fibulotalar and fibulocalcaneal ligaments (see Fig. 4). This permits an extreme varus of the os calcis and a shearing force on the medial malleolus. Indeed, in about 50% of the cases there is an associated oblique or almost vertical fracture of the medial malleolus which indicates a shearing mechanism of fracturing. The body of the talus rotates around the intact deltoid ligament and comes to rest posteromedially out of the ankle mortice with the fractured neck pointing superiorly and laterally (see Fig. 5). Here the talus may press on the neurovascular bundle, which is rarely injured primarily, but may be if pressure is not removed rapidly. The fracture patterns described and the displacements are the result of the usual mechanism of fracture. In high-energy injuries the forces may act in ways different to those described and as a result the fracture patterns and the displacements may vary.

Classification

Most widely accepted classifications are a combination of the classifications of Coltart [2] and of Hawkins [8]. The classification we have found useful is as follows:

- Fractures of the body of the talus
- Fractures of the neck of the talus

Type I: undisplaced fracture of the talar neck
Type II: displaced fracture of the neck with subluxation or dislocation of the subtalar joint
Type III: displaced fracture of the neck with subluxation or dislocation of the subtalar joint and ankle joint

- Subtalar dislocation
- Total dislocation of the talus

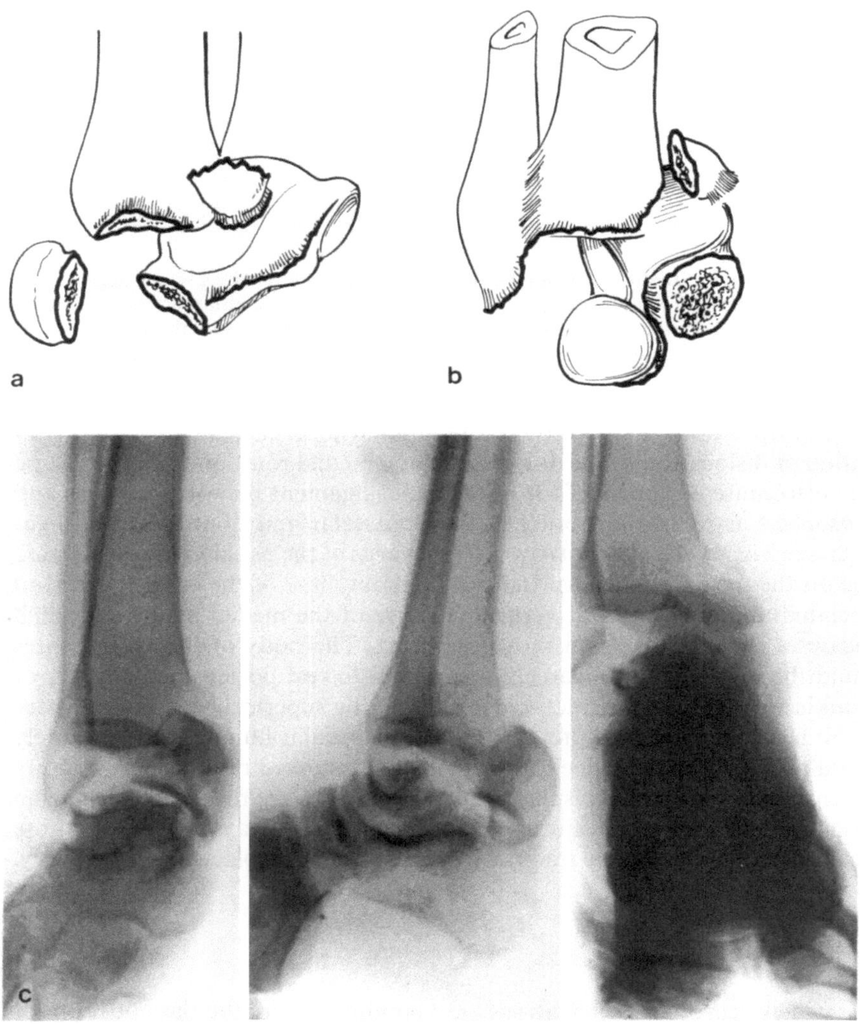

Fig. 5a–c. Type III: displaced fracture of the talar neck with posterior dislocation of the body of the talus. **a** Lateral and **b** anteroposterior diagrams showing a talar neck fracture with displacement of the body posteriorly and medially. Note the fracture of the medial malleolus, a common associated injury. **c** Oblique, lateral, and anteroposterior radiographs of an 18-year-old male with this injury

Hawkins has described as type IV a displaced fracture of the neck associated with a dislocation of the head and neck fragment from the talonavicular joint. The essence of this injury is the dislocation of the body from the ankle and the subtalar joints. It is for this reason that we feel that it does not warrant separation as a separate type.

Natural History of the Injuries

Fractures of the Body of the Talus

Simple undisplaced fractures through the body heal without problems if suitably immobilized and protected till union. Major violence may result in such severe fragmentation of the body of the talus that surgical reduction and fixation are impossible. In these cases the resultant malunion with varying degrees of avascular necrosis and collapse lead to incongruity of the ankle and subtalar joint and are usually associated with great disability. Secondary reconstructive procedures are almost always necessary.

Fractures of the Talar Neck

Type I

This is a fracture through the neck without displacement. The subtalar joint is not subluxed and there is no deformity of the foot. These fractures have an excellent prognosis if simply immobilized until union occurs. Vascular complications are exceedingly rare.

Type II

This is a fracture through the neck with displacement and subluxation or dislocation of the subtalar joint. Displacement of the neck cannot occur without displacement through the subtalar joint. Similarly, reduction of one is not possible without the other. Thus any residual displacement of the talar neck will result in subluxation of the subtalar joint with resultant disturbance of foot mechanics and osteoarthritis of the subtalar joint. The displacement through the subtalar joint is one of varus with medial displacement of the foot. Thus the medial soft tissues are almost always preserved even if there is an associated fracture of the medial malleolus. However, this does not rule out partial avascular necrosis, which has been reported with varying degrees of frequency: 33% [16], 36% [9] and 42% [8]. Total collapse of the body of the talus in this type of injury is exceedingly rare. Union of the neck occurs in almost 100% of the cases. Because of some preservation of blood supply revascularization will occur before collapse occurs. Thus, if reduction is anatomic the outlook should be excellent. Residual problems are usually caused by residual displacement with malunion of the neck and subtalar incongruity and disturbed foot mechanics. If any displacement is evident after an attempted closed reduction, an open reduction is mandatory. However comminution of the neck may make anatomic reduction extremely difficult. This explains in part the poor results associated with this injury.

Type III

This is a fracture through the neck of the talus with displacement of the body. This results in subtalar subluxation or dislocation and displacement of the body of the talus in the ankle joint. The body of the talus usually rotates about the intact deltoid ligament and comes to lie posteriorly and medially with the fractured neck pointing upwards and laterally. Avascular necrosis of the body in these injuries is almost 100% and plays a major role in the outcome. The cases which escape an avascular necrosis are those which retain the attachment of the deltoid ligament to the talus and with it the deltoid artery which supplies the medial one third of the body. The prognosis in type III injuries must be guarded. It is worse when the fracture is open.

Subtalar Dislocations

If recognized and reduced expeditiously this injury has a good prognosis.

Total Dislocation of the Talus

A complete dislocation of the talus is usually the result of a very violent inversion injury which causes an extrusion of the talus laterally. The dislocation is usually open and the talus is completely stripped of all soft-tissue attachment. Avascular necrosis is certain. Dead bone associated with an open wound does not bode a favorable outcome. The surgeon must face the decision of whether to attempt a salvage of the talus and risk greater sepsis or sacrifice the talus in an effort to decrease the likelihood of sepsis. In the series of Detenbeck and Kelly, who reported nine such cases, seven were open [6]. Eight of the nine developed sepsis. Seven of the nine had a talectomy. Five of the nine required a tibiocalcaneal fusion and one of the nine an amputation.

Treatment

In evolving the rationale for treatment we must consider the personality of the injury. Thus we must consider the patient factors such as age, concurrent disease, associated injuries, and patient expectation. Then we must consider the state of the limb. Lastly, in evaluating the injury itself the surgeon must put great emphasis on the state of the soft tissues. As already alluded to, the injury may be closed and on first examination appear quite benign. The surgeon must remember that these injuries are invariably the result of great violence and the injury to the soft tissues may not become manifest till a number of hours have passed. The associated swelling is usually great and fracture blisters the rule (see Fig. 6). Surgery through such tissues may prove disastrous.

Radiological Assessment

Anteroposterior lateral and oblique views of the hind foot are the standard views to order. To assess the subtalar joint Broden's views may prove to be useful, particularly in the operating room. In the clinical situation computer tomography (CT) is far more useful in assessing the subtalar joint as well as the fragmentation of the talus.

Timing

If the fracture is open immediate surgery is indicated. If the fracture is closed, careful assessment and planning are required. Type III fractures, in which the body is dislocated, or total dislocations of the talus constitute a surgical emergency. The dislocated talus may be pressing on the overlying skin, and in dislocations of the body the vessels responsible for the blood supply may be under stretch. In type II fractures a closed reduction should be performed as well as possible and surgery should be delayed until the swelling has subsided and the fracture blisters have dried up. Incisions should not be made through tense and swollen soft tissues, since skin necrosis and sepsis will be the outcome.

Surgical Approaches

The skin on the medial and lateral side of the foot must be handled with great care to avoid wound edge necrosis and infection. In order to avoid further damage to the precarious blood supply of the talus, stripping of soft tissues from the talus must be avoided. The surgeon must learn to do most of the surgical manipulation through the fracture and remember that in displaced fractures of the body of the talus the only remaining blood supply may be medial.

Medial

The medial approach is the preferred approach because it is more extensile. Occasionally, in more complex fracture patterns, it may have to be combined

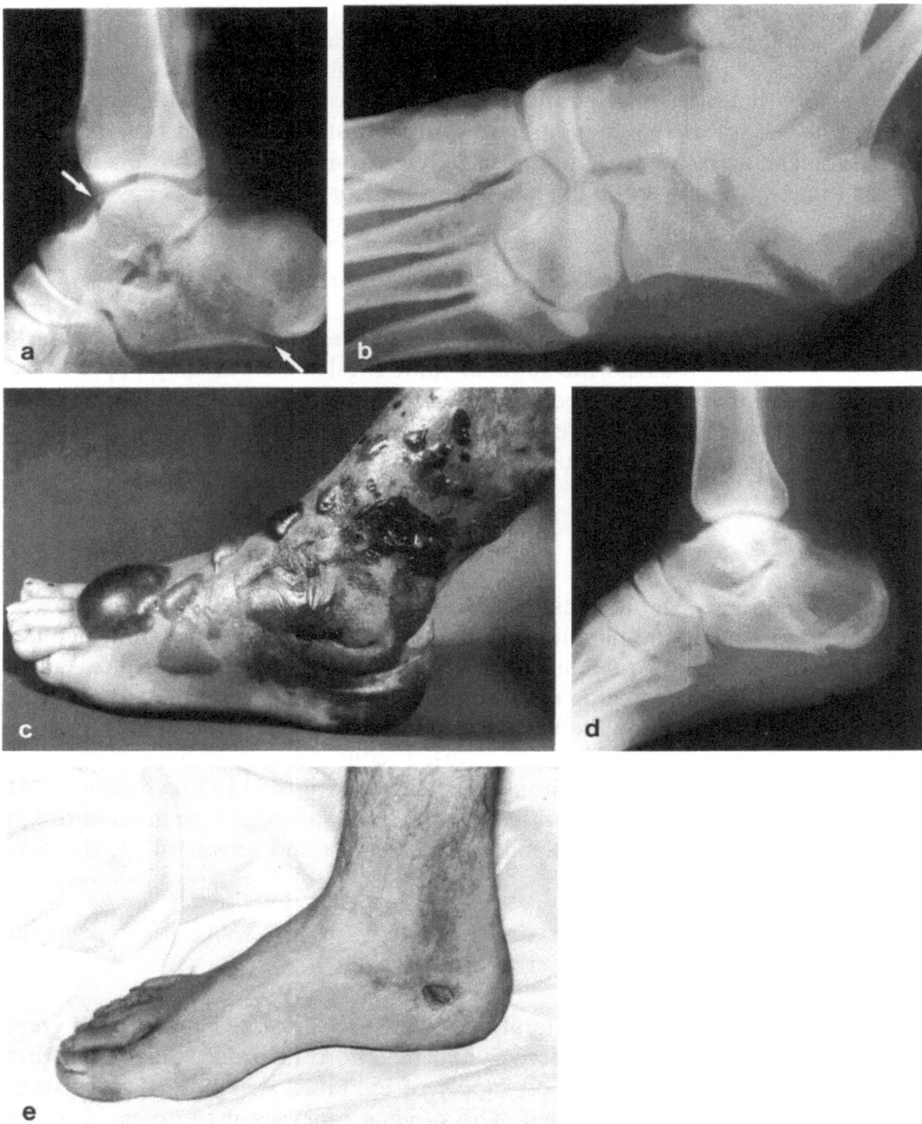

Fig. 6. Shearing injury to talus. This 32-year-old male had his foot caught in the jaws of a logging machine. His body was then rotated around the stabilized os calcis and talus, creating an open shear fracture through both bones. Within 48 h, massive fracture blisters and contusion were evident on the foot and ankle

with a lateral approach. The incision for the medial approach is made from the medial malleolus anteriorly along the superomedial margin of the neck out to the navicular. The capsule is then stripped from the superior and medial margin of the neck which will expose the fracture and allow its surgical manipulation. If the fracture extends into the body, or if the body is dislocated and the medial malleolus is not fractured, then it becomes necessary to carry out an osteotomy of the medial malleolus. The skin incision should then be extended more posteriorly and proximally to expose the malleolus. It is best to predrill and tap a screw hole for the fixation of the malleolus before its osteotomy. The osteotomy is then made slightly obliquely, sloping from above to end at the level of the ankle joint. It is best to make the cut most of the way with a small oscillating saw and then to complete it by inserting an osteotome into the cut and by fracturing through the subchondral bone and cartilage. Extreme care must be exercised not to damage the vessels coursing on the deep surface of the deltoid ligament and medial surface of the talus. If the body of the talus is trapped behind the medial malleolus, between it and the tendoachilles, and there appears to be no space for the body, the situation can be eased considerably by inserting the AO distractor on the medial side with one Schantz screw in the tibia and one in the os calcis. Distraction opens up the space between the tibia and the os calcis much more efficiently then manual traction and greatly eases the manipulative reduction of the displaced body.

Lateral

There are two lateral approaches to the talus. The oblique lateral approach affords excellent exposure of the neck and the subtalar joint but is more likely to result in wound edge necrosis (see Fig. 7). For this reason we are much more in favor of a liberal straight lateral incision which is made lateral to the extensor tendons. The extensor retinaculum is divided, which allows the retraction medially of all the tendons and of the neurovascular bundle. The ankle capsule, if not already ruptured, is then divided longitudinally. This gives an excellent exposure to the lateral aspect of the body and the neck as well as the anterior part of the posterior facet of the subtalar joint (see Fig. 8). As already alluded to above, in complex fracture patterns it may be necessary to make a

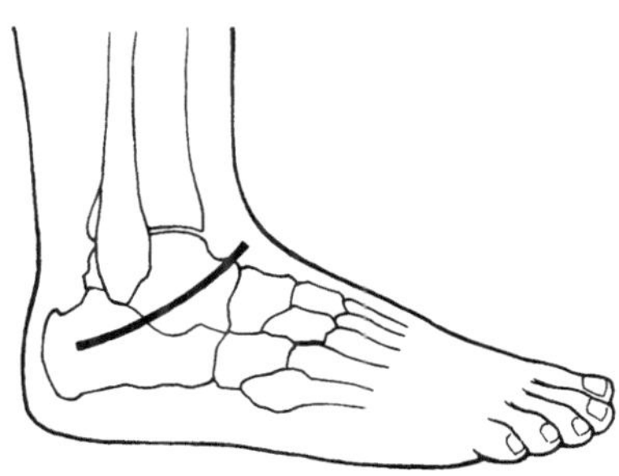

Fig. 7. Oblique lateral approach to the talus. (Adapted from [4])

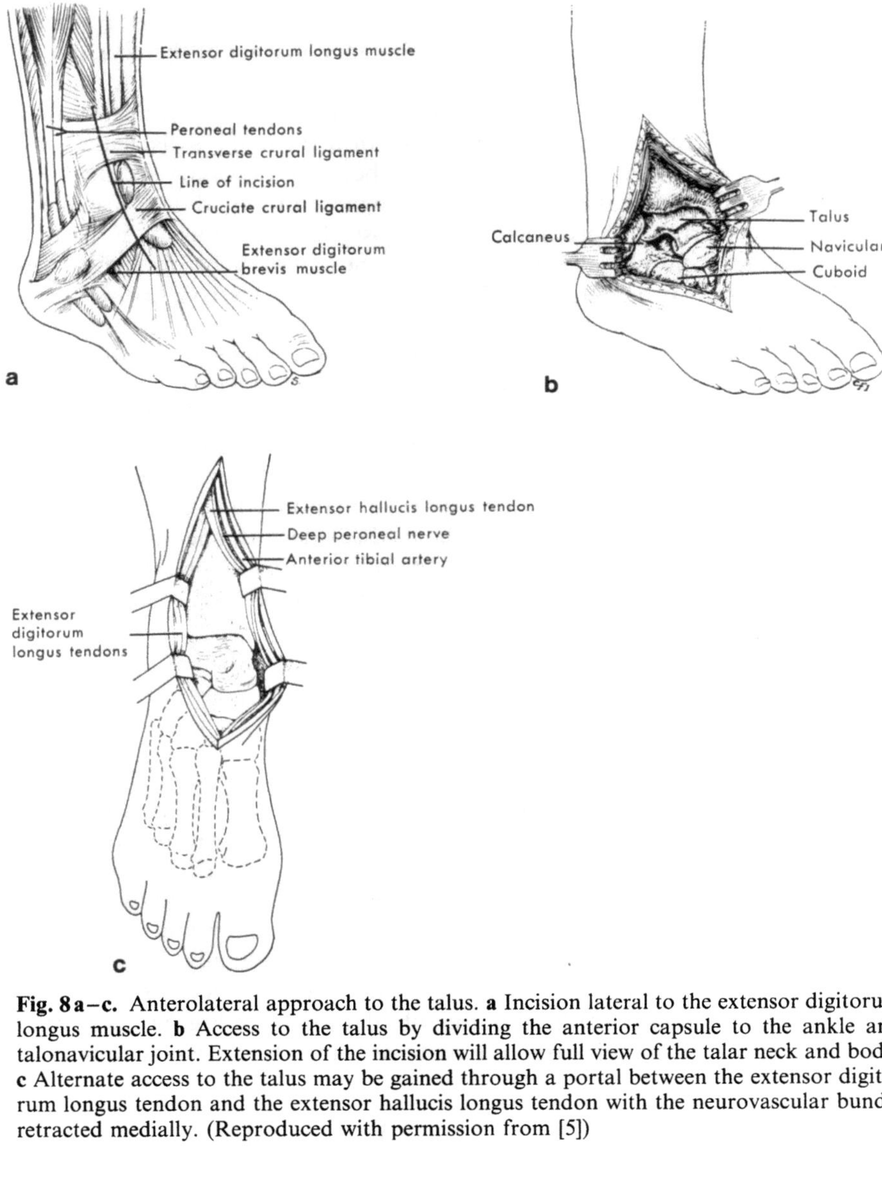

Fig. 8a–c. Anterolateral approach to the talus. **a** Incision lateral to the extensor digitorum longus muscle. **b** Access to the talus by dividing the anterior capsule to the ankle and talonavicular joint. Extension of the incision will allow full view of the talar neck and body. **c** Alternate access to the talus may be gained through a portal between the extensor digitorum longus tendon and the extensor hallucis longus tendon with the neurovascular bundle retracted medially. (Reproduced with permission from [5])

medial as well as a lateral approach in order to reduce the fracture accurately. If one is dealing with a multifragmentary fracture of the talar neck, where anatomic reduction is virtually impossible, then the lateral exposure with a view of the subtalar joint will allow the surgeon to reduce the subtalar joint anatomically. This will realign the head and the body of the talus in their proper relationship, which can then be maintained with appropriate internal fixation and a bone graft if necessary. If two incisions are made the surgeon must remember to leave a sufficiently wide bridge of skin between the two to avoid skin break down.

Internal Fixation

The internal fixation is best carried out with two 3.5-mm small cortex screws inserted from the neck into the body of the talus. If it is not possible to insert two screws then a screw and a Kirschner wire should be used to achieve rotational stability. It is usually possible to insert the two screws near the osteocartilaginous junction of the head, both on the medial side, or one on the medial side and one on the lateral side. It is rarely necessary to insert one of the screws through the cartilaginous covering of the head. If the screw is inserted through the cartilage the screw head should be recessed below the level of the cartilage. A screw can also be inserted from a posterolateral direction running anteromedially into the talar head. The advent of cannulated screws has made the insertion of such a fixation much easier. Kirschner wires alone should not be used for fixation because they do not provide sufficient stability. If the blood supply to the body of the talus is in question then we use pure titanium screws. This makes possible the subsequent use of magnetic resonance imaging (MRI) for the evaluation of the blood supply to the body of the talus. The cortex screws, whenever possible, should be inserted as lag screws to provide maximum stability. The surgeon should remember, however, that if the fracture of the neck is multifragmentary or if there is bone loss, the screws will have to be inserted without overdrilling the pilot holes, so that when tightened the screws will not exert a lag effect. Lagging the fracture together under such circumstances would lead to shortening of the neck, which would result in subtalar subluxation and all the problems of a malreduction.

Management of the Specific Fracture Types

Fractures of the Body

If undisplaced, the fracture of the body presents no particular problems. It simply requires immobilization in a below-knee nonwalking cast for 6–8 weeks until the fracture has united. The displaced fractures can present a major challenge. If the body is split, it may be possible to perform an open reduction and stable fixation. Most often, however, fractures of the body are the result of high-velocity injuries, and are so shattered that a reconstruction is not possible. Initially the limb should be immobilized to allow the swelling to subside. The decision must then be made whether to carry out a tibiotalar neck fusion or the Blair procedure, or to excise the body of the talus and carry out a tibiocalcaneal arthrodesis. If the shattered fracture of the body is associated with other injuries, such as a tibial plafond fracture, fracture of the os calcis and facture dislocation through the mid-foot, then an external fixator frame, should be considered as a temporary or definitive mode of fixation.

Fractures of the Talar Neck

Type I. If the fracture is undisplaced without subluxation of the subtalar joint, then the indicated treatment is simple plaster immobilization in a below-knee non-weight-bearing cast for a period of 6–8 weeks. The result should be a full return of function without the risk of avascular necrosis or subtalar arthritis. The surgeon must make sure, however, that no displacement has taken place and that the subtalar joint is in perfect alignment. Any displacement makes this a type II injury, which alters the treatment.

Type II. If the fracture is associated with any displacement of the neck (type II), then an anatomic reduction of the neck, which must restore its alignment and length, is essential in order to prevent any incongruity of the subtalar joint. This is rarely possible to achieve by closed means and an open reduction and internal fixation is almost always necessary. Although the complication of avascular necrosis has been reported with varying frequency (see above), it is invariably partial and is almost never associated with collapse of the body of the talus. The surgeon must make sure not to add to the vascular injury by injudicious manipulation of the talus from the medial side. If the fracture was not comminuted and stable internal fixation was possible, then plaster immobilization is not necessary. Weight bearing must be avoided till union has occurred, which usually takes 6–8 weeks. If the fracture was comminuted and the fixation achieved was not absolutely stable, then a below-knee non-weight-bearing cast is necessary for 6–12 weeks until union of the fracture has occurred. The appearance on a follow up X-ray at 6–8 weeks of a subchondral radiolucency, the so-called Hawkins sign, indicates the preservation of the blood supply to the body of the talus, and is a good prognostic sign.

Type III. A fracture dislocation of the body of the talus, whether open or closed, is a surgical emergency. The emergent nature of the open fracture is self-evident. In the closed injury the body of the talus may be pressing on the neurovascular bundle as it lies trapped and rotated behind the medial malleolus or its own vascular supply may be prejudiced by stretching of the remaining medial vessels. In the closed injury, a closed reduction may be attempted, but it almost always fails and an open reduction is necessary. The medial approach should be used. Over 50% of these injuries are associated with a fracture of the medial malleolus, which greatly facilitates the exposure. If the medial malleolus is intact then an osteotomy of the malleolus is necessary to gain access to the body of the talus. As already described, a distractor applied to the medial side may be helpful. Extreme care must be taken as the body of the talus is being manipulated not to strip any remaining soft tissue from the medial side of the talus as this may be the only remaining blood supply. The reduction achieved must be anatomic as in type II. We favor a stable internal fixation with screws as described. We do not believe that methods of revascularization such as subtalar fusion have any role to play in improving the rate of revascularization of the talus. Perhaps microvascular techniques with implantation of new vascular bundles into the body of the talus will become useful. To date there is no firm evidence to prove this. If a stable internal fixation was achieved there is no need for plaster immobilization for the neck fracture itself. It must be remembered, however, that type III injuries may be associated with ligamentous disruptions which would benefit from 6 weeks of plaster immobilization. The decision for plaster immobilization must therefore be made individually.

The open type III injury poses very difficult problems in management. The risk one faces is that the devitalized body of the talus in an open wound will add to the danger of sepsis. Once again the surgeon will have to individualize the treatment. We feel that if it is judged surgically safe it is best to preserve the body of the talus and treat it as above by anatomic reduction and stable fixation, with the exception, of course, that the wound is left open. If the surgeon feels, however, that the risk of sepsis is great, either because of the extent of damage of the soft tissues or the degree of contamination, and/or because of the duration of the interval between the injury and treatment, then it is best to sacrifice the body of the talus and perform a Blair type or a tibiocalcaneal type of fusion as soon as it is deemed safe to do so.

In type III injuries which are treated by open reduction and internal fixation, weight bearing should be withheld until the fracture of the neck has united. Thereafter we believe that full weight bearing should be allowed as there is absolutely no proof that non-weight-bearing has any preventive effect on the eventual collapse of the body of the talus which occurs as revascularization is taking place.

Late Reconstructive Procedures

Type II. A malunion with resultant subtalar arthritis and malposition of the foot cannot be treated with an in situ subtalar fusion. The malposition of the hind foot must be corrected at the time of surgery through the subtalar joint. Most of the time a triple arthrodesis is necessary to correct the associated problems.

Type III. In cases of avascular necrosis with collapse of the body of the talus, the most commonly performed procedures are either the Blair type of tibiotalar neck fusion or an excision of the body of the talus and a tibiocalcaneal arthrodesis. We prefer the later and prefer to do it from a lateral approach, combining it with an osteotomy of the lateral malleolus which greatly facilitates access to the talus, the distal tibia, and the os calcis.

References

1. Anderson HG (1919) The medical and surgical aspects of aviation. Oxford Medical Publications, London
2. Coltart WD (1952) "Aviator's astragalus". J Bone Joint Surg (Br) 34B: 545–566
3. Cooper A (1832) Treatise on dislocations and fractures of the joints. London, pp 341–342
4. Crenshaw AH (ed) (1971) Campbell's operative orthopaedics, vol 1, 5th edn. Mosby, St. Louis
5. Crenshaw AH (1980) Surgical approaches. In: Edmonson, Crenshaw AH (eds) Campbell's operative orthopaedics, 6th edn. Mosby, St. Louis
6. Detenbeck LC, Kelly PJ (1969) Total dislocation of the talus. J Bone Joint Surg (Am) 51A(2): 283
7. Haliburton RA, Sullivan CR, Kelly PJ, Peterson LFA (1958) The extra-osseous and intra-osseous blood supply of the talus. J Bone Joint Surg (Am) 40A: 1115–1120
8. Hawkins LG (1970) Fractures of the neck of the talus. J Bone Joint Surg (Am) 52A(5): 991
9. Kenwright J, Taylor RG (1970) Major injuries of the talus. J Bone Joint Surg (Br) 52B: 36–48
10. Kleiger B (1948) Fractures of the talus. J Bone Joint Surg (Am) 30A: 735
11. Lauro A, Purpura F (1956) La trabecolatura ossea e l'irroraxione sanguina nell'astragalo e nel calcagno. Minerva Chir 11: 663–667
12. Lexor E, Kuliga, Turk W (1904) Untersuchungen über Knochenarterien. Hirschwald, Berlin, Sect 4
13. McKeever FM (1943) Fracture of the neck of the astragalus. Arch Surg 46: 720
14. Montis S, Ridola C (1959) Vascolarizzazione dell'astragalo. Quad Anatomia Practica 15: 574
15. Mulfinger GL, Trueta J (1970) The blood supply of the talus. J Bone Joint Surg (Br) 52B: 160–167
16. Pennal GF (1963) Fractures of the talus. Clin Orthop 30: 53–63
17. Phemister DB (1940) Changes in bone and joints resulting from interruption of circulation. Arch Surg 41: 436
18. Sneed WL (1925) The astragalus: a case of dislocation excision and replacement; an attempt to demonstrate the circulation in this bone. J Bone Joint Surg 7: 384–399
19. Watson-Jones R (1946) Fractures and joint injuries, vol 2, 3rd edn. Livingstone, Edinburgh, pp 821–843
20. Wildenauer E (1950) Die Blutversorgung des Talus. Z Anat Entwicklungsgesch 115: 32

Late Results of Fractures and Fracture-Dislocation After ORIF

R. Szyszkowitz, W. Seggl, and R. Wildburger

Introduction

Displaced fractures and fracture-dislocations of the talus are challenging problems. Personal experience with talus fractures is usually limited because they represent only 0.14% [5] to 0.32% [6] of all fractures. For this reason to evaluate the well-known high percentage of permanent disability that results multicenter studies are important [2, 9–11].
The fact that more than three fifths of the surface of the talus is covered by articular cartilage, and the special arrangement of its blood supply [7], have a major influence on the fracture types and their outcome with respect to post-traumatic necrosis and arthrosis. To encompass all these variables we have reclassified all talar fractures into four types, combining the schemes of Hawkins [1], Weber [12], Marti [3, 4], and Kuner [2] (Table 1).

Patients and Methods

This study reports 108 fractures and fracture-dislocations of the talus which were treated by open reduction and internal fixation (ORIF). There were 80

Table 1. Classification of talus fractures. (After [1–4, 12])

Type		Circulation	Necrosis
I	Peripheral fractures: head, distal neck, processus fibularis, processus posterior, flakes	Intact	Very seldom (5%)
II	Central fractures without displacement: proximal neck, body (Hawkins I)	Mainly intact	Seldom (15%)
III	Central fractures with displacement and subluxation: proximal neck, body (Hawkins II)	Interosseous circulation interrupted, auxiliary circulation intact	Often (40%)
IV	Central fracture-dislocations and central comminuted fractures (Hawkins III and IV)	Interosseous and auxiliary circulation interrupted	Between 30% and 100% (av. 70%)

Table 2. Analysis of the present series of talus fractures by fracture type

Fracture type		Total	Closed	Open[a]		
				I	II	III
I	Peripheral	16	13	–	2	1
II	Central without displacement	26	22	–	1	3
	Proximal neck	12	10	–	–	2
	Body	14	12	–	1	1
III	Central with displacement	21	19	1	1	–
	Proximal neck	11	10	–	1	–
	Body	10	9	1	–	–
IV	Central fracture–dislocation and comminuted fractures	45	29	2	9	5
	Neck	31	23	1	6	1
	Body	14	6	1	3	4
		108	83	3	13	9

[a] *Types of open fracture: I*, the skin is pierced from within by sharp bone fragments. Basically these fractures can be regarded and treated as closed injuries; *II*, the skin is disrupted and crushed from without, with moderate damage to the skin, subcutaneous tissue and muscles; *III*, these fractures are compounded from without, with extensive necrosis of skin, subcutaneous tissue and muscle

male and 28 female patients with 83 closed and 25 open fractures of different degrees (Table 2). Most patients sustained their injuries in a traffic accident; the next largest category was injuries from falls. Sixteen patients sustained a peripheral fracture and 92 a central fracture or fracture-dislocation.

The fracture is usually exposed through an anteromedial approach. The skin incision begins proximal to the medial malleolus and runs in front of its anterior border in a straight line to the navicular bone. The tibialis tendons, the deltoid ligament, and the cutaneous nerves and the neurovascular bundle are carefully identified. Fractures of the body are exposed by splitting the capsule in front of the medial malleolus. The foot is then plantarflexed to expose and to reduce the fragments. After reduction and temporary fixation using Kirschner wires, the definitive fixation was usually achieved using two 4 mm cancellous screws. Better still, two 4 mm titanium lag screws or one cannulated 7.0 cancellous titanium screw allow MRI postoperatively.

If the medial cortex of the medial neck is too osteoporotic and comminuted, or in very distal fractures, one or two lag or positioning screws can be inserted through the cartilage of the talar head with countersinking of the screw heads. Initially, Kirschner wires alone in combination with a plaster cast were used. Later, however, lag and positioning screws became the fixation technique of choice because it avoids the necessity for a cast postoperatively and allows active motion of all joints under supervision of a physiotherapist (Table 3).

Table 3. Operative treatment

Operative treatment	Total	Peripheral fractures	Central fractures	Fracture-dislocations
Kirschner wire	25	4	9	12
Screw	60	9	28	23
Kirschner wire and screw	12	–	7	5
Open reduction and cancellous bone graft	4	2	2	–
Bone screw	1	–	1	–
Tibiotalar arthrodesis	1	1	–	–
Triple arthrodesis	3	–	–	3
Astragalectomy	1	–	–	1
Amputation	1	–	–	1
	108	16	47	45

A posterior incision parallel to the Achilles tendon was chosen in open fracture-dislocations, if the wound had to be extended, if the skin was badly contused anteriorly, or if interposition of the tibialis posterior and/or flexor hallucis tendon was suspected; it was also used in cases where there was only a posterior fragment. The femur distractor or an external fixator was used temporarily as a reduction and sometimes the medial malleolus had to be osteotomized to gain adequate exposure in order to achieve an anatomical reduction. Great care must be taken not to injure the deltoid branches of the tibialis posterior artery.

Whenever we use the dorsal approach we prefer cannulated 6 mm titanium screws. To avoid limitation of plantarflexion the screw head has to be placed close to the distal border of the posterior talus process. Postoperatively the possibility of compartment syndrome has to be kept in mind and the ankle must be splinted to prevent equinus.

Once the suction drains are removed (during the first 48 h postoperatively) and the dressing changed, active motion of all joints and full mobilization without weight-bearing are started under the supervision of a physiotherapist. The sutures are removed 12 days postoperatively and in type I and II fractures a below-knee walking-cast is usually applied for a further 4 weeks. Full weight-bearing without a walking-cast is allowed 6 weeks postoperatively provided radiographs indicate that union is progressing satisfactorily.

In type III and IV fractures a weight-relieving caliper is applied after removal of the sutures for a further 10 weeks. Full weight-bearing without the caliper is then allowed provided radiographs and MRI scans show no evidence of necrosis after bony union (which usually occurs 3 months after injury).

It is usually possible to detect the early signs of necrosis by comparing the follow-up radiographs with those of the normal side. Usually after dislocation or fracture-dislocation the body area becomes sclerotic or relatively dense radiologically compared with the neighbouring bones. Scintigraphy and scintimetry or, better, MRI should be performed. (Titanium screws can be left in place for MRI but steel screws need to be removed.) If the results indicate avascular necrosis, only partial weight-bearing should be allowed with the use of a caliper for up to 6 months. However, if radiography shows a subchondral translucency as a result of revascularization of the trochlea (Hawkins' sign) [1] and MRI reveals no signs of necrosis, full weight-bearing is allowed. Thirty-four percent of all patients with talus necrosis were asymptomatic and spontaneous revascularization of the necrosis occurred within 2 years in 21% [9]. Where MRI reveals suspicious fibrosis a CT study is necessary to evaluate the bony structure. Vascularized bone-block transfers using microsurgery should be considered for younger patients before collapse of the trochlea (and body). After high-energy trauma in some comminuted fractures of the talus, reconstruction, revascularization, and the prevention of severe post-traumatic arthrosis – and therefore a satisfactory functional end result – seem to be impossible. In these cases it is better to proceed to a primary arthrodesis or a primary reconstruction using an external fixator and screws, followed by an early secondary arthrodesis.

Results

Of 108 patients treated operatively late results were obtained in 87 from a follow-up after between 12 and 168 months (average 69 months). Of these, 11 had sustained a peripheral fracture, 38 a central fracture and 38 a fracture-dislocation.

Post-traumatic arthrosis was found in the tibiotalar (ankle) joint in 40% of patients and in the talocalcaneal (subtalar) joint in 53% (Table 4). In 8 patients secondary arthrodeses were performed. Usually these patients had not only painful post-traumatic arthrosis but also partial or total necrosis of the talus. The types of fusion performed were as follows: one tibiotalar arthrodesis, three tibiocalcanear arthrodeses, and four triple arthrodeses (Table 5). One amputation was necessary in a patient who sustained severe open fractures of the tibia, fibula, talus, and calcaneus with severe comminution.

Table 4. Severity of arthroses in relations to fracture type

Fracture type	Arthritis of:		All late results	%
	Tibiotalar joint	Talocalcaneal joint		
Peripheral	3	3	11 × 2	27
Central without displacement	4	6	20 × 2	25
Central with displacement	10	12	18 × 2	60
Fracture-dislocations	18	25	38 × 2	57

The multiplicator 2 under "All late results" means two joints, the tibiotalar and the talocalcaneal. In talus fractures there were always two joints, upper and lower ankle joint, to examine.

Table 5. Arthrodeses and amputations

	Number	Circumstances
Tibiotalar arthrodesis	1	After peripheral fracture
Tibiocalcaneal arthrodesis	1	After central fracture and infection
	1	After fracture-dislocation, body necrosis, and infection
	1	After fracture-dislocation and body necrosis
Triple arthrodesis	1	After fracture-dislocation
	1	After fracture-dislocation and infection
	1	After fracture-dislocation and bone screw
	1	After fracture-dislocation and body necrosis
Amputation at the middle of the tibia	1	After fracture-dislocation, primary triple arthrodesis, and infection

Table 6. Range of motion

Range of motion	Tibiotalar joint		Talocalcaneal joint	
	No.	%	No.	%
Normal	37	43	29	34
One third restricted	25	29	24	28
Two thirds restricted	15	17	13	15
Stiff	9	11	20	23

The ranges of motion of the tibiotalar and talocalcaneal joints are shown in Table 6. Six patients with peripheral fractures, 30 with central fractures, and 21 with fracture-dislocations had a more or less normal walking ability. Twenty-two of them (13 with fracture-dislocations and 6 with central fractures) had a limp, and 8 needed crutches. Walking capacity was normal in 8 patients with peripheral fractures, 33 with central fractures, and 24 with fracture-dislocations, it was limited in 1 patient with an peripheral fracture, 4 with central fractures and 11 with fracture-dislocations. Of all the patients only 6 had an extremely limited walking capacity.

The general assessments based on pain, motion, and the radiographic findings are given in Table 7 according to fracture type. As expected, the worst results were found after fracture-dislocations. Nevertheless, it was surprising to see many revascularized talus bodies.

Discussion

Displaced central fractures and fracture-dislocations of the talus are rare and associated with a high percentage of permanent disability. Early emergency

Table 7. Results relative to fracture type

Fracture type	Result			Total
	Very good	Good	Poor	
Peripheral	5	4	1	11
Central without displacement	10	8	2	20
Central with displacement	8	10	1	19
Fracture-dislocations	6	21	10	37
Percentage for all fracture types:	35%	49%	16%	100%

Table 8. Incidence of avascular necrosis

Fracture type	Avascular necrosis (%)		
	Schuind et al. [9]	Literature	Average
Peripheral	10	0–10	5
Central without displacement	24	0–24	12
Central with displacement	42	16–60	38
Fracture-dislocations	60	30–100	65

Table 9. Incidence of infection, arthrosis, and arthrodesis

Series	Infection (%)	Arthrosis (%)	Arthrodesis (%)
Schuind et al. [9]	4.9	38.5	15.5
Kuner et al. [2]	8.0	53.3	14.6
Szyszkowitz et al. (present study)	4.7	46.5	11.5

decompression of soft tissues by anatomical reduction – if necessary open – helps to reduce skin and bone necrosis and other complications. Stable fixation with lag or positioning screws, allowing functional treatment, leads to better fracture healing and revascularization of the fragments.

Kuner et al. [2], in a series of 262 talus fractures, reported about 20.7% avascular necrosis in 137 operatively treated central fractures. Analysis of the findings implies that the sooner anatomical reduction was achieved, the better were the final results. In central fractures Kuner recommended a nonweight-bearing time of 5 months, in accordance with the radiological and clinical assessment.

Schuind et al. [9] reported on 359 talar lesions with 267 talus fractures. The incidence of avascular necrosis in 136 operatively treated central fractures was 39.4%. One of the highest rates of avascular necrosis was reported by Hawkins

[1], with 52.6% in 57 cases. The literature reveals that the worst results regarding avascular necrosis were found after fracture-dislocations (Table 8). These findings are re-emphasized by the present series of 108 fractures and fracture-dislocations, which show an incidence of necrosis of 18.1% after ORIF. Schuind et al. [9] found only 18.5% avascular necrosis after anatomical reduction but 30.5% after non-anatomical reduction. Post-traumatic arthrosis in the ankle joint and subtalar joint after ORIF were found in 46.5% of cases in this study, in 53.3% of cases by Kuner et al. [2] and in 38.5% by Schuind et al. [9]. The incidence of infection and the percentage of patients requiring arthrodesis are also similar in the three studies (Table 9).

Conclusion

The results presented here on fractures and fracture-dislocations of the talus, as well as those reported in the literature, show clearly that early decompression of the soft tissues, anatomical reduction, and stable contact between fragments is very important in order to minimize damage to the blood supply and to promote revascularization and bony union of the displaced talar fragments. This can be achieved by early closed or open reduction and stable internal fixation with screws.

We recommend the use of cannulated titanium screws because it makes MRI possible. Compared with Kirschner wire fixation, interfragmentary compression with lag screws increases stability, leads to earlier union by allowing small vessels to cross the fracture plane [8], and provides for better revascularization. In comminuted areas positioning screws and autologous cancellous bone grafts may be necessary. Furthermore early functional postoperative treatment can be allowed, which also improves the circulation and prevents stiffness and atrophy of all tissues. Partial weight-bearing (10–20 kg) should be allowed a few days postoperatively.

In talus fractures developing avascular necrosis of the body, full weight-bearing should be delayed for 3–6 months or longer to allow revascularization. Clinical and radiological follow-up examination, including scintigraphy, scintimetry and MRI, contribute to a better postoperative understanding. Special follow-up interventions that need to be considered are: early removal of titanium or other screws, drilling, cancellous bone grafts in small necrotic areas, and vascularized bone-block transfer for the larger necrotic areas in younger patients before irreversible collapse of the trochlea occurs.

References

1. Hawkins LG (1970) Fractures of the neck of talus. J Bone Joint Surg [Am] 52:991
2. Kuner EH, Lindenmeier HL (1983) Zur Behandlung der Talusfraktur. Kontrollstudie von 262 Behandlungsfällen. Unfallchirurgie 9:35
3. Marti R (1971) Talusfrakturen. Z Unfallchir Versicherungsmed Berufskr 64:108

4. Marti R (1978) Talus- und Calcaneusfrakturen. In: Weber BG, Brunner C, Freuler F (eds) Die Frakturenbehandlung von Kindern und Jugendlichen. Springer, Berlin Heidelberg New York
5. Mockwitz J (1979) Ergebnisse nach konservativer und nach operativer Behandlung von Sprungbeinbrüchen. Hefte Unfallheilkd 135:51
6. Müller T (1980) Zur Problematik der Talusfraktur. Inauguraldissertation, University of Freiburg
7. Mulfinger GL, Trueta J (1970) The blood supply of the talus. J Bone Joint Surg [Br] 52:160
8. Schenk RK, Müller J, Willenegger H (1968) Experimentellhistologischer Beitrag zur Entstehung und Behandlung von Pseudarthrosen. Hefte Unfallheilkd 94:15
9. Schuind F, Andrianne Y, Burny F, Donkerwolcke M, Saric O (1985) Komplikationen nach Talustraumen. Aktuelle Traumatol 15:82
10. Szyszkowitz R, Reschauer R, Seggl W (1985) Eighty-five talus fractures treated by ORIF with five to eight years of follow-up study of 69 patients. Clin Orthop 199:97–107
11. Szyszkowitz R, Reschauer R, Seggl W (1983) Talusfrakturen. Unfallheilkunde 86:262
12. Weber BG (1976) Knöchel, Fußwurzel und Mittelfuß. In: Zenker R, Deucher F, Schink W (eds) Chirurgie der Gegenwart, vol 4. Urban and Schwarzenberg, München

Long-Term Results of Displaced Talar Neck Fractures

F. Behrens

Introduction

This review is based on a long-term study initiated by Dr. Thomas Comfort (Fig. 1), who was Chief of Orthopaedic Surgery at the St. Paul/Ramsey Medical Center in St. Paul, Minnesota, between 1968 and 1988. Early in his career Dr. Comfort recognized that the eclectic approach to fracture care that was prevalent in the United States after World War II caused too many unacceptable outcomes and did not lend itself to systematic analysis and improvement.

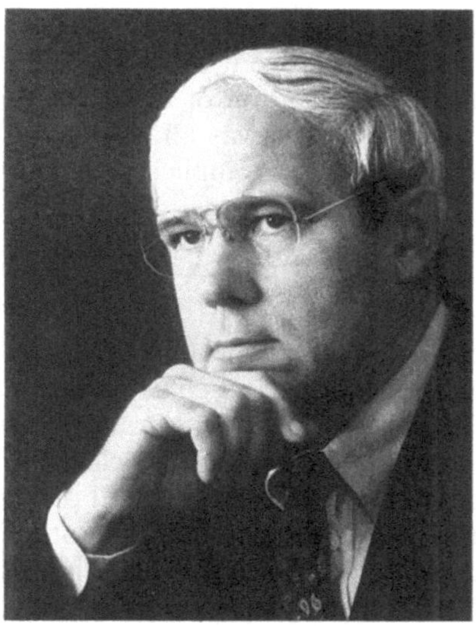

Fig. 1. Thomas H. Comfort, M.D.

He recognized quickly the revolutionary contributions of Gerhard Küntscher and the AO group and established one of the first orthopaedic services in the United States, devoted to the rigorous methods of operative fracture care. His broad experience and keen judgment made Tom Comfort a well-respected speaker at numerous American and European trauma courses, and at home, the University of Minnesota, he was the favorite teacher of many students and residents. With his untimely death in 1990, his students lost a generous and understanding friend, while his colleagues will miss his quiet wisdom and dry, self-effacing sense of humor.

The text that follows has been adapted, with few changes, from a study about talar fractures treated with internal fixation that was initiated by Tom Comfort and published in 1986 in *Clinical Orthopaedics and Related Research* [1] [1].

The displaced talar neck fracture has long perplexed surgeons. Talectomy [3, 5, 14] and local fusions [2, 11, 13] to speed revascularization are operations that have failed [7, 8]. Closed reduction and plaster fixation in equinus is still recommended, but with avascular necrosis, malunion, and non-union frequent [2, 3, 6, 10, 14, 16]. Sometimes primary tibiotalar fusion with excision of the body (the Blair procedure) has been suggested [12, 15]. Primary open reduction and internal fixation in displaced fractures is considered technically difficult with questions regarding the approach and method of fixation, and frequency of avascular necrosis and secondary arthrosis [5, 6, 16].

Here the long-term results of a series dominated by a policy of early open reduction and internal fixation (ORIF) through a medial approach are presented. The medial malleolus was osteotomized if it improved visualization or decreased the force required to effect reduction. The fixation was with medially inserted screws or Kirschner wires [8]. Plaster support and non-weight-bearing were used until bony union occurred. Protection from weight-bearing was continued in a weight-relieving brace if the dome failed to show disuse subchondral bone atrophy – an indication of avascularity. Weight-bearing protected from varus and valgus stress was allowed if the necrosis was partial. Local fusion was used only for late complications.

Patients and Methods

Thirty-six patients treated from 1968 through 1982 were reviewed. Twenty-six were re-examined, ten by telephone and chart review. The average time from fracture was 7 years. The ages were 7–57 years (average 25). All patients had complete fractures of the talar neck. They were classified by Hawkins' method with modification (Table 1). Hawkins defined all displaced neck fractures as category II in the series; however, his clinical photographs show slight displacement in some category I fractures. In this series, all category II fractures had malalignment of the posterior subtalar joint, and some category I fractures had vertical displacement upward of the distal fragment of a few millimeters (Table 2).

Preoperative assessment was made of the areas of comminution and the angle of the fracture line, particularly the involvement in the body or the subtalar joint. In 27 of 28 it was found that reduction could be obtained via a medial incision that started at the tuberosity of the navicular and continued posteriorly and superiorly into the line of the talus to pass over the medial malleolus (Fig. 2). The saphenous vein was ligated. Care was taken to identify the frac-

---

[1] The paper is reproduced here by kind permission of J. B. Lippincott, Philadelphia, PA.

Table 1. Hawkins' classification, modified

Classification	
I	Undisplaced tibiotalar or subtalar joint
II	Undisplaced tibiotalar, displaced subtalar
III	Displaced tibiotalar and subtalar joint
This was modified by adding:	
IV	Displaced talonavicular joint

Table 2. Distribution by Hawkins' classification

Classification	No.	Closed reduction	ORIF	Malleolar osteotomy
I	14	8	6	2
II	14	0	14	0
III	5	0	5	4
IV	3	0	3	0

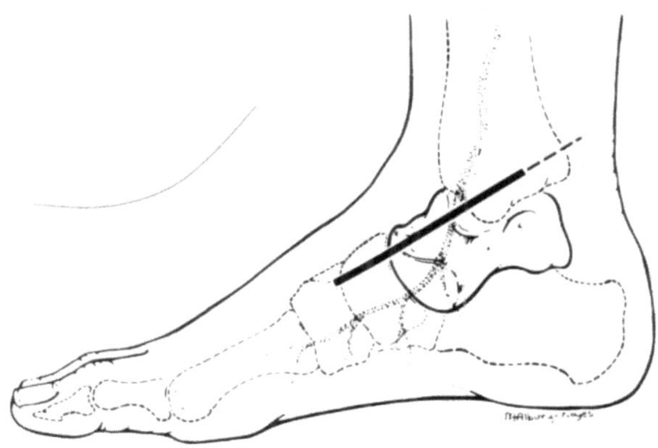

Fig. 2. The medial incision can be extended to allow medial malleolar osteotomy

ture without stripping tissue from the neck of the talus that could transmit blood supply. Also, the remaining attachments on the medial and posterior aspect of the body fragment were carefully preserved. A malleolar osteotomy increased the capacity of the ankle joint to allow reduction without heavy traction, leverage, or stripping of the fragments. Medial malleolar osteotomy was used to facilitate reduction in two Hawkins I fractures when the fracture line was posterior enough to involve a portion of the body that was obscured by the overlying tibial plafond. Also, four of five Hawkins III fractures had osteotomies to facilitate realignment, three of the medial malleolus and one of the lateral malleolus. The fragments were reduced and held with two Kirschner wires. The reduction position was confirmed with anteroposterior and lateral radiographs of the foot. If a lag screw was possible without displacing the fracture, it was added. Eleven patients were treated with screws, 11 with Kirschner wires. Operation was performed less than 12 h after injury in 18 patients, within 1–7 days in nine, and 17 days in one. One patient required a partial removal of the navicular to obtain a solid area of bone for the screw head. No posteriorly inserted screws were used [9]. A plaster cast to the knee, non-weight-bearing, was continued for 6 weeks. At that time a film out of plaster was analyzed for the presence of subchondral bone atrophy on the anteroposterior projection. Patients with total avascular necrosis were treated by continued non-weight-bearing in a short-leg cast or patellar-tendon-bearing brace. Those with partial areas of necrosis were allowed weight-bearing, but in a cast or brace. Type I fractures may not show subchondral atrophy. If the 6-week film did not show resorption, the film was then repeated at 12 weeks post-injury. If there was continued good bone structure, weight-bearing was allowed, and subsequent radiographs did not demonstrate areas of avascular necrosis. Healing times of the fractures out of all protection were from 9 to 74 weeks, averaging 29 weeks.

The protective brace was constructed so that weight relief was possible (Fig. 3). This required 5° of dorsiflexion to be built into the brace so that the patient walked with the knee in slight flexion. A patellar tendon pressure pad and a molded leather calf cuff relieved weight-bearing. For the weight-bearing mode, the brace was fitted with metal hinges to prevent medial and lateral loading stresses at the ankle and a molded foot plate to avoid inversion and eversion of the foot.

Results

Avascular necrosis was often present (10 of 12) and involved the partial width of the talus on the anteroposterior view (Fig. 4). There was no definite correlation between delay in operation and the degree of necrosis. Necrosis in one fragment was certain when the body was split. The presence of necrosis correlated with the degree of displacement. Type I fractures can be confusing. The talus may not show subchondral bone atrophy [2], but the only type I fracture to develop late sclerosis was a fracture that was delayed 1 ½ weeks to operation. Type II tended to show partial necrosis. Some necrosis was present in all patients with type III displacement. Partial necrosis and total necrosis were complicated by collapse at the fracture site only once, in a patient with body involvement and delayed operation. Partial necrosis was often followed by a good result, complete necrosis by a fair result (Table 3).

Malleolar osteotomy improved the visualization of reduction and the ease of reduction. It did not appear to interfere with the blood supply of the talus. The attached body fragment that had rotated on a vertical axis to face laterally retained medial blood supply, and the avascular necrosis was limited to the lateral aspect in three of the type III fractures.

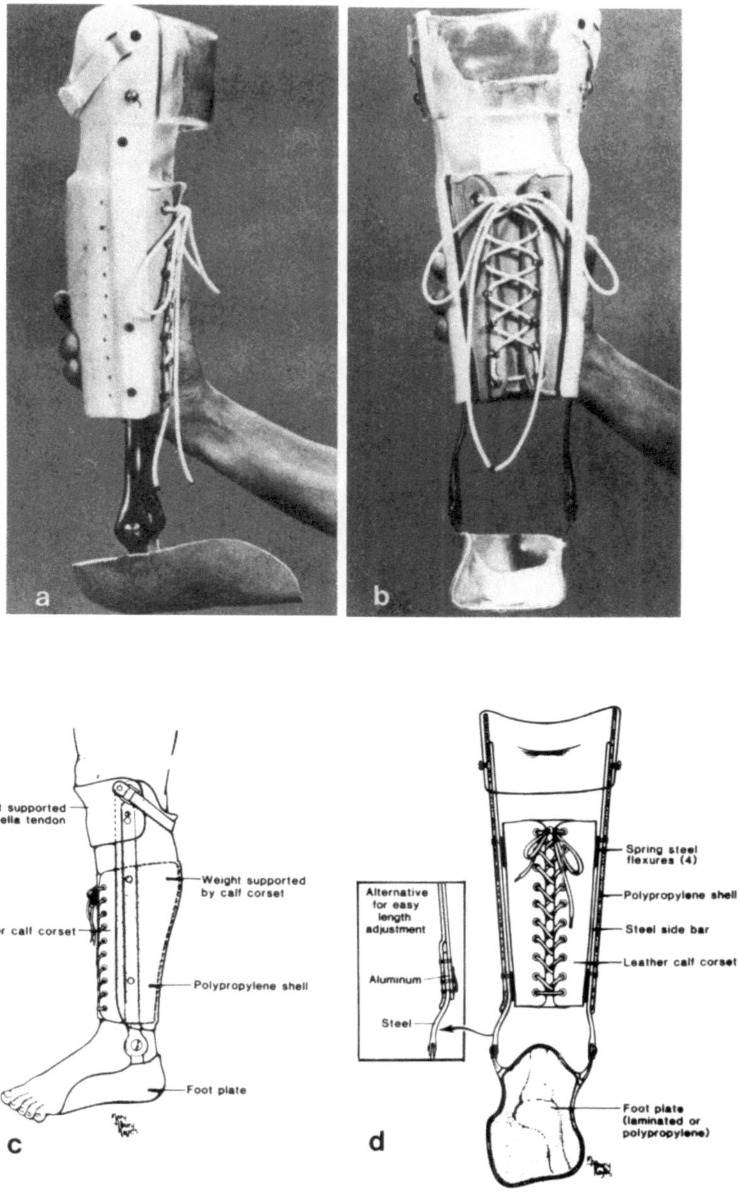

Fig. 3. a, b Protective brace with patellar-tendon-bearing top and lacer calf for leg suspension. Also, single-axis ankle and molded foot plate for weight-bearing mode, **c, d** Detail of the indirect attachment of the leather corset

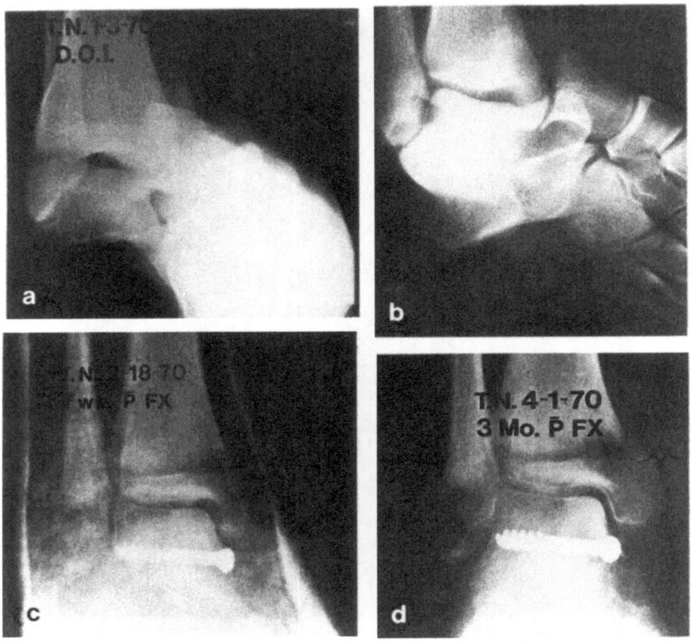

Fig. 4. a, b Details of injury, Hawkins II (talar neck fracture, subtalar joint dislocated, tibiotalar joint intact). **c, d** Seven weeks and 3 months after injury. Note that the lateral half of the talus is osteoporotic and, therefore, presumably vascularized. The medial half is denser because of lack of blood supply and failure of resorption of bone. **e–h** see p. 119

Table 3. Results by Hawkins' criteria

Classification	Excellent	Good	Fair
I	11	3	
II	3	2	1
III	2	3	
IV	2	1	

Table 4. Average motion in 26 patients

	Normal side (°)	Fractured side (°)
Plantarflexion	5.6	2.9
Dorsiflexion	44.0	35.0
Inversion	13.0	6.8
Eversion	6.0	2.8

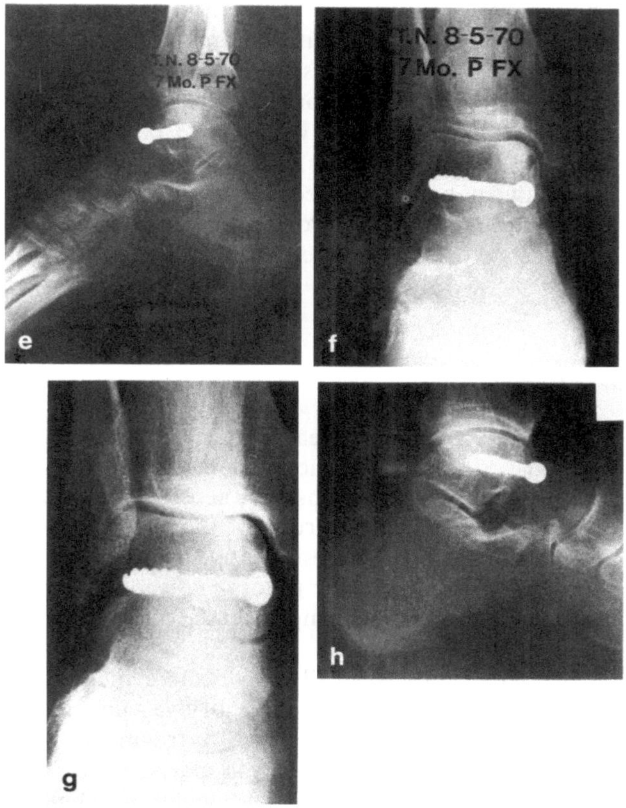

Fig. 4 *(continued)*. **e, f** Seven months after injury. There is no collapse despite weight-bearing. The leg was put in a brace with sturdy supports to avoid varus and valgus stress. The radiodense area is decreasing in size. **g, h** Thirteen years after injury. Hawkins' score 12, pain with sports and long walks

One patient required a later subtalar fusion. He had a 7-day delay in reduction and also a fracture that extended from the neck into the posterior subtalar joint that was reduced with a 1-mm stepoff. One patient, treated by closed reduction with subsequent slight shortening of the talus, developed a varus deformity and required a triple arthrodesis. Two patients developed a spontaneous subtalar fusion. Patients with fusions of the subtalar joint had good relief of subtalar pain and walked without a limp.

Seven patients complained of morning stiffness, three of swelling, and three of problems walking up hills. The 24 patients with radiographs demonstrated osteophytes and tibiotalar joint narrowing in eight ankle joints, three subtalar joints, and two talonavicular joints. No osteophytes were seen in 13 joints, and the late radiographs were not available in ten patients. Overall motion was well preserved in the ankle joint, decreased in the subtalar joint (Table 4).

The results were scored by the method of Hawkins. Six points were given for no pain, 3 for pain after fatigue, and 0 for pain on walking. Limp was rated 3 for none and 0 when present. Motion was graded at the ankle and subtalar joints: 3 points for full, 2 for partial, 1 for fusion, and 0 for deformity. Results were considered excellent with 13–15 points, good with 10–12 points, fair with 7–9 points, and poor with 6 or fewer.
All but two patients returned to work: 13 returned to heavy work, two changed from heavy work to light work, and nine continued in light work. Two patients previously working were retired.

Discussion

The long-term results of early open reduction and internal fixation appear favorable [8]. There were no incidents of malunion [18] or non-union, and no dorsal osteophyte resections were necessary [2]. The operation was technically demanding in that incongruity of the posterior subtalar joint would lead to arthrosis or fusion. The results appear preferable to a Blair fusion, although no series of such primary tibiotalar fusions has been performed. A medial malleolar osteotomy [13] improved the ease of exposure and reduction without complicating the healing.
While there is no statistically significant evidence that early operation was the cause, there was a low incidence of avascular necrosis. Early operation did allow easy reduction of the fracture fragments without additional stripping and accurate apposition of the vascularized neck to the remaining body. Easy reduction, which retained the retinacular attachments to the body, and apposition of a vascularized neck surface, may have provided blood supply to the body [16]. Also, it avoided problems with swelling, closure of the skin, or necrosis from the presence of displaced fragments seen with closed treatment [6, 13].
The series recognized the difference between partial and total necrosis [16] in that partial necrosis and residual bone would resist weight-bearing forces; therefore, non-weight-bearing was not necessary. It was considered important that varus and valgus stresses be avoided, because one segment of the bone was softer and, therefore, could have been damaged with inversion or eversion movements. The rigid hinges of the brace allowed vertical weight-bearing but not varus and valgus strains. This principle was recognized by Coltart [3] when he noted that weight-bearing in a short-leg cast did not lead to collapse of the fracture, and by Hawkins [7] who noted no subsequent problems with early weight-bearing.
Local fusions are useful in correcting deformity or subtalar arthrosis. Deformity is eliminated with accurate open reduction. There are advantages in delaying the fusion. Few patients become symptomatic. The local blood supply that would be damaged by the exposure for early fusion is preserved, and fusion, when necessary, will be performed in areas of revascularized bone,

which promotes early healing. There does not appear to be any reason to perform an early fusion in the absence of comminution of the body fragment. There was decreased subtalar motion. Rigid internal fixation followed by early motion might improve the problem, as it has in subtalar dislocation [4] without fracture. However, early motion without weight-bearing is known to lead to non-union [18].

Recommendations

1. Open reduction and internal fixation should be performed early.
2. Usually a medial approach is satisfactory.
3. A malleolar osteotomy is useful for incisional exposure.
4. Open reduction and internal fixation should be considered in displaced fractures when the joints are not subluxed, even though closed reduction may appear accurate.
5. Weight-bearing, protected from varus and valgus forces, is satisfactory for fractures with partial necrosis.
6. The brace needs a calf cuff and patellar tendon pad to be effective for non-weight-bearing.

References

1. Comfort TH, Behrens F, Gaither DW, Denis F, Sigmond M (1985) Long-term results of displaced talar neck fractures. Clin Orthop 199:81–87
2. Canale ST, Kelly FB Jr (1978) Fractures of the neck of the talus. J Bone Joint Surg [Am] 60:143
3. Coltart WD (1952) Aviator's astragalus. J Bone Joint Surg [Br] 34:545
4. DeLee JC, Curtis R (1982) Subtalar dislocation of the foot. J Bone Joint Surg [Am] 64:433
5. Dunn AR, Jacobs B, Campbell RD (1982) Fractures of the talus. J Trauma 6:443
6. Gillquist J, Oretorp N, Stenstrom A, Rieger A, Wennberg E (1974) Late results after vertical fracture of the talus. Injury 6:173
7. Hawkins L (1970) Fractures of the neck of the talus. J Bone Joint Surg [Am] 52A:991
8. Kenwright J, Taylor RG (1970) Major injuries of the talus. J Bone Joint Surg [Br] 52:36
9. Lemaire RG, Bustin W (1980) Screw fixation of fractures of the neck of the talus using a posterior approach. J Trauma 20:669
10. Lorentzen JE, Christensen SB, Krogsoe O, Sneppen O (1977) Fractures of the neck of the talus. Acta Orthop Scand 48:115
11. McKeever FM (1963) Treatment of complications of fractures and dislocations of the talus. Clin Orthop 30:45
12. Morris HD, Hand WL, Dunn AS (1971) The modified Blair fusion for fractures of the talus. J Bone Joint Surg [Am] 53:1289
13. Pantazopoulos T, Galanos P, Vayanos E, Mitsou A, Hartofilakidis-Garofalidis G (1974) Fractures of the neck of the talus. Acta Orthop Scand 45:296
14. Pennal GF (1963) Fractures of the talus. Clin Orthop 30:53
15. Penny N, Davis LA (1980) Fractures and fracture-dislocations of the neck of the talus. J Trauma 20:1029
16. Peterson K, Goldie IF, Irstram L (1977) Fracture of the neck of the talus. Acta Orthop Scand 48:696

Severe Foot Trauma in Combination with Talar Injuries

H. Zwipp

Severe foot trauma is often found in polytraumatized patients [3, 8–10]. General principles in the management of severe foot trauma have been advocated by Wright et al. [9]. These include: preserve circulation and sensation, preserve plantar skin and fat pads, encourage passive and active movement, prevent and control infection, maintain a plantigrade foot, and achieve bony union.

Definition

Our definition of severe foot trauma is based on a simple 5-point scoring system which provides 1 point for each involved fracture or fracture-dislocation level of the foot and ankle area (five levels) and 1 point for each degree of soft tissue trauma, considering an overall and degloving injury or a subtotal amputation as a fourth-degree lesion. Therefore by definition severe foot trauma should score a minimum of 5 points (Table 1).

Patient-Related Data

In a 20-year period (1971–1990) we analyzed 1558 fractures of the foot and ankle area, excluding metatarsal fractures. Five levels of involved fractures were distinguished. We treated 1112 fractures or fracture-dislocations of the pilon/ankle level, 117 central talar fractures, 208 intra-articular calcaneal fractures and 121 fractures and fracture-dislocations of the Chopart-Lisfranc area. A total of 149 cases were defined as severe foot trauma (Fig. 1). Of these 149 cases 31% were three-level fractures. Second- to third-degree open fractures were found in 24% of cases and second- to third-degree closed fractures in

Table 1. Definition of severe foot trauma

a.	Fracture/fracture-dislocation, levels 1–4	1–5 points
b.	Open/closed fracture/fracture-dislocation, first- to third-degree Overall/degloving/subtotal amputation, fourth-degree	*1–4* points
c.	Total of *a* + *b* (minimum)	5 points

35%. Urgent dermatofasciotomy was performed in 19% of cases, and primary partial or subtotal amputation in 9.4%.
Central talar fractures (Fig. 2) occurred in 41 of the 149 cases of severe foot trauma and in 32% of polytraumatized patients. There was a high percentage of open fractures in 18 of 117 cases (15.4%). In 6 closed fractures acute compartment syndrome had to be treated urgently (6%).
Concomitant fractures were found most often at the level of the ankle ($n=21$), calcaneus ($n=20$), cuboid ($n=8$) and navicular bone ($n=6$). Arterial transections were seen in 4 cases, neurotmesis in 2 cases and tendon ruptures in 5 cases (Fig. 5a, b). The cause of injury was most often a traffic accident ($n=71$).

Lessons Learned

Our experience of treating patients with severe trauma has taught us the following lessons:

1. Look at the condition of the whole patient. In stage 3 and 4 cases (Hannover polytrauma score) amputation should be done. In cases of severe barytrauma the degree of soft tissue and bone loss, sensation, and blood supply are looked for. The mangled extremity severity score [7] may be of help in judging these cases. However, our experience of using a primary modified Pirogoff amputation [6] in 6 patients was excellent (Fig. 3).
2. Be very aggressive in treating severe foot trauma by doing urgent radical debridement with the help of jet lavage. Redebridement or after-amputations should be done in a second-look operation within 24–36 h.
3. Use minimal osteosynthesis when fixing the fractures with Kirschner wires, 3.5 mm cortical screws and temporary tibiotarsal fixation for 3 weeks. This is achieved by placing a small Schanz screw into the first metatarsal and another in the fourth to keep the foot in a neutral position. Temporary use of semipermeable artificial skin has proven very successful (Fig. 4a, b).
4. Fix serial fractures from proximally to distally, except for talus fractures where fixation is preferred before the malleoli.
5. Cover large soft tissue defects within the first 3 days using a free flap. However, from our experience with 12 cases we learned that bone grafting and definite stable osteosynthesis should be done before tissue coverage with a free flap (Fig. 5).

We normally use the anteromedial, anterolateral, or posterolateral approach [5] to the talus. In open fractures and in cases of acute compartment syndrome the approach has to be modified or extended to relieve the involved compartments.
Figure 6 shows an extensive crush fracture sustained in a racing car accident, associated with dislocation posterolaterally. The dislocation can be clearly seen on the three-dimensional CT scan. The injury, which was treated as an emergency, required urgent decompression of the soft tissues, minimal osteosynthesis, tibiotarsal transfixation, and early subtalar arthrodesis after 10 days.

Case Reports

Case Report 1 (Fig. 7)

This is an example of real aviator's astragalus in a 40-year-old man. On the left side he sustained third-degree open total dislocation of the talus emerging out of the shoe with rupture of the posterior tibial artery (Fig. 7a, b). On the right side he sustained a second-degree open ankle fracture in combination with a Hawkins IV fracture-dislocation (Fig. 7c). After radical debridement, open reduction, and minimal osteosynthesis one can see a well-reconstructed foot on both sides (Fig. 7d, e). Temporary tibiotarsal transfixation was performed on both sides (Fig. 7d–f) as well as secondary skin grafting. After 3 years a severe arthritis of the ankle joint developed on the side of the Hawkins IV lesion (Fig. 7g). On the left side the foot looks flattened; however, it has relatively good function (Fig. 7h).

Case Report 2 (Fig. 8)

This is an example of severe three-level trauma (ankle, calcaneus, Chopart) with a blow-out fracture of the calcaneus and dislocation of the whole talus, and a second-degree open wound (Fig. 8a). The hindfoot was reconstructed using minimal osteosynthesis with Kirschner wires. In order to minimize trauma to the soft tissue temporary tibiotarsal transfixation for 3 weeks was used (Fig. 8b). The radiological and clinical outcome after 1 year is relatively good (Fig. 8c, d).

Case Report 3 (Fig. 9)

This example shows severe three-level trauma with a second-degree open wound. This is typical of the high-energy traumas that we have been seeing with increasing frequency over the last 5 years. There is severe ankle fracture with impaction of the medial pilon corner, talar neck fracture, and intra-articular calcaneal fracture (Fig. 9a, b). Debridement was followed by screw fixation of the talar neck fracture, screw fixation of the malleoli, and finally screw fixation of the calcaneus and temporary tibiotarsal transfixation for 3 weeks (Fig. 9c, e). Skin grafting was done after 10 days (Fig. 9d). After 8 months the radiographs still look quite good (Fig. 9f). After 2 years progressive posttraumatic arthritis at the level of the ankle joint can be seen but no subtalar arthritis (Fig. 9g); function remained relatively good.

Talus-Related Results

According to our modified Hawkins [2] and Marti [4] classification 21 patients had a type 4 fracture, 17 of whom sustained severe foot trauma. The type 4 fracture still seems to be the most problematic. Of the 21 cases there were 7 with avascular necrosis, 2 with septic necrosis, and 7 with severe arthritis of the ankle and/or subtalar joint. The last complication was especially common after attempted initial closed reduction, inadequate operative technique, or a delay before operation of more than 6 h.

Conclusion

The following general conclusions can be drawn from our experience with severe foot trauma:

1. Do primary partial/total amputation in severe polytrauma/barytrauma, preferably using the transmetatarsal or Pirogoff amputation
2. Do urgent radical debridement, dermatofasciotomy and open reduction
3. Do minimal osteosynthesis with Kirschner wires, 3.5 mm cortical screws, and temporary tibiotarsal transfixation for 3 weeks
4. Do, in serial fractures, open reduction and internal fixation first of the talus, then of the malleoli, calcaneus, Chopart's and, lastly, Lisfranc's joint
5. Do realignment of the lateral and medial column of the foot and fill larger bony defects temporarily with polymethylmethacrylate beads
6. Do temporary wound closure with artificial skin
7. Do second-look operations with redebridement and/or amputation within 24–48 h
8. Do an early free flap within the first 3 days, with definite fixation and bone grafting if needed
9. Do secondary wound closure skin grafting and early arthrodesis, when needed, within the first 10 days
10. Do early physiotherapy and partial weight-bearing after 3 weeks

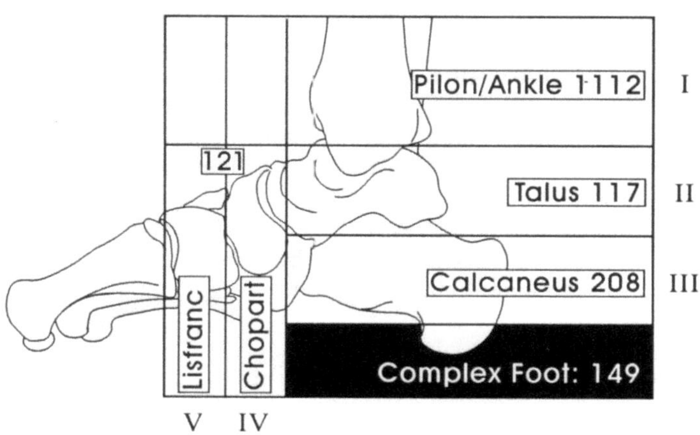

Fig. 1. Foot and ankle fractures treated at Hannover Medical School from 1971 to 1990 ($n=1558$)

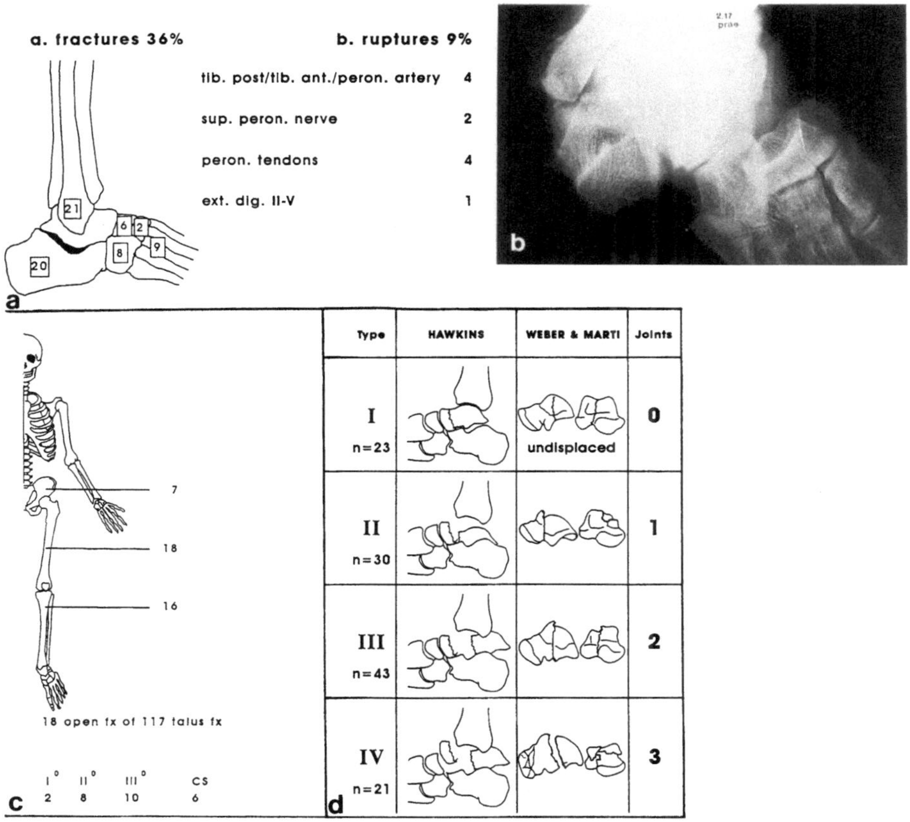

Fig. 2a–d. Involvement of concomitant lesions in 117 central talar fractures. **a** Concomitant lesions in the foot area. **b** Example of a total dislocation of the talus ($n=3$), one of the 41 cases of severe foot trauma in combination with talar injuries. **c** Distribution of 18 open fractures in 117 cases. There were 6 cases of acute compartment syndrome (CS) in 99 closed fractures. **d** Fracture classification modified after [1, 2, 4] (117 central talar fractures)

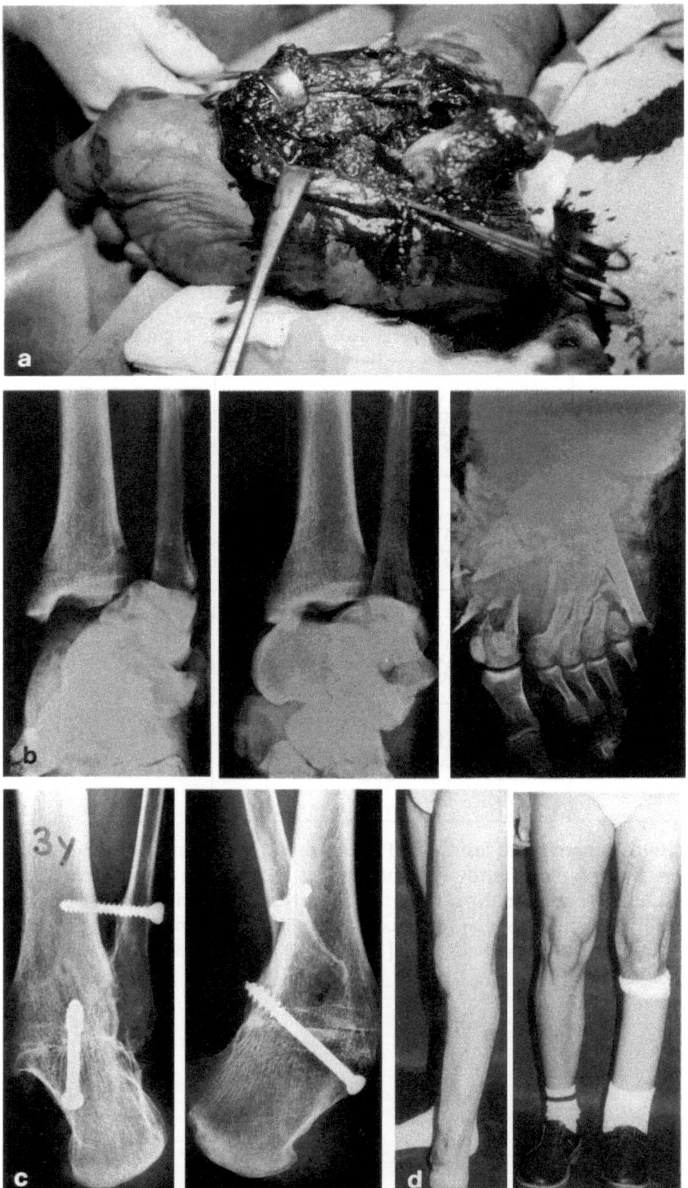

Fig. 3a–d. Third-degree open severe foot trauma in a polytraumatized 28-year-old patient (Hannover polytrauma score: PTS III). **a** Soft tissue situation. **b** Lower leg fractures with ankle disruption, talar dislocation, complex Chopart/Lisfranc lesion, and metatarsal fractures. **c** Three years after primary Pirogoff amputation. **d** Normal leg length with stable soft tissue of the weight-bearing stump

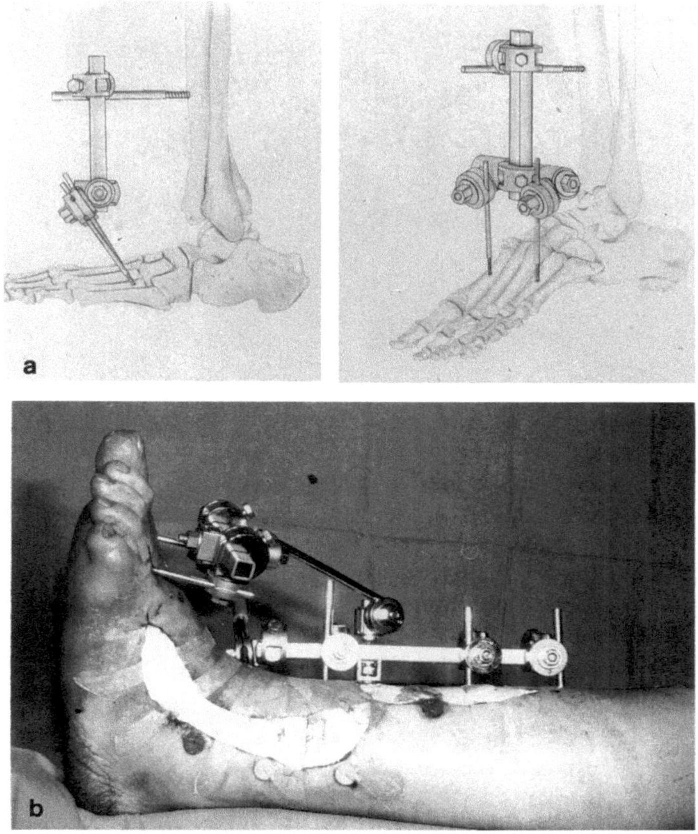

Fig. 4. a Temporary transfixation in severe foot trauma. **b** Tibiotarsal transfixation in combination with a lower leg fracture; skin defects temporarily covered with artificial skin

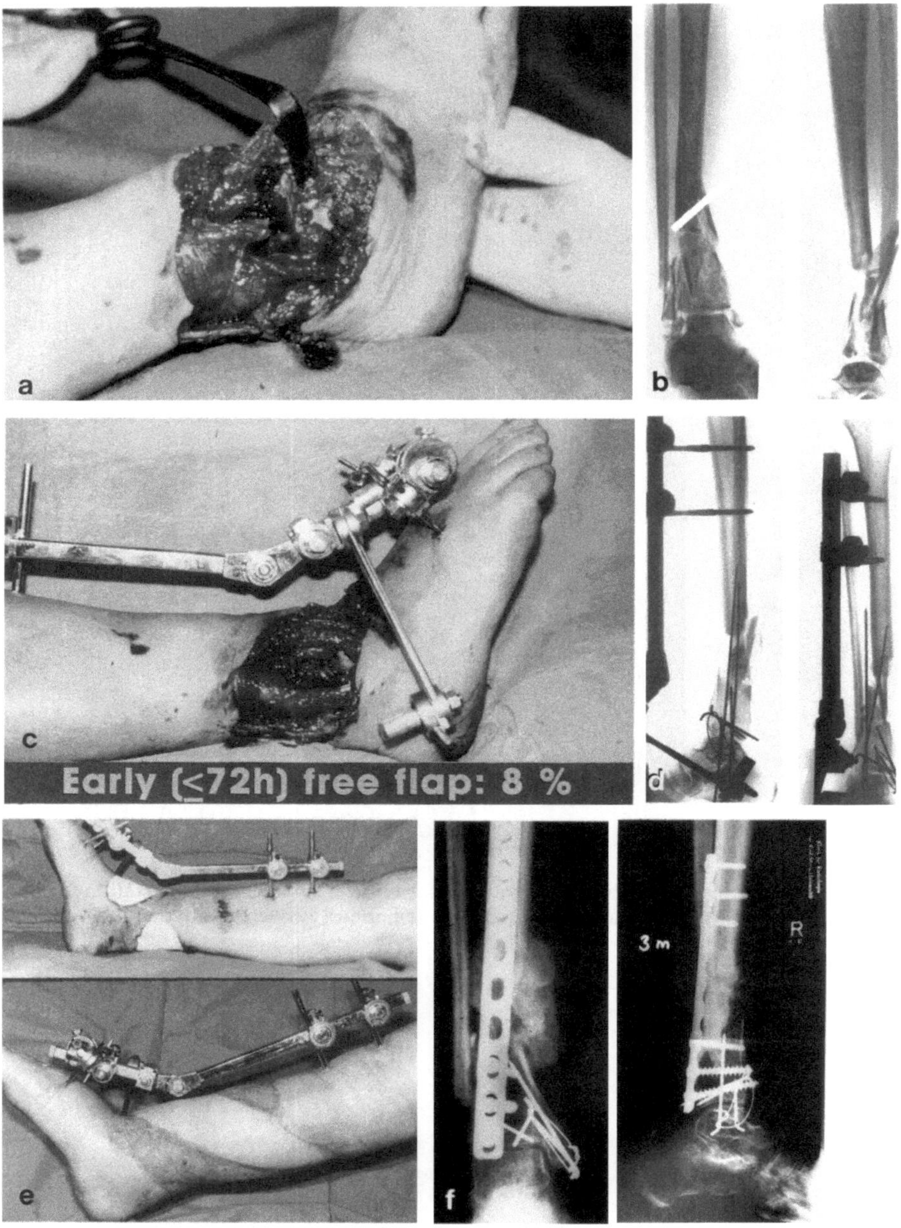

Fig. 5 a–f. Complex pilon fracture in a 42-year-old woman who was involved in road traffic accident in which her foot and ankle were crushed between two cars. **a** Third-degree open pilon fracture with soft tissue and bone loss. **b** Pilon fracture (C3), and partial bony defects of the fibula and tibia. **c, d** After radical debridement, resection of the distal fibula, joint reconstruction with minimal hardware, and temporary tibiotarsal transfixation with additional support of the hindfoot. **e** Redebridement after 36 h, and decision for performance of a free flap within 72 h (*above*). Free latissimus dorsi flap (6 weeks postoperative) after initial temporarily artificial skin grafting (*below*). **f** Three months after dorsal LC-DC plate fixation and bone grafting

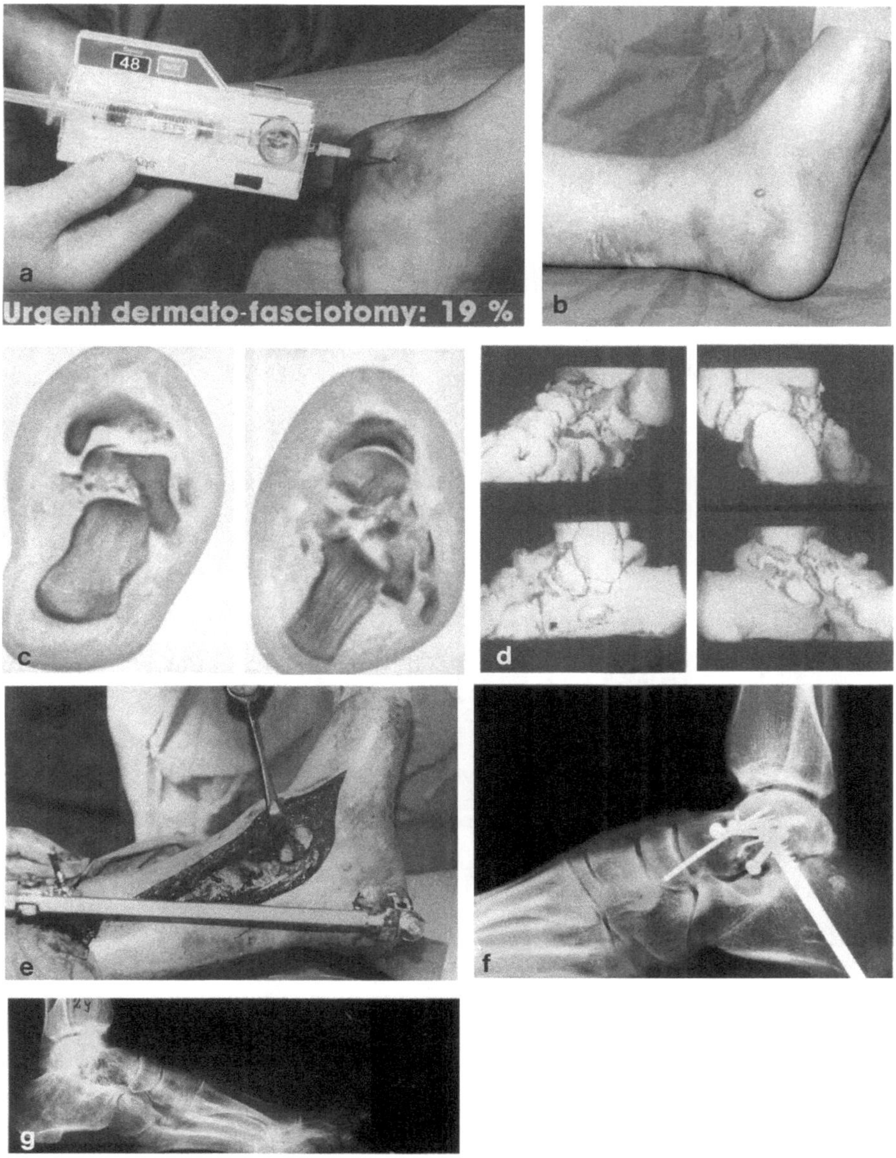

Fig. 6a–g. Acute compartment syndrome in a talar crush fracture (type 4 Weber/Marti) sustained by a 41-year-old man in a car racing accident. **a** Example of monitoring in acute compartment syndrome. **b** Three hours after injury there was rapid blistering of the skin. **c** CT scan done as an emergency shows the laterally dislocated burst fracture of the body. **d** Three-dimensional CT scan shows clearly the dorsolateral dislocation of the burst talar body. **e** Acute decompression of the soft tissues by a long anteromedial incision with splitting of the superior and inferior extensor retinaculum, minimal osteosynthesis of the talus with Kirschner wires and screws, and temporary use of an external fixator. **f** Early subtalar fusion after 10 days. **g** Weight-bearing lateral radiograph after 2 years

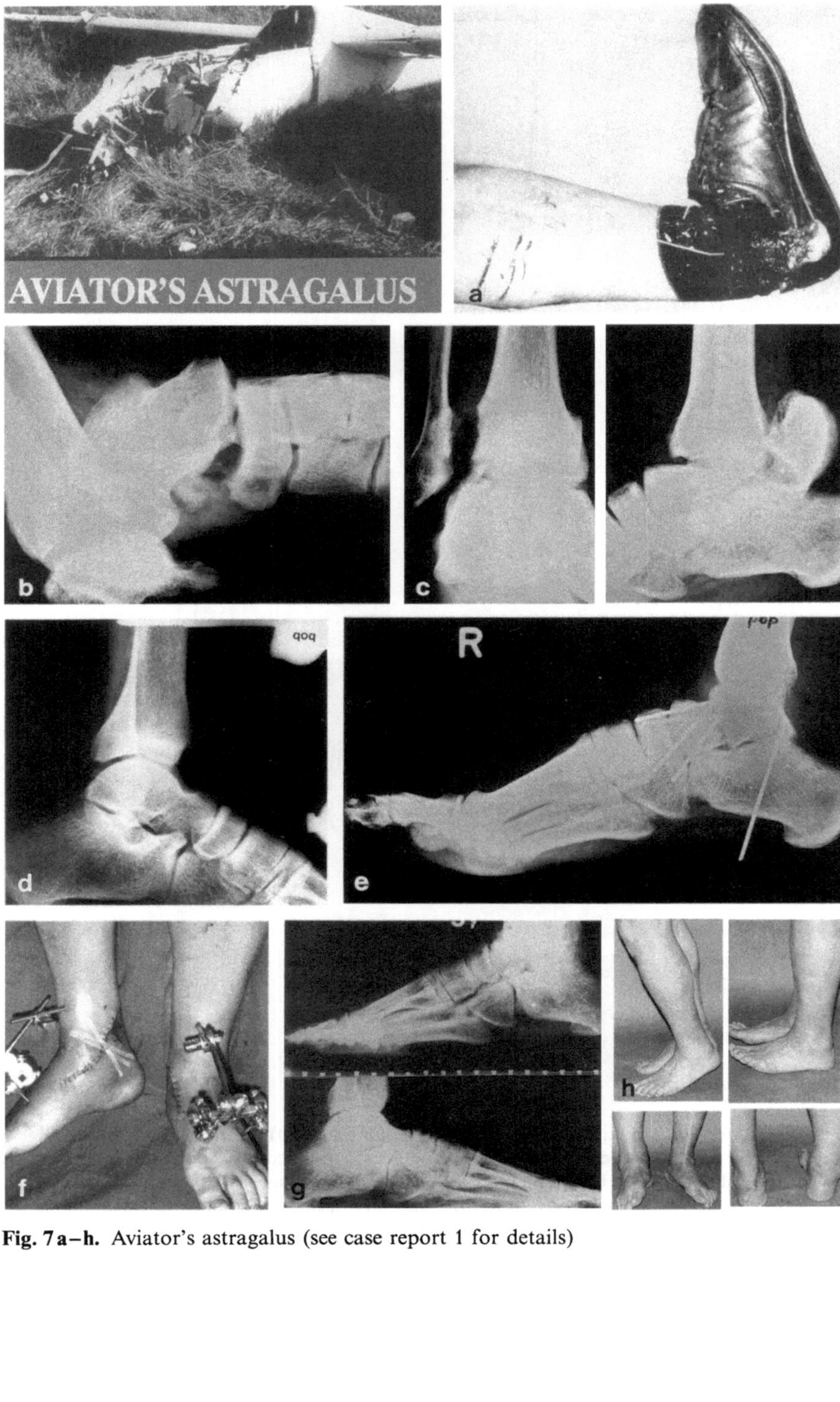

Fig. 7 a–h. Aviator's astragalus (see case report 1 for details)

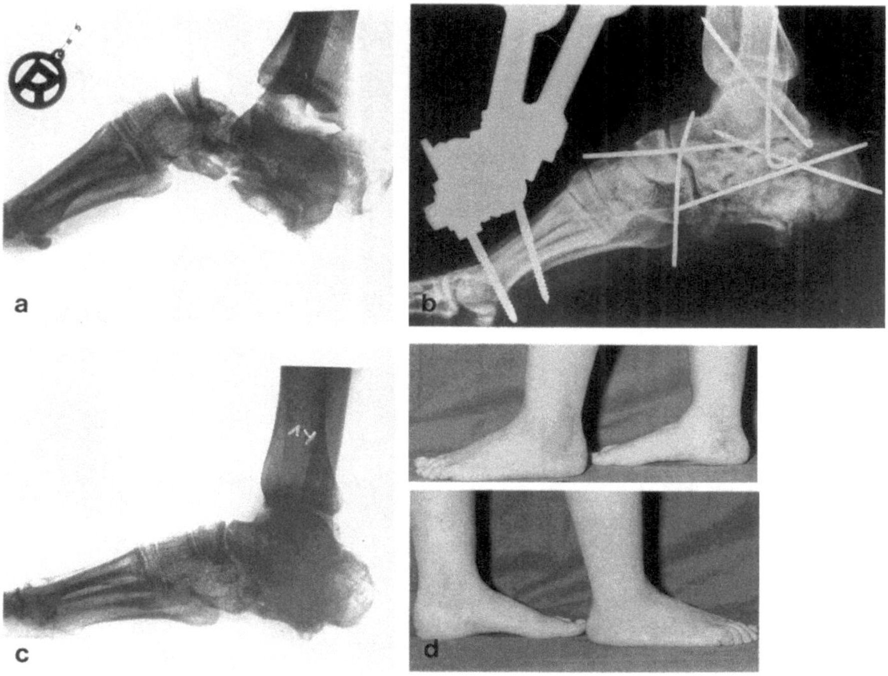

Fig. 8 a–d. Three-level trauma (ankle, calcaneus, Chopart joint) with a second-degree open wound in a 40-year-old woman after a fall from 10 m (see case report 2 for details)

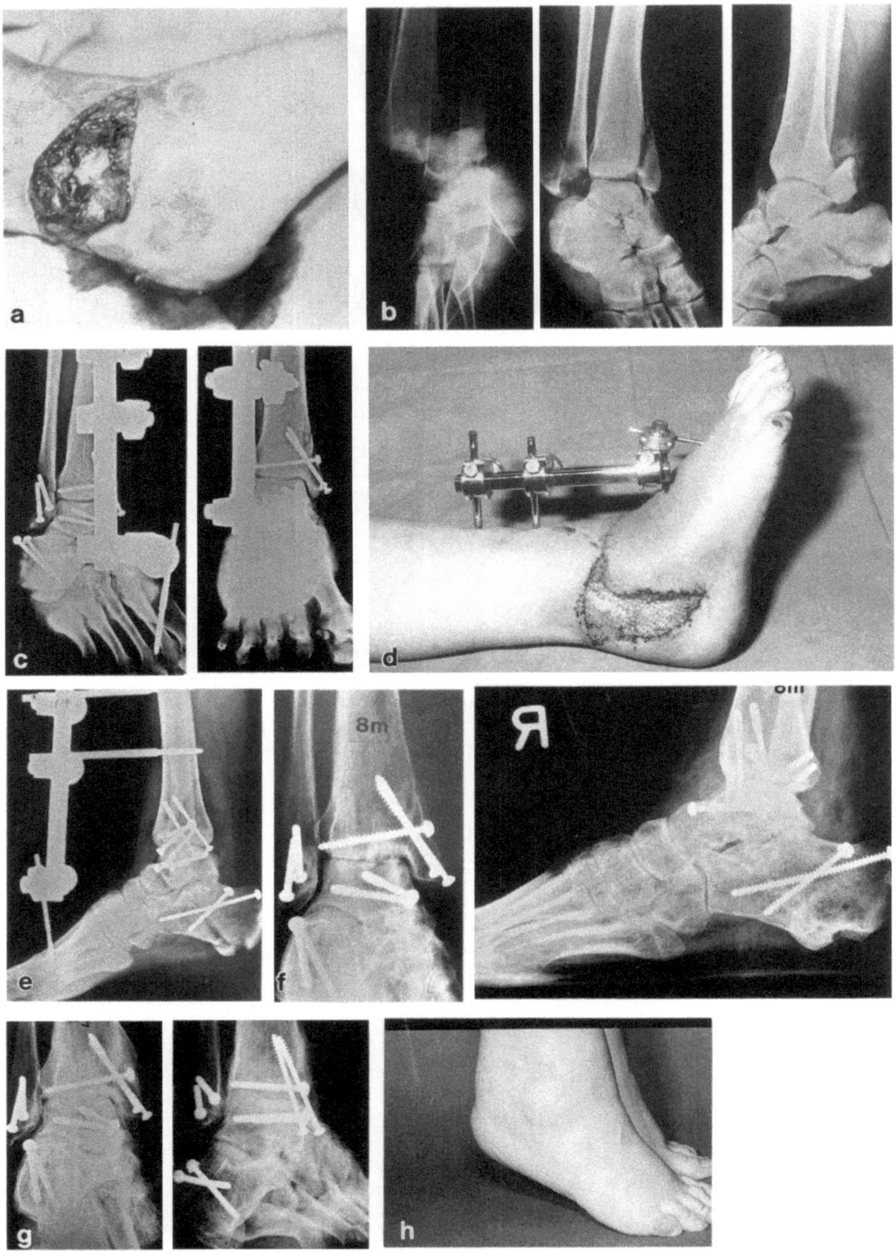

Fig. 9 a–h. High-energy trauma at three levels (ankle, talus, calcaneus) with a second-degree open wound sustained by a 45-year-old woman in a high-speed car accident (see case report 3 for details)

References

1. Canale ST, Kelly FB Jr (1978) Fractures of the neck of the talus. Long-term evaluation of seventy-one cases. J Bone Joint Surg [Am] 60:143
2. Hawkins LG (1970) Fractures of the neck of talus. J Bone Joint Surg [Am] 52:991–1002
3. Heckmann JD, Champine MJ (1989) New techniques in the management of foot trauma. Clin Orthop 240:105–114
4. Marti R (1978) Talus- und Calcaneusfracturen. In: Weber BG, Brunner CF, Freuler F (eds) Die Frakturenbehandlung von Kindern und Jugendlichen. Springer, Berlin Heidelberg New York
5. Mayo KA (1987) Fractures of the talus: principles of management and techniques of treatment. Techniques Orthop 2/3:42–54
6. Pirogoff NI (1864) Grundzüge der allgemeinen Kriegschirurgie. Vogel, Leipzig
7. Swiontkowski MF (1990) Limb reconstruction or primary amputation in massive lower extremity trauma? The development of a decision making scale. AO/ASIF Dialogue III
8. Tscherne H (1987) Management der Verletzungen am distalen Unterschenkel und Fuß. Langenbecks Arch Chir 369:539
9. Wright J, Worlock P, Hunter G et al. (1987) The management of injuries of the midfoot and forefoot in the patient with multiple injuries. Techniques Orthop 2/3:71–79
10. Zwipp H, Tscherne H, Berger A (1989) Rekonstruktive Fußchirurgie nach Komplextraumen des Fußes. Unfallchirurg 92:1–15

Complications of Talar Fractures

E. L. F. B. Raaymakers

Non-union

Dunn et al. [4] reported a frequency of non-union of 13% after conservative treatment of central talus fractures. In the proceedings of the Reisensburger Workshop, 12 years later, this complication is not even mentioned [3].
Since the introduction of open reduction and stable internal fixation as the routine treatment for displaced fractures it has become a hard job indeed to create a non-union in this well-vascularized cancellous bone. The same is true for the peripheral fracture types: the osteochondral fracture of the dome [2] and fractures of the posterior and lateral processes of the talus [10].
Once there is a non-union of a body/neck fracture open reduction and screw fixation should be carried out. Attention has to be paid to the correct length of the talus. Especially in longstanding non-unions continuous motion at the fracture site causes osteolysis and loss of substance, which necessitates interposition of a corticocancellous graft between the fragments in order to regain the correct length of the talus and avoid incongruency of both the talocrural and talocalcaneal joints.
Removal of the fragment in the case of non-union of an osteochondral fracture of the dome is the treatment of choice [1, 8]. Only large pseudarthrotic fragments of the lateral process, which have the insertion of the anterior talofibular ligament, are reduced and fixed with a screw. Frequently the fragment is small and is excised [11]. Traction of the posterior talofibular ligament is always the cause of a fractured posterior process. In order to restore the stability of the ankle refixation of a pseudarthrotic posterior process is mandatory.

Arthritis

Sixty percent of the surface of the talus consists of cartilage which is divided into seven articular facets. Almost every talus fracture is an intra-articular fracture; sometimes two joints are involved by the same fracture. Even minor malunions cause incongruency arthritis and it is therefore understandable that arthritis is the main complication after talus fractures.
The lateral process of the talus is extremely sensitive to malreduction as it forms part of both the ankle and subtalar joint. However, only a very large fragment can malarticulate with the fibula, independent of the position of the

foot. Thus this fracture is, in fact, a problem of the subtalar joint. On the basis of the poor results of conservative treatment Mills and Horne [10], among others, advocates internal fixation of large fragments, which involve both the ankle and subtalar joints. Small fragments, involving only the subtalar joint, and comminuted fragments should be excised. Our experience with six cases (Table 1) confirms Mills' philosophy. Our small series shows that we were not very successful. We tried to reconstruct ambitiously small fragments and could not obtain an anatomical reduction in a single case.

Table 1. Results of operative treatment of fractures of the lateral process of the talus

Operative treatment	Result
Screw fixation ($n=5$)	Malreduction ($n=5$) Subtalar arthritis ($n=3$) Subtalar + ankle arthritis ($n=1$)
Excision ($n=1$)	Full recovery

Fracture of the posterior process is caused by traction of the posterior talofibular ligament. The lesion presupposes a rupture of both other lateral ligaments and is therefore combined with a dislocation of the talus from the ankle mortise. A fracture of the posterior process involves only the subtalar joint and, if malreduced, gives rise to a talocalcaneal arthritis, as we experienced in our only case. Statistics on this fracture are not available, because the lesion is very rare or at least rarely diagnosed.

Correct reduction of peripheral fractures is probably not so easy and excision should be considered, provided the stability of the ankle joint is not jeopardized.

The remarkably high frequency (21%) of post-traumatic arthritis after non-displaced fractures reported by Burri and Rüter [3] in their survey of 206 central talus fractures could be explained by the supposition that not all these fractures were really undisplaced. As Watson-Jones showed [14], it is easy to fail to appreciate slight subtalar dislocation of the talar body. If this dislocation is not reduced, subtalar arthrosis is inevitable. A very pronounced example of this "optical illusion" is shown in Fig. 1. The gross subtalar dislocation was not recognized. A little excuse for this mistake was that the distal fragment of the talus together with the navicular bone and probably the whole medial bow of the foot shifted proximally. Therefore, the usual gap between the talar fragments was absent in this case. For this reason the reduction of this fracture gave no difficulty at all as the body of the talus was still dislocated. Again this was not recognized on the postoperative radiograph. The gross incongruency of the subtalar joint resulted in a very painful arthritis, which made a partial triple fusion necessary within 5 months.

The typical fracture mechanism of central fractures is a forceful dorsiflexion of the ankle. The anterior rim of the tibia acts as a chisel, cracking the neck of

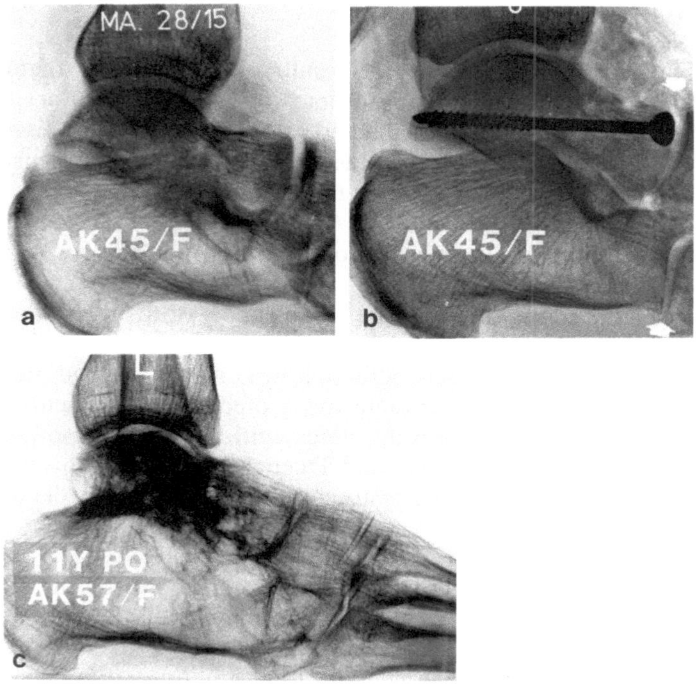

Fig. 1. **a** Central fracture of the talus with dislocation of the talar body (see text). **b** Screw fixation. The subtalar dislocation still exists. **c** Eleven years after a partial triple fusion slight degenerative changes are found in the ankle joint, causing some pain

the talus outside the ankle joint. Less well known is that 90% of so-called neck fractures run into the posterior talocalcaneal joint. This was observed already by Ombredanne in 1902 and confirmed by Grond [5]. Therefore a distinction between neck and body fractures seems to be artificial. Furthermore it explains why the subtalar joint is the main focus of posttraumatic arthritis in many series [9, 13]. Another important point is that these authors report a remarkably high percentage of ankle joint arthritis. An explanation for this finding could be that in the Marti/Weber classification, used by them, comminuted fractures were combined in one group with fracture-dislocations. However, sagittal, impression, and comminuted fractures are, in fact, the counterparts of the pilon fracture. They have their own pathology and have a greater impact on the ankle joint than on the subtalar joint. If we analyse this group of lesions separately, at least in our series, the percentage of ankle arthritis after a real central fracture falls dramatically from 28% to 12%.

Avascular Necrosis

Hawkins [6] reported on the results of conservative treatment of displaced talus fractures and fracture-dislocations. He found a very high frequency of avascular necrosis (42% and 91% respectively). The figures for the same fracture types, published in the proceedings of the Reisensburger Workshop [3], are 36% and 16%. They refer to fractures that were treated with open reduction and osteosynthesis. Anatomical reduction and stable internal fixation accelerate revascularization and limit the number of clinically obvious cases of avascular necrosis.

It is a misconception that the blood supply of the talus is poor. In spite of its large articular surface and lack of muscle attachments, the talus is well supplied with blood vessels, although in narrowly defined areas. Extensive soft tissue damage is therefore always a precursor of avascular necrosis. On the other hand triple fusion interferes with the blood supply as well, but never causes necrosis. Mulfinger and Trueta [12] explained this phenomenon by the numerous intraosseous anastomoses they were able to demonstrate inside the talus.

The diagnosis of avascular necrosis depends on radiological changes which occur only when disuse, caused by non-weight-bearing and/or immobilization, has produced porosis of the surrounding vascular bone. The relative increase in density of avascular bone can be detected 6–8 weeks after the fracture. This phenomenon is particularly liable to misinterpretation, especially on the lateral radiograph. Due to the overlapping density of both malleoli the suggestion of necrosis is easily created.

On the other hand partial necrosis of the talar body does not produce enough changes on the lateral radiograph to be detected. Bilateral anteroposterior radiographs are therefore essential for checking whether avascular necrosis is developing. The most accurate method of determining the extent of body involvement is magnetic resonance imaging (MRI). Hawkins [6] described a useful sign which indicates viability of the body of the talus. If there is subchondral "bone atrophy" – a zone of radiolucency recognized between 6 and 8 weeks after injury – this indicates bone resorption and establishes beyond doubt that the vascular supply of the talus is intact or is being restored.

Once avascular necrosis is diagnosed a strict regime of non-weight-bearing without immobilization is advised. Under these conditions revascularization has to be waited for under MRI control at 6-month intervals. In the majority of recent articles on this subject periods of non-weight-bearing of up to 2 years are advocated [7, 13]. With this regime secondary collapse of the talar body is rare, although exact figures are not available.

Collapse of the talus is, however, frequent under septic conditions. In this connection open fractures have a bad reputation. Figure 2 illustrates a bilateral open fracture-dislocation of the talus. Because of an overwhelming infection on the left side after conservative treatment, a below-knee amputation was carried out 2 weeks after the accident. The fracture on the right side was reduced and fixed with Kirschner wires. After a total of ten operations the

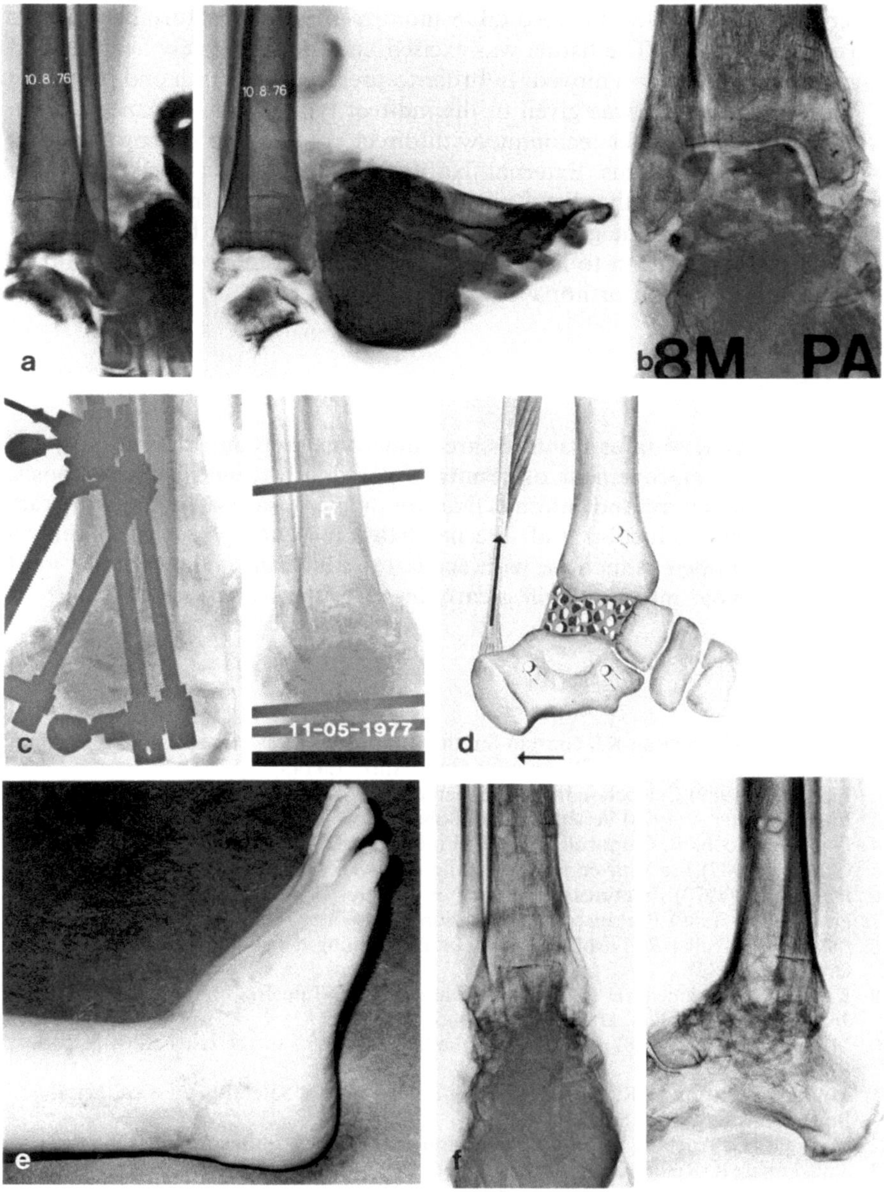

Fig. 2. **a** Bilateral open fracture-dislocation of the talus sustained by a 42-year-old woman in a road traffic accident. **b** Eight months after the accident there is septic necrosis of the talar body. **c** Scheme of a tibiocalcaneal fusion with preservation of the shape of the foot. **d** Nine months after the accident. Tibiocalcaneal fusion with a cancellous bone graft. **e** Eighteen months after the accident. **f** Two years after the accident

patient was referred to our hospital, 8 months after the fracture, with septic necrosis of the talus. The fistula was excised and the completely necrotic and fragmented talar body removed. In order to preserve leg length and the shape of the foot preference was given to the indirect type of tibiocalcaneal fusion over the somewhat safer technique with direct contact and compression between tibia and calcaneus. External fixation, the method of choice in infected cases, was used, with the distal pins in the calcaneus and metatarsals. The primary cancellous bone graft was followed 3 months later by an additional one. The fusion went on to healing and the patient could walk without pain with the support of an orthopaedic shoe.

Conclusions

Complications after talus fractures are numerous and concern especially the subtalar joint. Improvement of results is possible through early diagnosis, anatomical reduction and internal fixation, and excision of peripheral fractures if internal reduction and internal fixation is not possible. In central fracture types open reduction, with accurate reduction of the subtalar joint and care to avoid infection, will greatly improve the results.

References

1. Anderson IF, Crighton KJ, Grattan-Smith T, Brazier D (1989) Osteochondral fractures of the dome of the talus. J Bone Joint Surg (Am) 71:1143–1152
2. Biedert R (1989) Osteochondrale Läsionen des Talus. Unfallchirurg 92:199
3. Burri C, Rüter A (1978) Verletzungen des oberen Sprunggelenkes. Hefte Unfallheilk 131
4. Dunn A, Jacobs B, Campbell R (1966) Fractures of the talus. J Trauma 6:443
5. Grond J (1947) Fractuur en luxatie van de talus. Thesis, University of Amsterdam
6. Hawkins L (1970) Fractures of the neck of the talus. J Bone Joint Surg [Am] 52:991
7. Hendrich V (1989) Frakturen und Luxationen des Talus. Unfallchirurg 92:110
8. Ittner G, Jaskulka R, Fasol P (1989) Zur Behandlung der flake fracture des Talus. Z Orthop 127:183
9. Kuner E, Lindenmeier H (1983) Zur Behandlung der Talusfraktur. Kontrollstudie von 262 Behandlungsfällen. Unfallchirurg 9:35
10. Mills H, Horne G (1987) Fractures of the lateral process of the talus. Aust NZJ Surg 57:643
11. Mukherjee S, Pringle R, Baxter A (1974) Fracture of the lateral process of the talus. J Bone Joint Surg [Br] 56:263
12. Mulfinger G, Trueta J (1970) The blood supply of the talus. J Bone Joint Surg [Br] 52:160
13. Szyszkowitz R, Reschauer R, Seggl W (1985) Eighty-five talus fractures treated by ORIF with five to eight years of follow-up study of 69 patients. Clin Orthop 199:97
14. Watson-Jones R (1976) Fractures and joint injuries. Churchill Livingstone, Edinburgh London New York, S 1183

PART III · CALCANEAL FRACTURES

Biomechanical Considerations in the Hindfoot

S. T. Hansen, Jr.

Introduction

An examination of normal hindfoot function puts into perspective the advantages of anatomic internal fixation for both talar and calcaneal fractures. Almost all talar fractures involve the subtalar or the talocalcaneal joints directly or indirectly. Intra-articular calcaneal fractures, which account for at least 70% of all calcaneal fractures, are commonly treated by internal fixation and, by definition, always involve the subtalar joint.

The biomechanical considerations for the hindfoot are presented in two sections in this chapter. In the first section, potential damage and functional loss in the subtalar joint resulting from either talar or calcaneal fractures are discussed. The topic of discussion in the second section is restoration of normal calcaneal anatomy in order to preserve calcaneal function following major intra-articular calcaneal fractures. Specificially, these functions include the calcaneus acting as a lever arm, as a vertical support or foundation, and as a horizontal support of the lateral column of the foot.

Functions of the Subtalar Joint

Perhaps the most important function of the subtalar joint is to cushion impact during gait by converting the internal rotatory forces the tibia produces between heel-strike and foot-flat into pronation in the foot. Internal rotation in the leg and the talus increases the talocalcaneal angle in the foot and softens the normal arch, allowing it to drop and absorb impact (Figs. 1, 2). In effect, the arch of the foot acts as a leaf spring. During relaxed standing in a neutral position, the subtalar joint, the arch, and the heel place little stress on surrounding muscles and ligaments (Fig. 3). Conversely, during the foot-flat to toe-off phases of gait, external rotation in the tibia is transmitted through the talus and the subtalar joint, the foot is supinated, the talar head is twisted laterally up and over the calcaneocuboid joint, and the midfoot becomes more rigid (Fig. 4). When the heel, the midfoot, and the forefoot are locked, the foot acts as a long lever powered by the gastrosoleus muscle (Fig. 5). In this position, the foot is capable of a strong push-off or acceleration, actions that are very important for moderate to rapid walking.

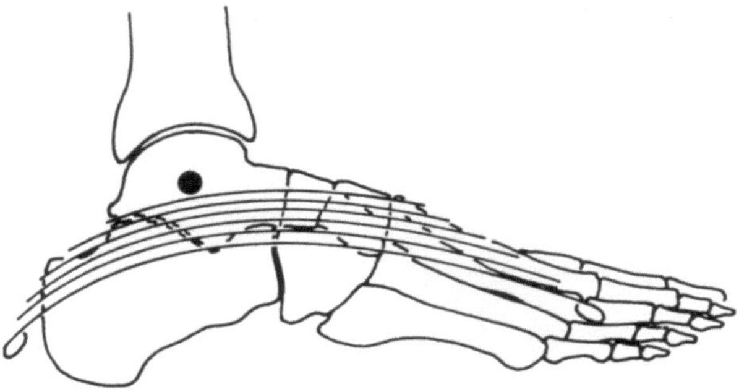

Fig. 1. The arch of the foot functions as a leaf spring. The bony and ligamentous structures of the foot are capable of softening through the arch when the tibia is internally rotated and locked onto the dome of the talus. This position, known as pronation, allows the foot to rotate laterally under and in front of the talus. Pronation occurs at the beginning of the weight-bearing portion of the gait cycle as the foot strikes the ground and accepts body weight. At this moment, the arch of the foot functions as a leaf spring

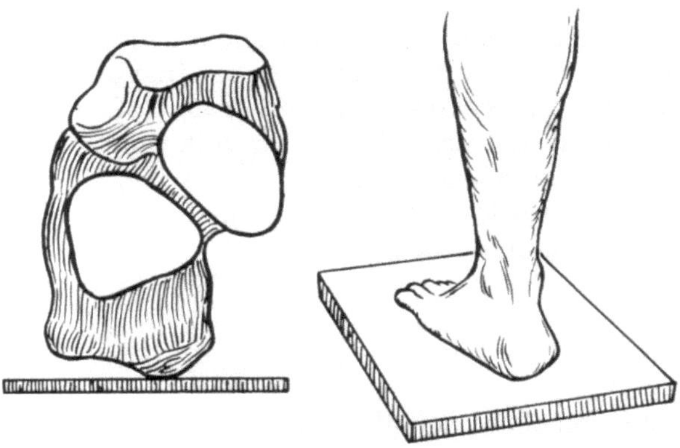

Fig. 2. *Left:* The head of the talus and the anterior calcaneus are visualized at the calcaneal facet of the calcaneocuboid joint (Chopart's joint) during pronation. The calcaneus and the midfoot have rotated laterally to the talus through the subtalar and talonavicular joints. The midfoot softens to allow the spring action during the impact of body weight. *Right:* The foot is seen from a posteromedial view. The arch is lowered and the heel is in slight valgus, a position defined as pronation

The second major function of the subtalar joint is to adapt the foot to uneven surfaces by means of inversion and eversion. These actions protect the ankle or tibiotalar joint, which essentially is a gliding joint in the sagittal plane, from stresses produced by medial and lateral tilt. Long-term studies of subtalar and triple arthrodeses reveal that significant ankle arthrosis occurs when the subtalar joint cannot cushion or protect the ankle from medial and lateral tilt stresses. Without inversion and eversion through the subtalar joint, children

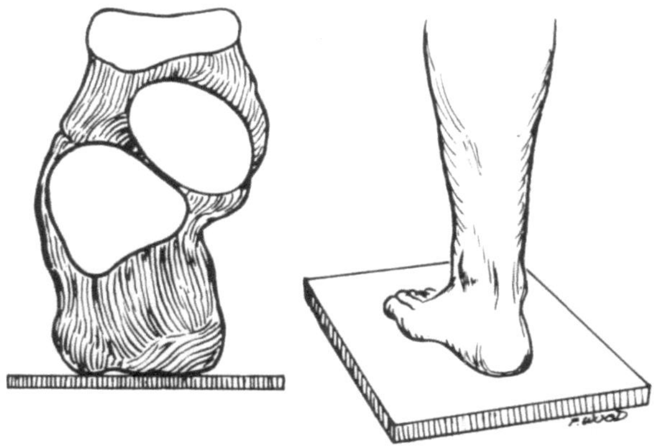

Fig. 3. *Left:* The relationship of the talus and the calcaneus are seen in Chopart's joint during a neutral mid-stance position. *Right:* A foot with a normal arch and with the heel in a neutral position is seen from a posteromedial view

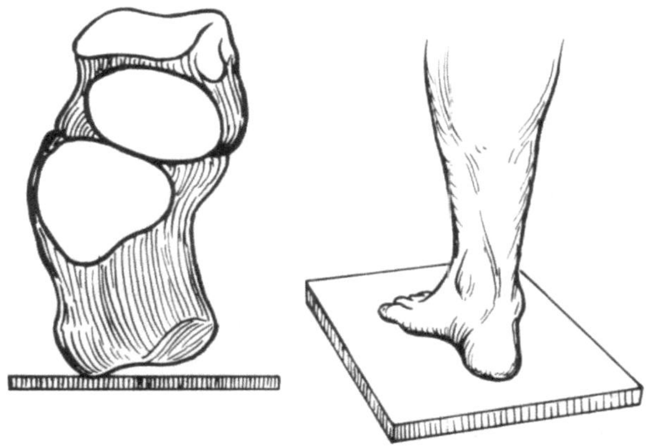

Fig. 4. *Left:* The tibia and the talus are rotated externally during the late stance phase while the foot is fixed on the ground. The talus rotates over the calcaneus and the midfoot stiffens or locks. The foot becomes a lever arm for push-off using the gastrocsoleus muscle as a motor. *Right:* Supination of the hindfoot is slightly exaggerated when the heel is in varus and the arch is high during push-off

with congenital subtalar fusions or coalitions can develop "ball-and-socket" ankle joints from stresses on the ankles.

In practical terms, these findings suggest that patients without a functional subtalar joint should avoid jobs or sports which entail much walking and should work primarily on level surfaces. In addition, they should wear shoes with thick, soft rubber heels to cushion gait and beveled heels and toes to shorten the lever arm of the shoe working against the leg musculature.

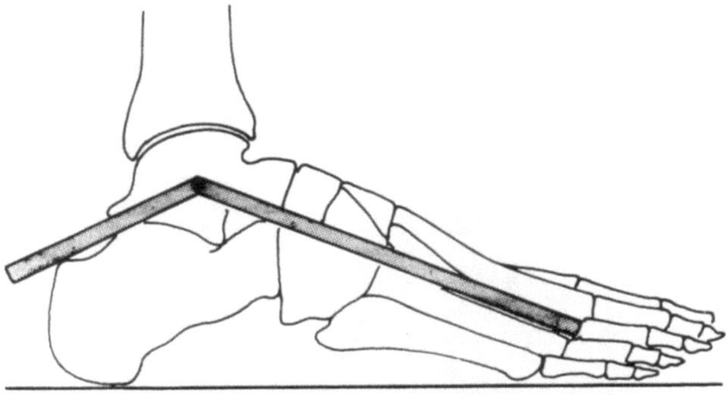

Fig. 5. The foot as a lever arm. Normal foot function demands both a normal subtalar joint, which allows hindfoot supination and locking of Chopart's joint, and normal architecture of the calcaneal body

Hindfoot Functions Related to Normal Calcaneal Anatomy

The calcaneus provides three principal functions for normal gait:

1. It acts as a lever arm that is powered by the gastrosoleus mechanism. During normal function, this lever arm is extended through the midfoot and the forefoot by normal subtalar supination (Fig. 5).
2. It provides a foundation or a vertical support for body weight transmitted through the tibia, the ankle, and the subtalar joints (Fig. 6).
3. It provides support for and maintains the length of the lateral column, which affects abduction and adduction of the midfoot and the forefoot (Fig. 7). Lateral support indirectly assists the foot with supination and allows strong push-off during gait.

To function efficiently as a lever arm, the calcaneus must maintain an anatomic fulcrum or hinge point in the mid-body of the talus, and it must interact normally with its motor, the gastrosoleus muscle. High-energy calcaneal fractures can markedly disrupt these anatomic relationships. The gastrosoleus muscle is functionally weakened when the subtalar joint is disrupted and the heel rides upwards.

The calcaneus functions as a vertical support or foundation for body weight transmitted through the leg. Normal alignment is necessary under the weight-bearing line of the tibia to prevent tilting and eccentric weight distribution. If the body of the calcaneus is displaced laterally, it may impinge under the fibula and the lateral plafond. Eccentric weight bearing may cause actual tilt and produce tension on the medial soft tissues. When the body is displaced into varus alignment, pressure is increased on the medial part of the ankle joint and tension is noted in the lateral ligaments. This may predispose the ankle to lateral sprain and eventually produce an actual tilt of the talus in the mortice and secondary arthrosis in the ankle. Talar dorsiflexion can be seen during

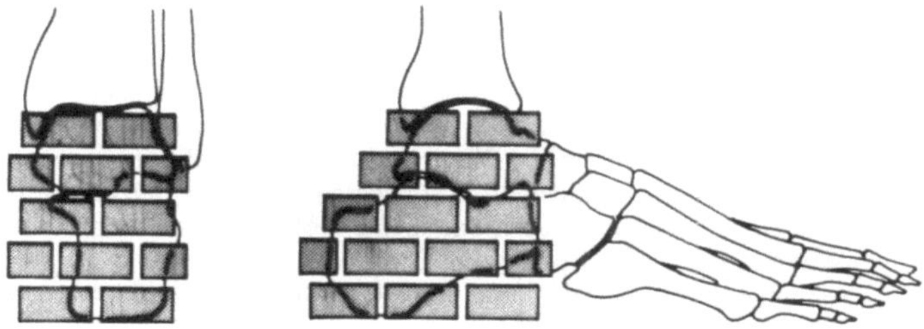

Fig. 6. The hindfoot as a foundation for weight bearing. Like any weight-bearing structure, the hindfoot must be aligned with the weight-bearing forces and be of adequate height and strength to withstand the loads placed on it. If the calcaneus collapses, the articulation of the talus with the tibial mortice will be disrupted. A straight collapse will push the talus into dorsiflexion in the ankle mortice; a collapse with lateral or valgus displacement will cause a lateral tilting moment, place tension on the deltoid ligamentous structures and excessive compression under the lateral tibial plafond, and transfer excessive weight to the fibula. Varus displacement is uncommon, but tilting of the heel into varus can occur with lateral calcaneal displacement. Varus malalignment may occur with an occult deep posterior compartment syndrome and posterior tibial muscular contracture following a talar or calcaneal fracture. Varus malalignment at the ankle has the opposite effect, causing tension on the lateral ligaments and compression in the medial plafond

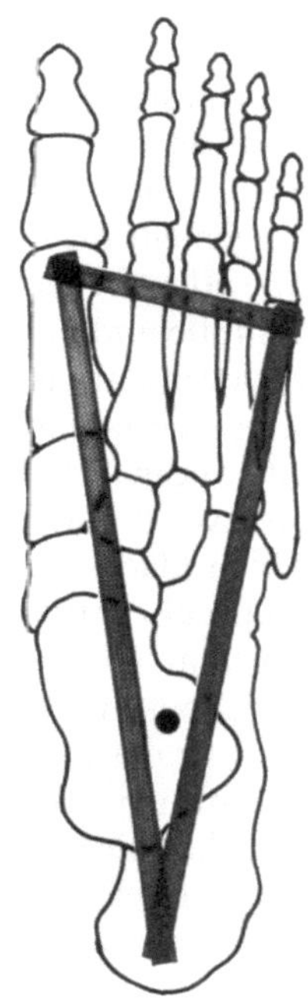

Fig. 7. The calcaneus as a support in the lateral column. The normal length of the calcaneus is as important to maintaining the length of the lateral column (the calcaneus, the cuboid, and the fifth metatarsal) as the length and position of the talus is to maintaining the medial column (the talus, the navicular, first cuneiform, and first metatarsal). Shortening of the lateral column allows the foot to drift laterally from underneath the talus and precludes the capability of locking the Chopart's joint. The resulting functional losses include persistent pathologic pronation, weak push-off, and secondary pain and arthrosis

Fig. 8a–f. Radiographs of the left hindfoot in a patient who had suffered a severe fall and landed on the point of the heel. **a, b** Lateral (**a**) and axial (**b**) radiographs taken 2 years after the fall. Note that the posterior body is crushed and displaced dorsally and laterally in relation the talus and the subtalar joint. The fibula is slightly obscured but, in fact, the calcaneus is impinged under the fibula and has displaced the peroneal tendons. In addition, the overall length of the calcaneus is shortened from an extension or dorsiflexion deformity in the calcaneocuboid joint as is the lateral column. The talus is dorsiflexed in the ankle mortice and is not aligned properly with the midfoot. In this case, the subtalar joint could not be salvaged, but the heel could be restructured and realigned to salvage some function. **c, d** Lateral (**c**) and axial (**d**) radiographic views taken post-operatively reveal osteotomies of the heel in two planes. Alignment, declination from the talus, and longitudinal length have been restored with translation and bone-block grafts. Stabilization is provided by fully threaded positioning screws instead of compression screws. Cancellous bone chips have been added to cancellous block grafts to stimulate union. The patient was positioned with the affected side up to allow access to the ipsilateral posterior iliac crest for bone-graft harvesting. A lateral extensile incision was made to expose the entire calcaneus and subtalar joint for the surgery. **e, f** The axial (**e**) and lateral (**f**) radiographs show the same patient several months later. The two screws at the corner of the heel caused irritation and were removed after satisfactory union had been achieved. The patient was markedly less symptomatic and was able to return to work as a farm laborer. The length of the lateral column is adequate enough to align the midfoot and forefoot correctly. The ankle is capable of dorsiflexion, medial-lateral tilt forces are balanced, and the gastrosoleus muscle has adequate strength. The patient is unable to adapt well to uneven surfaces and must wear supportive shoes with thick cushioned heels and supportive insoles to cushion gait

neutral stance on a lateral radiographic projection when the calcaneal foundation has been shortened by impaction of the body of the talus into the calcaneus. When pronounced, this condition can produce anterior and dorsal impingement or, eventually, arthrosis in the ankle.

The effect of the axial length of the calcaneus on the lateral column of the foot is subtle and not generally recognized, yet it is very important. When a transverse fracture in the anterior calcaneus shortens and subsequently causes the lateral column of the foot to shorten, the midfoot and the forefoot are forced into abduction through Chopart's joint, the naviculocuneiform joint, or possibly even Lisfranc's joint. Abduction results in lateral peritalar subluxation, which places increased tension on the posterior tibial tendon and can cause eventual rupture or failure of the tendon. If failure occurs, lateral and dorsal peritalar subluxation are increased. The resulting malalignment forces the calcaneus into a very lateral position and severely compromises its function as a vertical support. Subsequently, the sinus tarsi is impinged laterally and tension is increased on the medial structures, including the deltoid ligament and the calcaneonavicular ligaments.

Surgical restoration of normal calcaneal anatomy is amply justified whenever it is feasible. Surgery has two goals:

1. Reconstruction of the articular anatomy of the subtalar joint, which cushions gait and protects the ankle by adapting the foot to uneven surfaces
2. Restoration of normal calcaneal anatomy, which is essential for normal hindfoot function during all weight-bearing activities

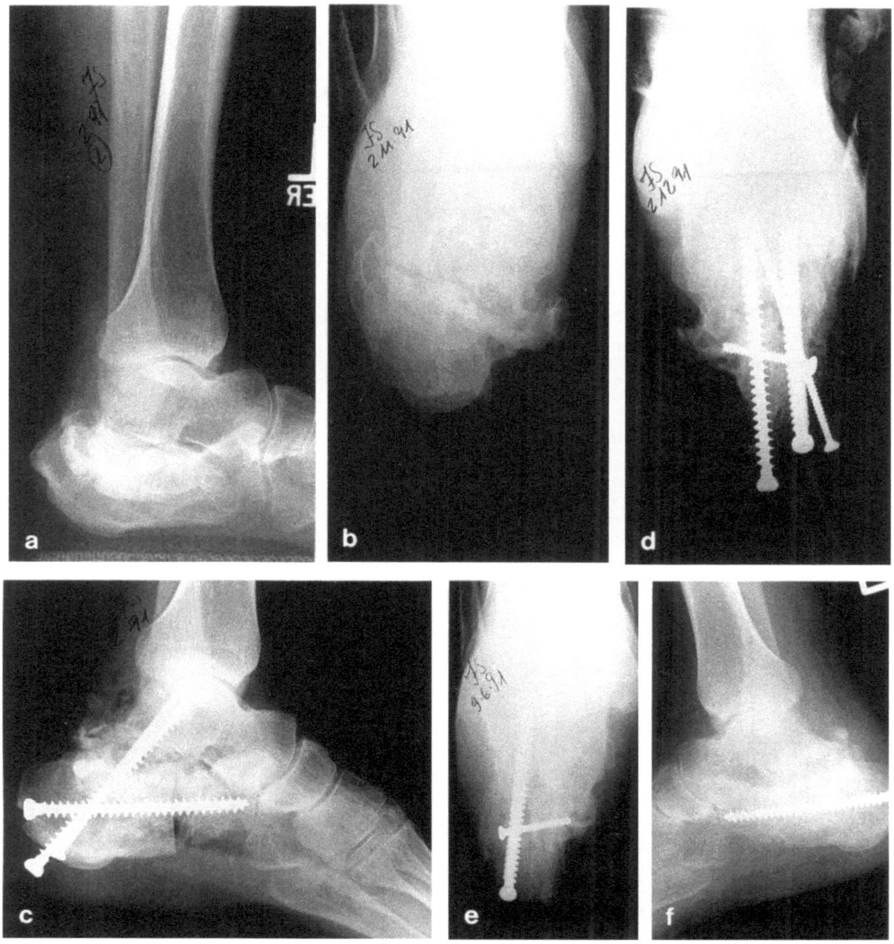

Further Reading

1. Mann RA (ed) (1986) Surgery of the foot. Mosby, St Louis, Chap 1
2. Root (ed)

Calcaneal Fracture

H. Tscherne and H. Zwipp

Historical Review

The development of the treatment of calcaneal fractures clearly shows the close relationship between diagnostic means and consequent action, i.e., the feasibility of surgery. Three main phases can be recognized.

The *conservative period* was caused by the lack of radiological diagnostic means. It began with Hippocrates (460–385 B.C.) and included Lisfranc (1790–1847) and Hoffa (1859–1907) as well as other renowned late-nineteenth-century surgeons. These doctors had to rely on clinical diagnosis. Their treatment recommendation consisted of elevating the foot, applying moist bandages, and 3 weeks of bedrest.

The second, *semi-operative period* started only at the beginning of the twentieth century. Until this began, however, there was the precocious development of a traction device by the American Clark in 1855 [5] and the pioneer work on open repositioning by Bell in Edinburgh in 1882 [2]. The advent of the semi-operative phase doubtless resulted from the fact that radiological detection of fracture pathology was now possible.

Goff [11], in his excellent review of 156 reports on the treatment of calcaneal fracture from 1720 to 1936, described 41 different semi-open techniques which were advocated in the period between 1905 and 1936. These included the insertion of a kangaroo tendon or a silver wire, the bolting in of a bone plate, and astragalectomy. Other methods were also practised, such as external hammer modeling [6], diverse traction methods, early subtalar arthrodesis, and double or triple arthrodesis.

Lenormant et al. [14] and Palmer [19] were the first to recognize the necessity of lining an impacted depression fracture of the posterior facet with bone chips. Böhler [3] amended his therapeutic procedure in calcaneal fracture more often than that for any other fracture. Because of numerous infections, which he saw in other hospitals as a result of the procedure according to Palmer, Böhler himself soon returned to the semi-operative procedure according to Westhues [23]. There remained general uncertainty with regard to the therapeutic procedure up to the end of the 1970s, with surgeons vacillating between primary functional treatment [20], early arthrodesis [10], and modifications of the Westhues method.

Although pioneers such as Leriche [15] and Judet et al. [13] introduced primary screw or plate osteosynthesis of the calcaneus, the third, *surgical period* using open anatomical reduction and primary osteosynthesis commenced only at the beginning of the 1980s. This was made possible by the advent of new imaging methods such as CT which allowed better detection of the fracture pathology and provided the basis for new surgical strategies. Numerous authors have since applied to calcaneal fractures the same principles of surgery as those appropriate to any other joint fracture, i.e., restoration of the articular surface and the external form by means of stable osteosynthesis and early functional postoperative treatment.

Anatomy

The calcaneus is the largest tarsal bone of the foot. Three bony processes emanate from its main mass:

1. The powerful sustentaculum tali, which is rendered very stable biomechanically by its trabecular structure, and which constitutes the inner column for support of the talus owing to its position on the medial side. Because of its extremely strong ligamentous connection with the talus it practically never loses its fixed positional relationship with the talus.
2. The calcaneal tuberosity which is the most massive process extending dorsal. In its upper dorsal half it accommodates the strong insertion of the powerful triceps surae tendon.
3. The lateral peroneal trochlea, which is the smallest process on the lateral side and forms the fixed groove for the two peroneal tendons together with the peroneal sulcus and the retinacula.

Altogether, the calcaneal bone cannot be compared with any geometrical figure. The thickness of the cortical layer is very variable. Under the posterior facet an area of more highly condensed bony substance roughly 1 cm wide is to be found. In 1911 Destot [8] termed this the calcaneal thalamus. The cortex is thickest in the region of the angle of Gissane and in the sustentaculum (Fig. 1).

On the other hand, in other places (for example on the lateral side) the cortical layer is very thin, so that it often and very easily breaks out and is designated as the lateral bulge or the lateral wall expansion.

The trabecular structure of the calcaneus develops in response to the tractional and pressure forces. However, somewhat lateral to the calcaneal sulcus there is an almost triangular area in which the cancellous bone trabeculae are poorly developed and which is not subjected to normal loading. This area (Fig. 2) is called the trigonum calcis [7], the pseudocyst triangle [1], or the neutral triangle [12]. The last designation indicates that the calcaneus is subject to less stress at this point under physiological weight bearing.

The three major joint facets of the calcaneus are the posterior facet, the medial and anterior facet (which are fused in 20% of cases according to our own cadaver studies, and which are to be regarded as a functional unit), and the calcaneocuboid articular surface.

The short but very thick ligaments of the calcaneus do not readily rupture. This applies in particular to the extremely strong interosseous talocalcaneal ligament, which extends into the sinus and tarsal canal.
The "tuberosity-joint angle", a term inaugurated by Böhler, has decreased somewhat in clinical importance since the introduction of CT, since this angle may be quite normal in numerous intra-articular depression fractures even if the posterior facet has been destroyed.

Pathomechanics of Fracture

In 1843 Malgaigne [16] was already able to show very graphically the classical tongue-type fracture corresponding to the later description of Essex-Lopresti [9]. In 1948 Palmer [19] described the typical development of the "joint depression fracture" according to Essex-Lopresti in his original paper, with a coronal section such as we are familiar with today from CT. An axial force initially leads to a shear fracture, which passes through the posterior facet and forces the posterolateral fragment to undergo a parallel lateral displacement with continued force. The posterolateral portion of the talus acts like a hammer on the posterior facet and impacts this into the posterolateral fragment, with break-out of the lateral wall. With reduction of the force, the posterolateral fragment then sinks with the impacted posterior facet. This results in a typical depression fracture with a step in the joint.
In 1952 Essex-Lopresti [9] distinguished between these two types of intra-articular fracture (Fig. 3). He coined the term "primary fracture line", which begins exactly in the angle of Gissane, and arises exactly where the fibular process of the talus can strike the calcaneus like a chisel. In this way the anteromedial anterior main fragment supporting the sustentaculum and the posterolateral main fragment comprising the posterior facet are produced in the first stage of the action of force. Considered from the calcaneal surface, the fracture may come to lie laterally, through or anteromedially to the posterior facet [22]. The position of this oblique sagittal fracture depends on the position of the foot at the time of compression. In valgus position it tends to be displaced laterally, in the neutral position it passes through the joint, and in varus position it passes anteromedial to the posterior facet (Fig. 4). If the compression energy has not yet dissipated, secondary fractures result. Depending on the position of the foot, cranial parts of the calcaneal tuberosity of various sizes can be fractured. In a joint depression fracture the compressed fragment is very short and the fracture line passes directly behind the posterior facet (Fig. 3 a). In the tongue-type fracture there is an elongated cranial fragment, and the fracture line passes into the tuberosity dorsally (Fig. 3 b).
According to experimental investigations by Thorén [21], a joint-depression-type fracture tends to arise in a dorsally flexed foot, whereas a tongue-type fracture is more likely in a plantarflexed foot. This could not be confirmed by our own experimental investigations carried out on 40 cadaver feet. No tongue-type fractures were produced even in plantar flexion. It must be as-

sumed, therefore, that these occur only in the living as a result of the extreme reactive traction of the Achilles tendon at the calcaneal tuberosity at the moment of distribution of compression energy. Burdeaux, in a clear description in his 1983 paper [4], was able to show very convincingly that two axis conditions in particular are very relevant for the development of fracture in the calcaneus:

1. The load axis of the leg is not situated centrally, but is shifted medially, excentrically above the calcaneus.
2. The longitudinal axis of the calcaneus is rotated outwards in relation to the longitudinal axis of the talus. In falls from a great height there is hence always an initial shear fracture which leads to the development of the "sustentacular main fragment" which McReynolds [17] designated as the key fragment, since it always remains firmly attached to the talus and enables the medial wall of the calcaneus to be remodeled anatomically with a medial approach, so that the axis of the hindfoot can be exactly reconstructed (Fig. 5).

In addition to the observations of Burdeaux [4], our own meticulous analysis of more than 200 axial and coronal CT scans has shown that the majority of intra-articular calcaneal fractures are 4-fragment (36%) or 5-fragment (48%) fractures. The five main fragments are the sustentacular fragment, the tuberosity fragment or tuber or body fragment, the posterior facet fragment or lateral joint fragment, the anterior process fragment, and the anterior facet fragment. The number of calcaneal joint facets involved is closely correlated with the number of fragments. The posterior facet is almost always fractured. The calcaneocuboid articular facet is additionally fractured in 59% of cases, and the medial or anterior facets of the talocalcaneal joint are additionally involved in 18%.

Our own fracture classification (Fig. 6) scores, for example, a simple extra-articular fracture such as the duck bill fracture as a 2-fragment/0-joint fracture (=2 points), an isolated depression fracture of the calcaneocuboid articular facet as a 2-fragment/1-joint fracture (=3 points), and a "blow-out fracture" as a 5-fragment/3-joint fracture (=8 points). The additive point system (Table 1) scores open and closed fractures (open grade 1 to open grade 3) with an additional 1–3 points for better comparability of the severity of the fracture and the damage to the soft tissue. The increase in severity of the injury in consequence of a zone comminution of one of the main fragments or an

Table 1. Example of a Hannover calcaneal fracture score

	Points
5-fragment/3-joint fracture	8
Soft tissues (third-degree injury)	3
1 comminuted fragment or additional foot fracture	1
(max)	12

additional fracture such as a concomitant tarsal fracture is taken into consideration by an additional point.

A 5-fragment/3-joint fracture can thus attain a maximum of 12 points: besides the 8 basic points, 3 points are added for the third-degree soft tissue damage, as well as comminution point for the or an additional tarsal fracture. The pattern of fracture distribution of our cases on the additive point system shows, that fractures with 6–9 points predominate, accounting for 69% of cases (Fig. 7). The soft tissue damage was graded most frequently as closed grade I (70.1%). We had 20.3% second- and third-degree closed and 9.6% open fractures.

Besides our own classification, a ±200 point score has been suggested. This comprises 36 criteria including 7.5% subjective, 60% clinically objective, and 32.5% radiological criteria including CT after removal of the implants. It thus provides the essential basis for comparability of fractures in multicenter studies.

Our own analysis indicates that our fracture classification along with the additive point system has a high predictive value with regard to the success of surgery. It can, for example, be stated that patients with a score of 6 points may expect excellent results, patients with a score of up to 8 points will very probably have a good result, patients with between 8 and 10 points are likely to have a satisfactory result, and patients with 11 to 12 points can only expect a poor result (Fig. 8).

With regard to the analysis of accidents, it remains to be mentioned that compared with the rest of the literature our patients sustained a very much higher proportion of their calcaneal fractures in road traffic accidents (53%) compared with falls from a great height (43%) and other causes (4%).

It was striking with regard to the pathomechanism of high-energy injuries in traffic accidents, that in the majority of cases the front of the car interior sustained the impact and that the foot had been wedged between the pedals in some cases.

Pathomorphology of the Injuries

If untreated, an intra-articular calcaneal fracture leads to substantial problems as a rule. These are described below:

1. The incongruence of the posterior facet reported in 62% of cases by Böhler [3] occurred in 84% of our own patients. If untreated, in the majority of cases this necessitates a later subtalar arthrodesis.
2. According to Winkler [27], patients with calcaneal fractures which show incongruence of the calcaneocuboid joint in addition to destruction of the posterior facet give rise to the group with the highest retirement rate (40% reduction of earning capacity). Such fracture types can be demonstrated in 59% of our own patients.
3. Owing to the talus breaking into the calcaneus, dorsal tilting of the talus occurs as a rule, especially in tongue-type fractures. As a consequence of

this, the broad talar trochlea becomes located in the ankle mortise and constitutes a severe prearthrotic deformity of the ankle joint, which is manifested as an impingement of the talus against the anterior edge of the tibia in the initial stage.
4. The static bony problem is characterized by a plump deformity of the calcaneal part of the foot due to fracture manifested by a reduction in height and length as well as a broadening, which can additionally be exacerbated by development of a varus and, in particular, a valgus position of the hindfoot. In addition to the disturbed biomechanics, a lateral bulge can lead to impingement of the peroneal tendon, which is especially painful when the malleolus rides on this (abutment syndrome).
5. Dynamic imbalance is present, especially when the tuberosity fragment with the insertion of the triceps tendons remains too cranial, so that there is relative shortening of this muscle.
6. The bolt function of the plantar aponeurosis is lost in the collapse of the tuberosity fragment in relation to the anterior process fragment, so that there is additional prearthrotic deformity in the calcaneocuboid joint in this regard.

Methods of Diagnosis

Besides the standard lateral and axial radiographs of the calcaneus and the tarsal bones, and an anteroposterior view of the ankle joint, "Broden" radiographs are very valuable for the detection of subtalar joint involvement. Comparison radiographs of the healthy calcaneus mainly serve to visualize the physiological plane of the subtalar joint and the Böhler and Gissane angles as compared with those on the surgical side.
The axial CT scan shows length, width, and the cuboidal joint; the coronal CT scan demonstrates height, axis, and the subtalar joint. An additional three-dimensional CT scan provides even more information on the outward arrangement of the fragments.

Indications for Surgery

The aims of treatment are:

1. Restoration of height, length, width and axis of the calcaneus
2. Anatomical reconstruction of all joint surfaces
3. Restoration of function by stable osteosynthesis

Open reduction and stable internal fixation to permit functional aftertreatment is therefore necessary in all intra-articular fractures with relevant joint displacement and in all extra-articular fractures with unacceptable positioning, shortening, and broadening of the calcaneus.

Contraindications are excessive comminution, unfavourable soft tissues, unreliable patients, and general contraindications (e.g., arteriosclerosis, diabetic vascular diseases, HIV positive). In cases with contraindications for surgery we recommend either the procedure according to Westhues [23] or the purely conservative procedure according to Omoto [18].

Surgical Procedure

Fixation Devices

Various devices can be used for internal fixation of calcaneal fractures. We use 3.5 mm AO cortical screws and H plates of different sizes, but the 3.5 AO reconstruction plates or ⅓ tubular plates also work well. Kirschner wires are necessary for preliminary fixation.
Some surgeons prefer the indirect reduction technique using an external fixator or distractor. We use the direct reduction technique and insert a Schanz screw through the heel into the tuberosity fragment. It is necessary to know where the greatest bone density is in order to get the optimal screw-hold. There is a very dense bone under the articular surfaces of the calcaneocuboid joint and the thalamus, on the tuber, but it is densest bone at the angle of Gissane.

Approaches and Surgical Techniques

We use three surgical approaches and procedures for the treatment of calcaneal fractures: the medial approach, the bilateral approach, and the extended lateral approach. In all approaches the soft tissue requires that the incision goes straight through the skin and subcutaneous tissues, leaving them attached so as to maintain blood supply to the skin. A meticulous atraumatic surgical technique prevents wound healing problems.

Medial Approach

The medial approach, modified after McReynolds (Fig. 9a) starts with an 8-cm straight incision following Langer's lines and running between the medial malleolus and the sole. The incision is carried down to the subcutaneous tissue and fascia (Fig. 9b). The abductor hallucis muscle is retracted caudally and the tibial neurovascular bundle is identified (Fig. 9c). It is snared and retracted upward or downward as needed (Fig. 9d).
This medial approach is ideal for simple 2- or 3-fragment fractures. The body fragment can be reduced against the stable sustentacular fragment, which restores the strong contour of the medial wall anatomically.

Bilateral Approach

If the subtalar joint is involved an additional lateral modified Palmer approach is performed (Fig. 10). This gives a good access to the subtalar joint, allowing bone grafting if necessary, and reduction and fixation of the anterior process. The peroneal tendons with their sheaths are identified and retracted caudally as far as necessary. The tarsal sinus is exposed and the subtalar joint is explored whilst applying a slight varus stress.
The lateral joint fragment, which is frequently found to be impacted and tilted in valgus angulation, is elevated to its anatomical position. It is fixed with Kirschner wires and definitively with two screws to the sustentaculum, which is easily palpable through the medial incision. Cannulated screws make this procedure easier. Lag screws must be used with their screw heads countersunk. The resulting bony defect beneath the lateral joint fragment should be filled with bone graft. The lateral bulge is eliminated with digital pressure, allowing the peroneal tendons to move free. The anterior fragment is reduced, if necessary, and fixed with a 60–70-mm long neutralization screw inserted percutaneously through the tuberosity fragment towards the calcaneocuboid joint. The last step is the final fixation of the restored medial wall with a four-hole H plate (Fig. 11).
The bilateral approach makes anatomical reduction on the medial and lateral side possible, prevents tendon impingement, and minimizes lateral soft tissue damage. It is used mainly with simple 3–4-fragment/1–2-joint fractures (Table 2).

Extended Lateral Approach

In fractures with gross comminution, or comminution of the sustentacular fragment, the medial approach offers no advantages. In these severe cases the extended lateral approach is prefered.
The L-shaped incision starts 4 cm above the lateral malleolus halfway between fibula and Achilles tendon, goes straight down to the heel and curves anterior-

Table 2. Steps of the bilateral procedure

1. Medial approach
Schanz screw
Reduction (tuberosity fragment to sustentaculum)
Kirschner wire
2. Lateral approach
Reduction and screw fixation (posterior fragment to sustentaculum)
Bone grafting
Reduction of lateral wall
3. Medial
H plate fixation

ly to the calcaneocuboid joint on a halfway line between the tip of the malleolus and the sole (Fig. 12a). The most important principle of the extended lateral approach is to raise a full-thickness flap consisting of all tissue layers down to the bone: the skin, all soft tissues, the periosteum (which includes the peroneal tendons), the sural nerve, and the detached calcaneofibular ligament. The peroneal tendons must be mobilized as far distally as possible if the calcaneocuboid joint is to be visualized (Fig. 12b). When the flap is raised care has to be taken not to jeopardize its vascularity. With this approach the widened lateral wall is visualized and moved aside to expose the posterior facet. The lateral fracture sides can be reduced under direct vision while the medial sustentacular fragment and the medial wall are held and reduced indirectly.

As soon as the calcaneus is exposed the first step is the insertion of a Schanz screw into the tuberosity (Fig. 12c). By pulling this screw backwards and downwards the fragment is reduced and Kirschner wires were temporarily inserted from the posterior into the sustentacular fragment, as well as into the talus. The second step is the reduction and preliminary fixation of the lateral joint fragment in combination with bone grafting. The third step is the reduction of the anterior process fragment and the cuboidal facet. In the fourth step the lateral wall is reconstructed. When all fractures have been reduced and fixed with Kirschner wires (Fig. 12d) radiographic controls should confirm the reduction. The definitive fixation is made with a double or triple H plate (Fig. 12e). Normally the lateral wall is flat; only the peroneal tubercle may be prominent and must be removed. Because of the flat wall the plate should not be bent, to prevent varus angulation. The incision is closed carefully using atraumatic sutures with a small drain under the flap and a soft compression dressing.

Aftertreatment

Postoperatively the foot should be elevated for some days. On the first day the patient is started on active circumrotatory excercises of the foot, including dorsal flexion and plantarflexion as well as pronation–supination excercises, performed under the supervision of a physiotherapist. At all other times a short-leg removable cast is worn until wound healing is complete. The cast holds the foot at right-angles to avoid equinus.

From the fifth day on the patient is ambulated and allowed touch weight-bearing in order to activate the muscle pump. This reduces venous stasis and swelling. The patient is discharged without a cast and restricted to partial weight-bearing for 6–12 weeks, depending on the fracture configuration and on the amount of the bone grafting performed. A course of outpatient physiotherapy is followed. Full weight-bearing is usually possible after 12–16 weeks, and heavy work or sports activities after 4–6 months (Table 3).

Table 3. Scheme of postoperative care

- Elevation of foot, short-leg cast
- Immediate range of motion exercises
- Partial weight-bearing after 6–12 weeks
- Progress to full weight-bearing at 12 weeks
- Hard work and sports allowed after 4–6 months
- Hardware out after approx. 1 year

Table 4. Postoperative complications ($n = 187$)

Complication	*n*	%
Wound edge necrosis	16	8.5
Hematoma (evacuated)	5	2.6
Soft tissue and bone infection	4	2.1
Non-union	3	1.6

Results

In this prospective study 157 out of a total of 187 of our patients were followed up for a minimum of 6 months after the operation (average 3.8 years). Details of two case reports are given in Figs. 13–16. In accordance with the changes in our own surgical procedure, the learning curve, and the changes in the indications for surgery associated with this, there are three chronological groups of patients. In comparison with our results from the first group (1983–1985), the patients in the second group (1986–1988) showed a marked increase in results classified as excellent or good. The fewer excellent and good results in the third group (1988–1990) are attributable to the fact that there were more 5-fragment/2–3-joint fractures (57%) being treated compared with the earlier groups (19%) as we extended the indications [25].

In the 187 operations, wound margin necrosis was the most frequent complication (8.5%); there was no significant difference in frequency between the three approaches. In the early postoperative phase, hematomas which had to be evacuated were found in 2.6% of cases. A deep soft tissue and bone infection occurred in four cases (2.1%). In one case, this could only be controlled by a latissimus dorsi transfer and in three cases by partial or total calcanectomy (Table 4).

Three cases with postoperative pseudoarthrosis (1.6%) have been treated successfully in the meantime by reoperation with cancellous bone grafting and lag screw osteosynthesis. In the entire prospective series a subtalar arthrodesis has been performed in four patients. This has been recommended to further three patients, corresponding to a rate of post-traumatic arthritis totalling 3.7%. Subtalar fusion is then performed in a well-reconstructed hindfoot, as part of our surgical philosophy.

Conclusion

The operative treatment of calcaneal fractures requires a meticulous surgical technique. Atraumatic soft tissue handling, thorough understanding of biomechanical principles and classification, and three-dimensional anatomical knowledge are essential prerequisites for surgeons in this field. We believe that a "reducible" fracture without severe soft tissue damage, treated by stable osteosynthesis that allows immediate functional aftertreatment, will result in a good or excellent outcome in the majority of cases.

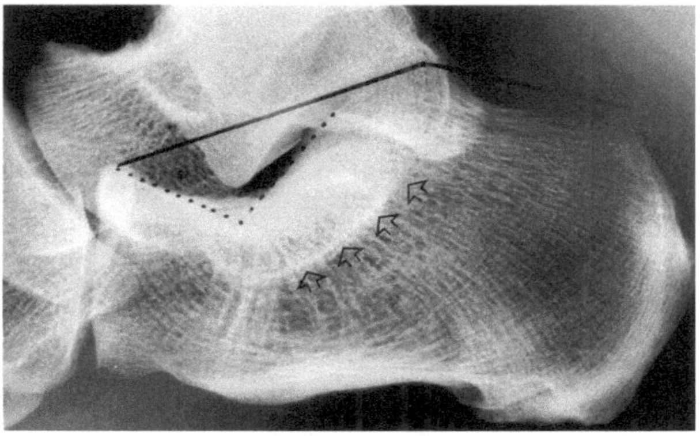

Fig. 1. Calcaneal thalamus (*arrows*), angle of Gissane (*dotted line*), and angle of Böhler (*continuous line*)

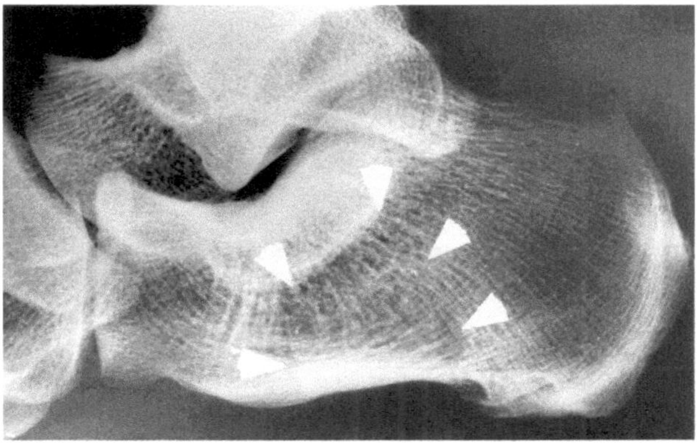

Fig. 2. Trigonum calcis

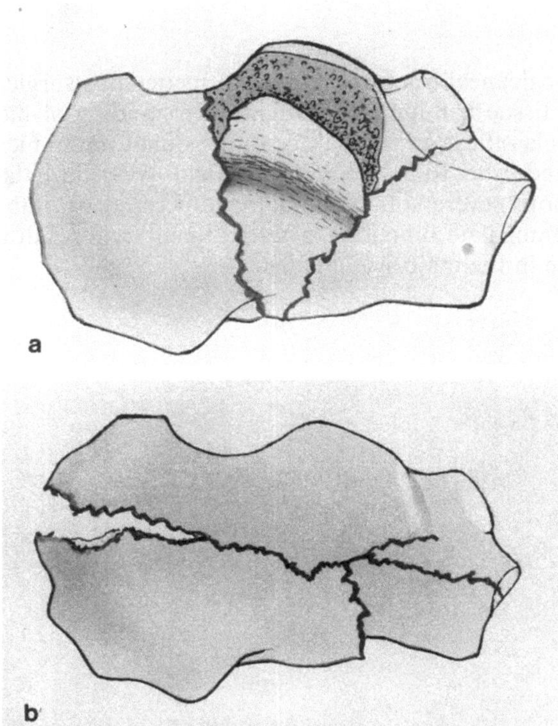

Fig. 3. **a** Joint-depression-type fracture. **b** Tongue-type fracture

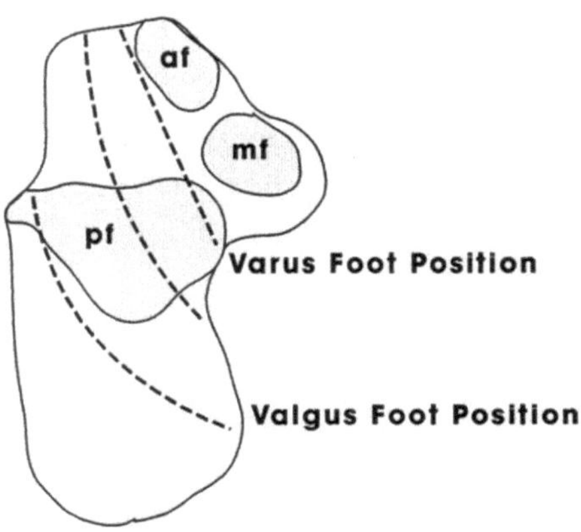

Fig. 4. Course of the fracture line, depending on the position of the foot. *af,* anterior facet; *mf,* middle facet; *pf,* posterior facet

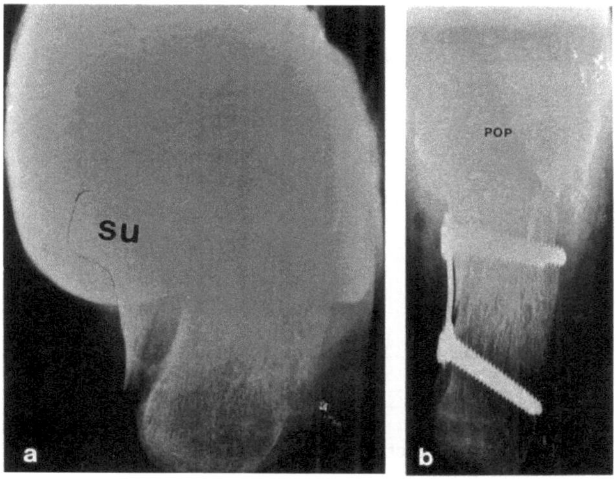

Fig. 5. **a** Sustentacular main fragment (*su*), which is the key fragment according to McReynolds. **b** Anatomical realignment by a medial approach and H-plate fixation

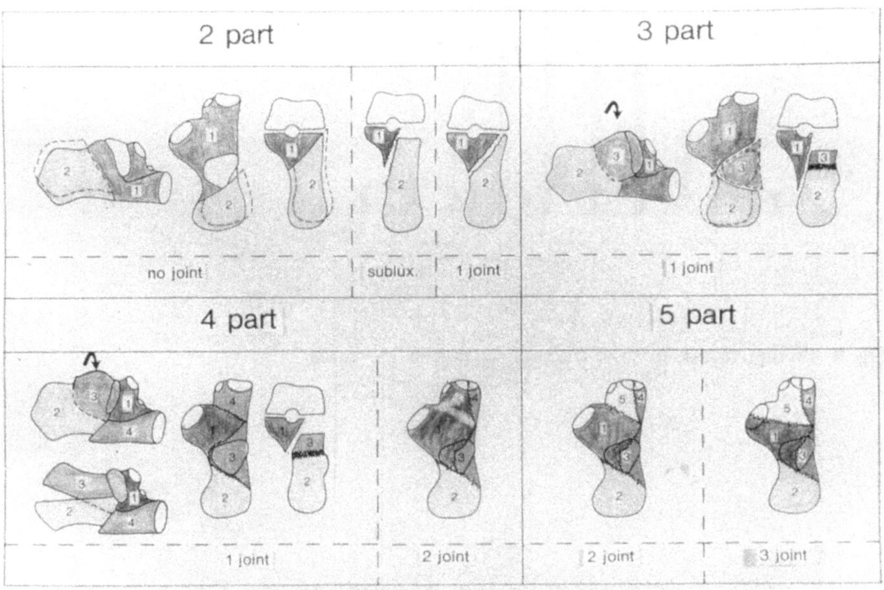

Fig. 6. Hannover calcaneal fracture classification: *x* fragments/*y* joints. *1*, sustentacular fragment; *2*, tuberosity fragment; *3*, posterior facet fragment; *4*, anterior process fragment; *5*, anterior facet fragment

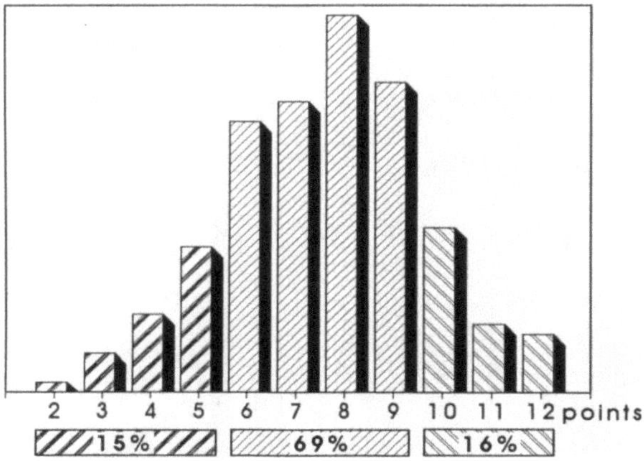

Fig. 7. Pattern of fracture distribution in 187 cases. Numbers are points on the Hannover calcaneal fracture score

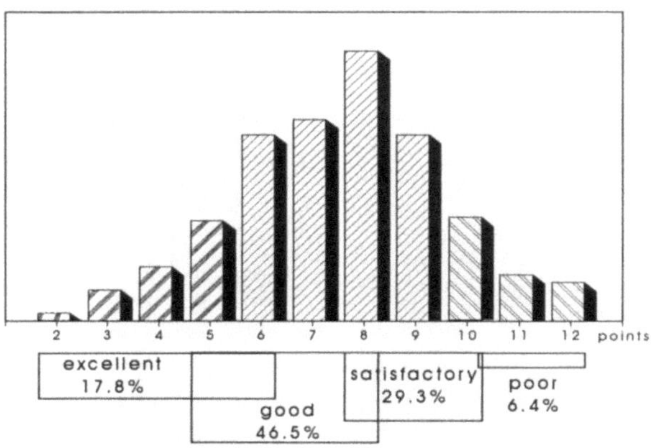

Fig. 8. Predictive value of the fracture scoring in 157 cases

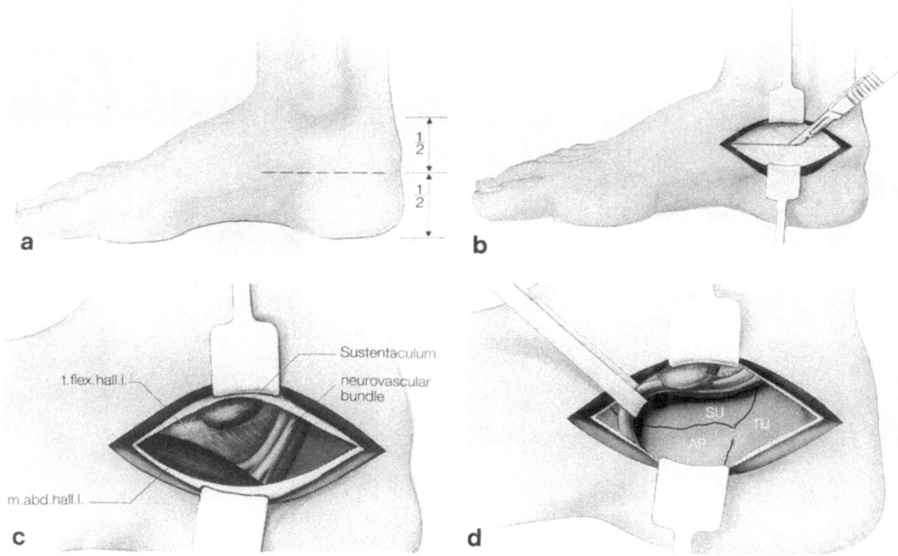

Fig. 9a–d. Medial approach, after McReynolds. *m. abd. hall. L.*, abductor hallucis muscle; *t. flex. hall. L.*, flexor hallucis longus tendon; *AP*, anterior process; *SU*, sustentacular fragment; *TU*, tuberosity fragment

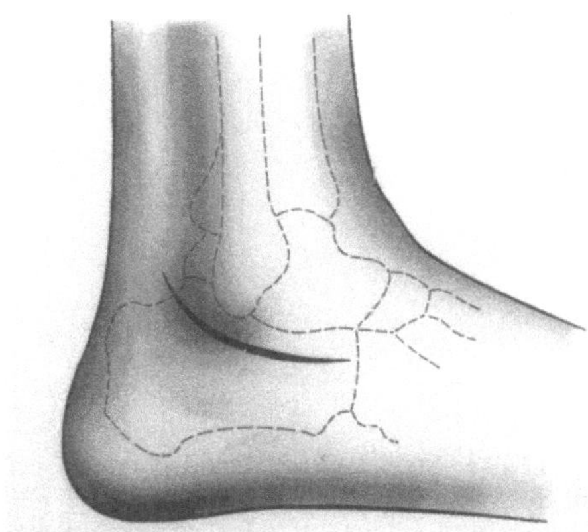

Fig. 10. Modified lateral approach. (After Palmer)

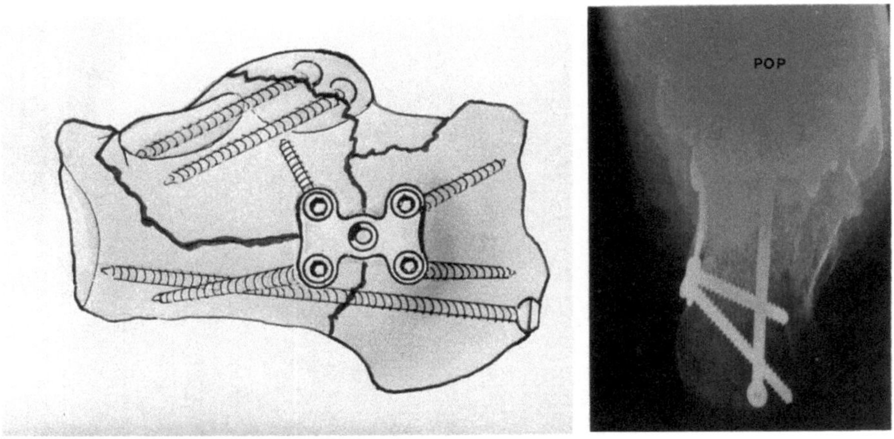

Fig. 11. Scheme of the bilateral procedure

Fig. 12 a–e. Steps of the extended lateral procedure. **a** Method of incision. **b** Raising a full-thickness flap consisting of the sural nerve, the peroneal tendons, and the detached calcaneofibular ligament. **c** Insertion of a Schanz screw, and pulling the tuberosity fragment backwards, downwards, and laterally to reduce it towards the sustentacular fragment. **d** After reduction of the posterior facet and the anterior process fragment all fragments are temporarily fixed with Kirschner wires. **e** After radiographic control (lateral axial, and 20° Broden view) the triple H plate achieves stable fixation ▶

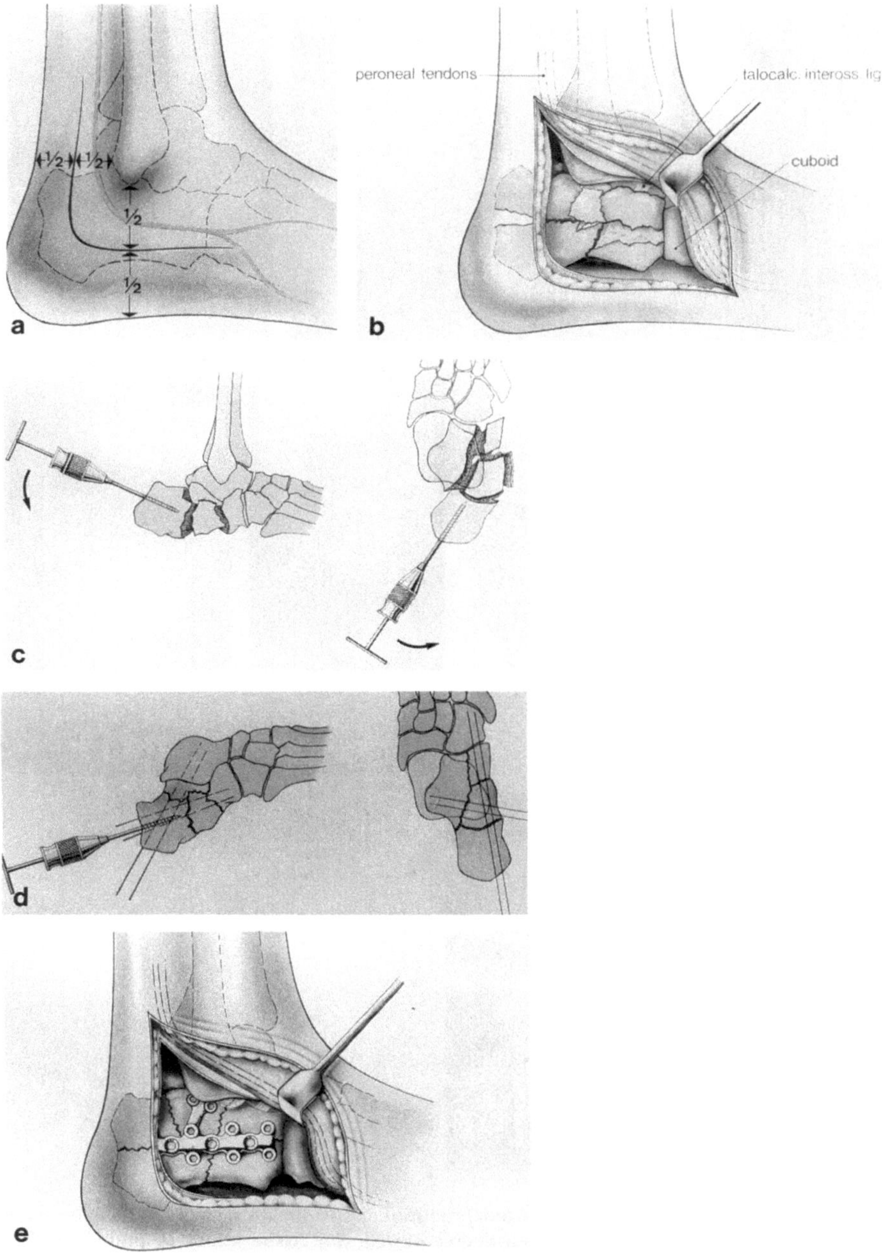

½
½
½
½
a
peroneal tendons
talocalc. inteross. lig
cuboid
b
c
d
e

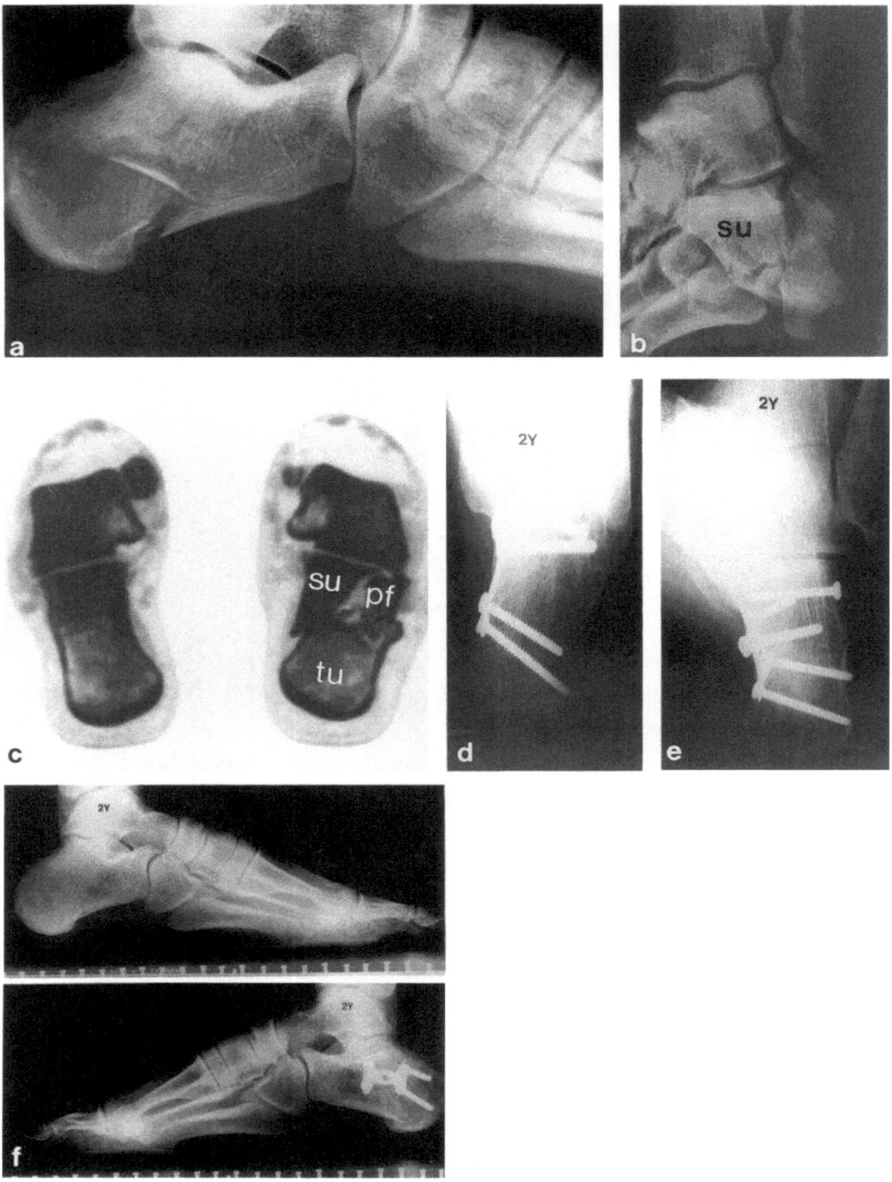

Fig. 13 a–f. Case report 1. A 49-year-old practitioner sustained a typical joint depression fracture (4 fragment/1 joint) with first-degree closed soft tissue injury (6 points). **a** The subtalar joint appears uninvolved on the lateral radiograph. **b** The Broden view shows the fracture of the joint surface and a large sustentacular key fragment. **c** In the coronal CT scan the extent of joint involvement as well as the flattening, varus deformity, broadening, and the lateral bulge can be seen. **d, e** The axial view 2 years after bilateral procedure shows no deformity, the Broden view no step of the subtalar joint. **f** In the weight-bearing lateral view the foot is normal in shape. *pf*, posterior fragment; *su*, sustentacular fragment; *tu*, tuberosity fragment

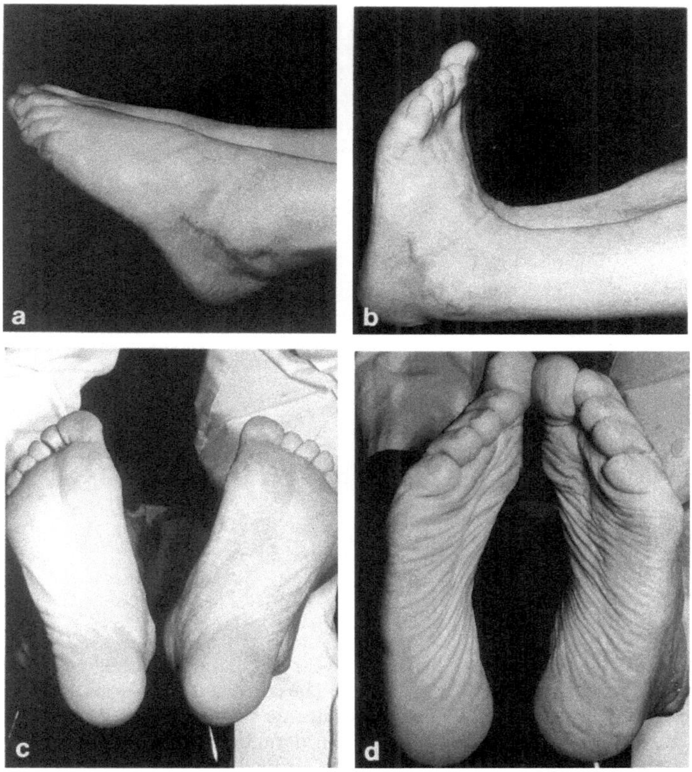

Fig. 14 a–d. Case report 1. Full function of ankle (**a, b**), subtalar and Chopart joint (**c, d**). The 2-year follow-up score 176 points, which classifies as an excellent result

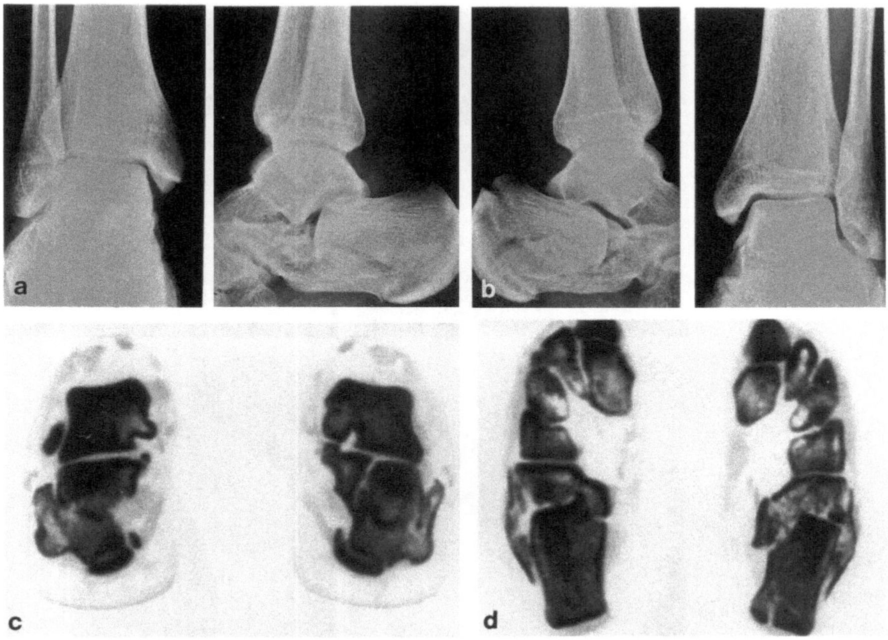

Fig. 15 a–d. Case report 2. **a, b** A 20-year-old marathon athlete sustained a bilateral tongue-type fracture after a fall from a wall. **c** The coronal CT views show on the right side the intact but tilted posterior facet, and on the left side a relatively small sustentacular fragment. **d** The axial CT views clearly demonstrate the lateral buldge on both sides and comminuted anterior process fragment

Fig. 16 a–g. Case report 2. **a** After an extended lateral procedure on both sides the Broden views 18 months postoperatively indicate the intact subtalar joint and the realigned axis. **b** In the lateral weight-bearing radiographs the normal architecture of both feet can be seen. **c** Normal trabecular patterns of the os calcis are visible after hardware removal. **d, e** The coronal and axial CT scans respectively show the subtalar joint free from degenerative arthritis, and the normal height, length, and width of the calcaneus. **f, g** The 2-year follow-up shows full range of motion of both feet. The follow-up score was 182 for the right side and 177 points for the left, both of which are excellent results ▶

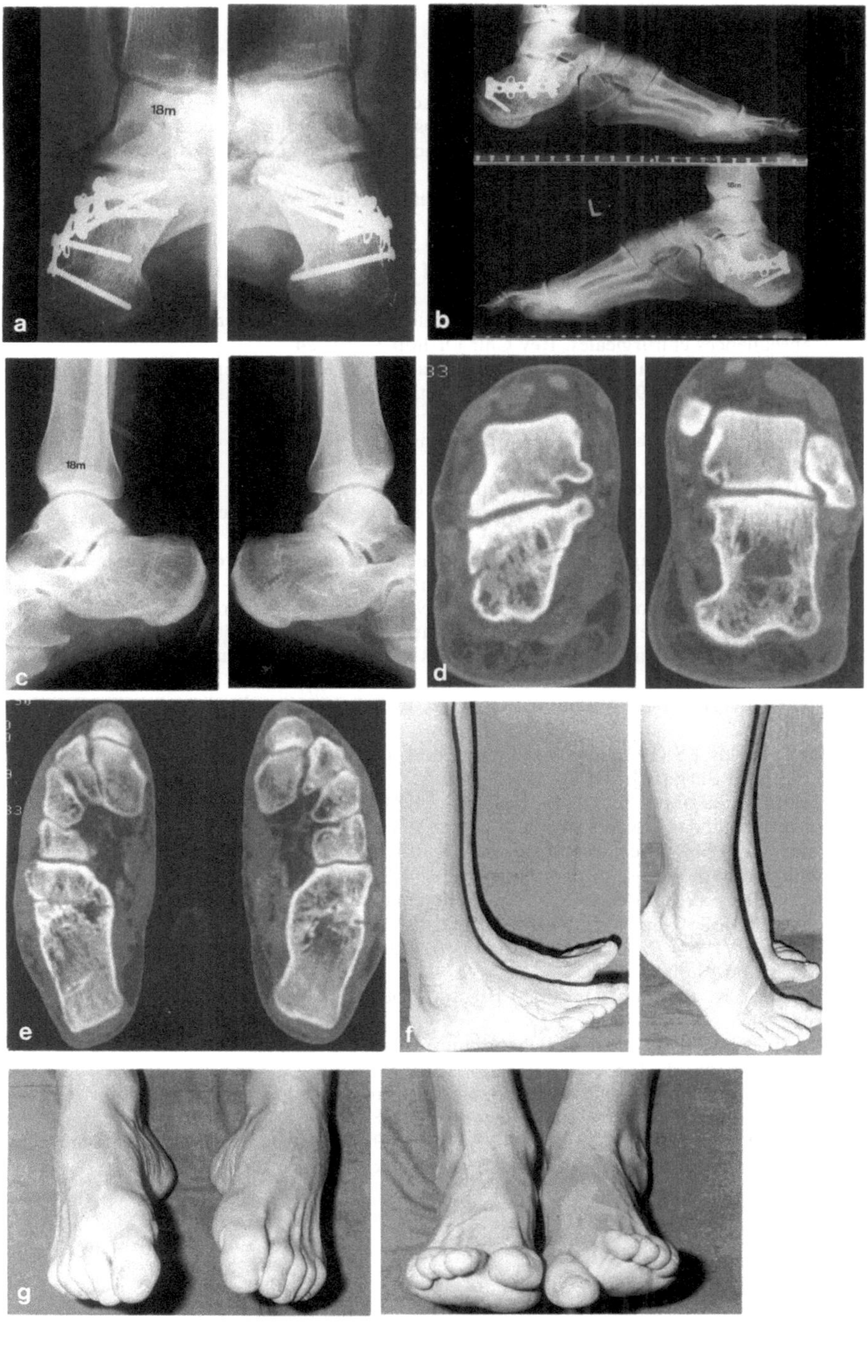
18m
18m
L
18m

References

1. Belenger M, Van der Elst E, Lorthioir J (1951) Les fractures du calcanéum. Leur traitement et le traitement des séquelles. Acta Orthop Belg 17:58–67
2. Bell C (1882) Compound fracture of the os calcis. Edinburgh Med J 27:1100
3. Böhler L (1957) Technik der Knochenbruchbehandlung, vol 2, part 2, 12th/13th edn. Maudrich, Vienna, p 2145
4. Burdeaux BD (1983) Reduction of calcaneal fractures by the McReynolds medial approach technique. Clin Orthop 177:87–91
5. Clark G (1855) Fracture of the os calcis. Lancet 1:403
6. Cotton FJ, Henderson FF (1916) Results of fractures of the os calcis. Am J Orthop Surg 14:290–298
7. Courty A (1945) Étude sur l'architecture du calcanéum. Considérations physiologiques. Conséquences chirurgicales. Rev Chir Orthop 31:10–24
8. Destot E (1911) Traumatisme du pied et rayons X. Masson, Paris
9. Essex-Lopresti P (1952) Mechanism, reduction technique and results in fractures of the os calcis. Br J Surg 39:395–419
10. Gallie WE (1943) Subastragalar arthrodesis in fractures of the os calcis. J Bone Joint Surg 25:731–736
11. Goff CW (1938) Fresh fractures of the os calcis. Arch Surg 36:744–765
12. Harty M (1973) Anatomic consideration in injuries of the calcaneus. Orthop Clin North Am 4:179–183
13. Judet R, Judet J, Lagrange J (1954) Traitement des fractures du calcanéum compartant une disjunction astragalocalcanéenne. Mem Acad Chir 80:158–160
14. Lenormant C, Wilmoth P, Lecoeur P (1928) A propos du traitement sanglant des fractures du calcanéum. Bull Mem Soc Nat Chir 54:1353–1355
15. Leriche R (1929) Traitement chirurgical des fractures du calcanéum. Bull Mem Soc Nat Chir 55:8–9
16. Malgaigne JF (1843) Mémoire sur la fracture par écrasement du calcanéum. J Chir (Paris) 1:2
17. McReynolds LS (1972) Open reduction and internal fixation of calcaneal fractures. J Bone Joint Surg [Br] 54:176–177
18. Omoto H, Sakurada K, Sugi M, Nakamura K (1983) A new method of manual reduction for intraarticular fracture of the calcaneus. Clin Orthop 177:104
19. Palmer I (1948) The mechanism and treatment of fractures of the calcaneus. Open reduction with the use of cancellous grafts. J Bone Joint Surg [Am] 30:2–8
20. Rowe CR, Sakellarides HT, Sorbie C, Freeman PA (1963) Fractures of the os calcis: long-term follow-up study of 146 patients. JAMA 184:920–923
21. Thorén O (1964) Experimental os calcis fractures on autopsy specimen fractures. Acta Chir Scand [Suppl] 70:11
22. Warrick CK, Bremner AE (1953) Fractures of the calcaneum. J Bone Joint Surg [Br] 35:33–45
23. Westhues H (1934) Eine neue Behandlungsmethode der Kalkaneusfraktur. Arch Orthop Unfallchir 35:121–128
24. Winkler W (1986) Technische Orthopädie im Rahmen der Rehabilitation von Patienten mit Calcaneusfrakturen. Orthop Schuhtechnik 8:390
25. Zwipp H, Tscherne H, Wülker N, Grote R (1989) Der intraartikuläre Fersenbeinbruch: Klassifikation, Bewertung und Operationstaktik. Unfallchirurg 92:117–129

The Results of Operative Treatment of Displaced Intra-articular Calcaneal Fractures Using a CT Scan Classification

R. Sanders, P. Fortin, T. DiPasquale, A. Walling, D. Helfet, and E. Ross

Introduction

Displaced intra-articular fractures of the calcaneus remain a diagnostic and therapeutic dilemma. The classification of these fractures has been frustrated in the past by limitations of radiographic technique. In 1975, Soeur and Remy reported on their operative experience with these fractures [26]. Unique to their discussion was a classification based on the number of bony fragments as determined by plain radiographic views. First-degree fractures were nondisplaced shear fractures with widening of the joint surface. Second-degree included secondary fracture lines, resulting in a minimum of three pieces, two of which were articular. Illustrations in their text indicated that the posterior main fragment could be broken into three fragments: lateral, middle, and medial. Third-degree fractures were highly comminuted, but unfortunately the authors did not specify whether the comminution referred to the calcaneal body or the articular surface of the posterior facet.

Since 1986 we have treated displaced intra-articular calcaneal fractures according to an operative protocol. This was designed to determine whether an anatomical reduction through a lateral approach alone could be consistently obtained and maintained with a plate and lag screws without the use of bone graft. Analysis of results required that similar fracture patterns be compared. Therefore, in a logical progression from the classification of Soeur and Remy, CT scan classification was developed based on the number and location of articular fracture fragments. We now report our results using this CT classification.

Classification

The classification system is based on the coronal section CT scan alone (Fig. 1). All coronal sections were analyzed, but the classification arbitrarily used that section with the widest undersurface of the posterior facet of the talus. The talus was divided into three equal columns by two lines: A and B. These two lines divided the posterior facet of the calcaneus into three potential pieces: a medial, central, and lateral column. (The term "central" is used in place of Soeur and Remy's "middle" to avoid confusion with the "medial" fragment.) A third fracture line, C, corresponding to the medial edge of the

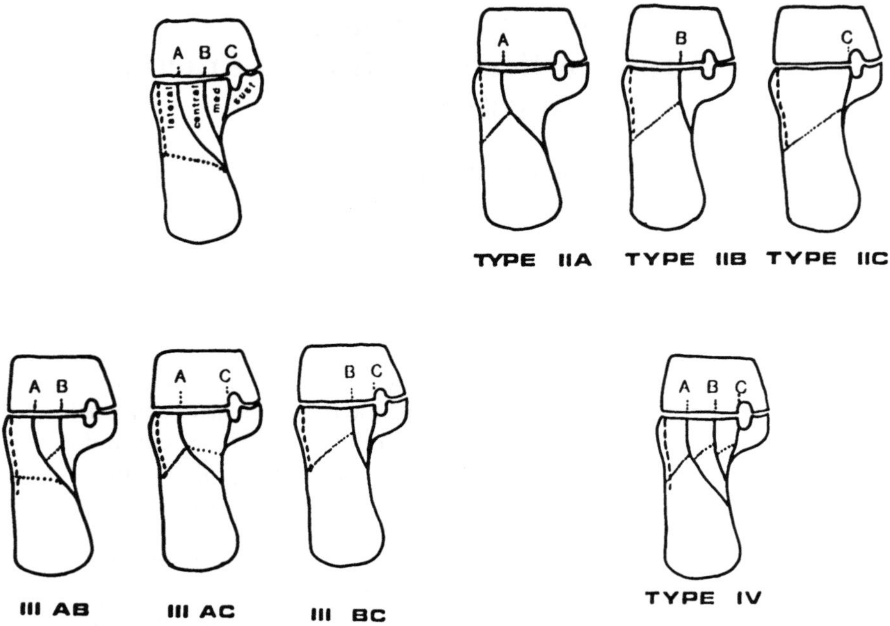

Fig. 1. The CT scan classification of intra-articular calcaneal fractures

posterior facet of the talus, separated the posterior facet from the sustentaculum and resulted in a total of four potential pieces.

All nondisplaced articular fractures, irrespective of the number of fracture lines, are considered type I fractures. These benefit from nonoperative intervention unless the body itself is severely displaced.

Type II fractures are two-part fractures of the posterior facet, similar in appearance to a split fracture of the tibial plateau. Three types – II A, II B, and II C – exist, based on the location of the primary fracture line. As the fracture line moves medially, intraoperative visualization of joint reduction will become more difficult.

Type III fractures are three-part fractures that feature a centrally depressed fragment, similar to a split depressed tibial plateau or die-punch distal radial fracture. Types include III AB, III AC, and III BC. As the fracture lines move medially, the reduction will become more difficult, with a III BC being the hardest to reduce and hold.

Type IV fractures, or four-part articular fractures, are highly comminuted. Often, more than four articular fragments exist. If the majority of these pieces are significantly displaced from one another operative reduction is essentially futile.

Materials and Methods

CT Scanning

CT scans were performed on a Philips Tomoscan 60 TX scanner with a third-generation software package to minimize scatter. The patient is positioned in the supine position, with the hips and knees flexed. The feet are kept together with the plantar surface resting on the table [17]. Both feet are routinely scanned for comparison. A lateral digital radiograph (scout film) is obtained and the position is modified until the coronal sections are truly perpendicular to the posterior facet. Smith and Staple have recommended an extension piece to aid in positioning, but we have not found this necessary [25]. Once the scout film is correct, contiguous 3-mm-thick sections are obtained from the posterior calcaneus to the navicular. The patient is then asked to extend the hips and knees, and a second scout is obtained for transverse (axial) CT scanning. Once correctly positioned, 3-mm-thick sections are taken from the plantar surface to the talus. These two views, at 90° to each other, allow the surgeon a graphic representation of the fractured and normal calcaneus.

Indications for Surgery

All patients with 3 mm or more of articular displacement in the posterior facet were treated operatively according to protocol, except in the following situations: (1) open fractures or fractures in patients with life-threatening injuries that precluded early intervention; (2) soft tissue compromise, such as blistering, which prevented timely surgery; (3) severe peripheral vascular disease; and (4) severe infirmity.

Operative Treatment

Timing of Surgery

Surgery was performed within the first 3 weeks after injury to prevent difficulties with reduction secondary to early consolidation of the fracture. Surgery was not attempted until after swelling in the foot and ankle had significantly decreased, to avoid the complications of wound breakdown postoperatively [11]. Because this may take 7–14 days, immediate application of ice and elevation on a Böhler-Braun frame was mandatory. If this was not accomplished, the window of time for fixation was lost and nonoperative treatment was elected.

Positioning

The patient was placed in the lateral decubitus position on a translucent table or cardiac pacemaker insertion board (pacer board) so that fluoroscopy could be used intraoperatively. After exsanguination the tourniquet was inflated to 300 mmHg. A bolster under the medial malleolus allowed the heel to fall into slight inversion, thus improving visualization of the subtalar joint.

Incision

Originally, the calcaneus was approached through a standard Kocher lateral incision. Because problems with the sural nerve developed, a modified right-angled approach, as advocated by surgeons at the University of Washington, Seattle, was employed. In this modification the incision is made more posterior and inferior to avoid damaging the sural nerve, which is then brought anteriorly with the skin flap. The incision is extensile, and may be taken as far distally as the calcaneocuboid joint and as far proximally as needed, thus allowing the fixation of any associated ankle fractures simultaneously [8, 15]. To avoid the sequelae of peroneal tendonitis and devascularization of the anterior skin flap, the peroneal tendons are left in their sheath. The sheath is stripped off the lateral wall of the calcaneus subperiosteally [8, 15]. It is then freed subperiosteally from the lateral malleolus until it can be shifted anteriorly over the malleolus as one unit. The sheath is held subluxed anterior to the fibula by the use of two Kirschner wires, one in the fibula and one in the talus. This retracts the peroneal tendons and also obviates the need for manual retraction of the anterior skin flap. This "no-touch" technique has the advantage of preventing subsequent scarring of the tendons and vascular compromise to the anterior flap.

Joint Reduction

The calcaneofibular ligament is identified, sharply cut off the calcaneus, and retracted anteriorly. The lateral wall is subperiosteally cleaned of soft tissue to maximize the inferior skin flap. The wall is then gently pried laterally to expose the fracture fragments. After clot removal, the posterior facet is evaluated. The depressed fracture fragment is first rotated out from within the body of the calcaneus. This immediately decompresses the lateral wall. After identification of all remaining articular fracture fragments, preliminary reduction of the facet is obtained using Kirschner wires. In order to align the fragments properly with respect to rotation, visualization of the anterior and posterior aspects of the facet is necessary; this may require excision of the fat immediately behind the posterior facet. Gissane's angle is carefully evaluated, as this is the key to the anterior reduction.

As the articular fracture line moves medially, or if several articular fracture lines exist, visualization of joint reduction becomes exceedingly difficult. This is primarily due to the fact that once the lateral articular surface is reduced, the joint cannot be adequately opened to visualize the reduction. Therefore, intraoperative fluoroscopic Broden's views are obtained to aid in this assessment [24]. The fluoroscope can be left on for a sweep of the joint when reduction is believed to be anatomical. When the reduction is satisfactory, Kirschner wires are exchanged for 3.5 mm lag screws which are angled to obtain purchase into the constant sustentacular fragment. Washers should be employed as needed [15].

Reduction of the Body

Attention is then turned to reduction of the tuberosity fragment. Through the lateral approach this can most easily be accomplished by placing a small periosteal elevator across the fracture line, and levering the body against the medial edge of the sustentacular fragment (the spike), thereby correcting length and width. An axial spike or transverse traction pin is placed into the tuberosity fragment to assist reduction if necessary [2, 15, 18, 23, 26]. This maneuver to correct body alignment may need to be performed before joint reduction, if varus tilt of the lateral fragment of the posterior facet exists. Unless this is corrected, the body will prevent articular surface reduction. A Harris heel view is obtained intraoperatively, either by fluoroscopy or plain film to assess reduction. Once satisfactory, an anterior cervical AO plate (H plate) is used to reduce the body and buttress the lateral wall. Intraoperative fluoroscopic or plain lateral radiographs are also obtained to assess height and angulation.

Closure and Postoperative Management

If acceptable, closure is performed over a drain and final films are taken. The leg is placed in a bulky Jones dressing. The drain is removed on postoperative day 2; the dressing on day 3. A removable short leg cast is then put on, and subtalar motion begun. This is the most important aspect of the patient's postoperative care.

Repeat CT scans in both the coronal and transverse planes are then obtained to evaluate the reduction. Sutures should be left in place for 3 weeks to minimize the chance of wound dehiscence. The patient is kept non-weight-bearing for 8 weeks, with progressive weight-bearing being started after that. Full weight-bearing is allowed by 3 months.

One hundred and twenty calcaneal fractures were treated between January 1986 and December 1989. All fractures that were diagnosed as extra-articular on plain films were excluded from CT scanning and treated nonoperatively. Eighty-five fractures were subsequently scanned. Of these, 68 had an intra-articular component. There were 10 type I fractures: all were treated nonoperatively. The remaining 58 fractures demonstrated intra-articular displacement and were treated operatively. There were 40 type II, 12 type III, and 6 type IV fractures.

Radiographic follow-up examination was performed in the immediate postoperative period and again at 1 year. Included were plain radiographs, Broden's views and CT scans in both coronal and transverse planes. These films were

Table 1. Maryland Foot Score

1. Pain	
a) None, including with sports	45
b) Slight, no change in ADL[a] or work ability	40
c) Mild, minimal change in ADL[a] or work	35
d) Moderate, significant decrease in ADL[a]	30
e) Marked, during minimal ADL[a] (e.g. bathroom, simple housework). Stronger, more frequent analgesics	10
f) Disabled, unable to work or shop	5
2. Function	
A. *Gait*	
1. Distance walked	
a) Unlimited	10
b) Slight limitation	8
c) Moderate limitation (2–3 blocks)	5
d) Severe limitation (1 block)	2
e) Indoors only	0
2. Stability	
a) Normal	4
b) Weak feeling – no true giving way	3
c) Occasional giving way (1–2 per month)	2
d) Frequent giving way	1
e) Orthotic device used	0
3. Support	
a) None	4
b) Cane	3
c) Crutches	1
d) Wheelchair	0
4. Limp	
a) None	4
b) Slight	3
c) Moderate	2
d) Severe	1
e) Unable to walk	0
B. *Functional activities*	
1. Shoes	
a) Any type	10
b) Minor concessions	9
c) Flat, laced	7
d) With orthotics	5
e) Space shoes	2
f) Unable to wear shoes	0
2. Stairs	
a) Normally	4
b) With banister	3
c) Any method	2
d) Unable	0
3. Terrain	
a) No problem with any surface	4
b) Problems on stones, hills	2
c) Problems on flat surfaces	0

Table 1 *(continued)*

3. Cosmesis	
a) Normal	10
b) Mild deformity	8
c) Moderate	6
d) Severe	0
e) Multiple deformities	0
4. Motion	
(Ankle, subtalar, midfoot, metatarsophalangeal)	
a) Normal	5
b) Slightly decreased	4
c) Markedly decreased	2
d) Ankylosed	0
Total points: 100 (Maximum)	

[a] ADL, activities of daily living.

assessed for return of body height, width, and length, for anatomical reduction of the articular surface of the posterior facet and the calcaneocuboid joint, and for restoration of Böhler's and Gissane's angle.

The Maryland Foot Score was used for clinical evaluation (Table 1). Initially, absolute subtalar motion was assessed using a goniometer, after the method of Inman, but the inability to stabilize this device and also obtain maximal dorsiflexion of the ankle prevented the collection of consistently reproducible data [13]. Motion was therefore evaluated according to the method of Morrey et al., where heel jog is clinically estimated as a percentage of the normal limb [20]. Return to previous occupation, change of occupation, or total disability was also noted.

Finally, a statistical analysis of the data was performed using the Chi-squared test.

Results

Follow-up was possible in 60 cases: 10 type I, 34 type II, 10 type III, and 6 type IV fractures. All type I fractures were treated nonoperatively and had an excellent result.

The results of follow-up of the 50 operative cases are shown in Table 2. Reduction of body height, length, and width were 98%, 100%, and 110% of normal respectively, regardless of fracture type. Böhler's and Gissane's angles were reduced within 5° of normal in all but one case.

Thirty-two of the 34 type II fractures (94%) had an anatomical reduction of the articular surface. Despite this, three patients had a poor result and five were failures requiring subtalar fusions. In all these cases, arthrogram, CT scan, and inspection of the joint at time of fusion verified an anatomical

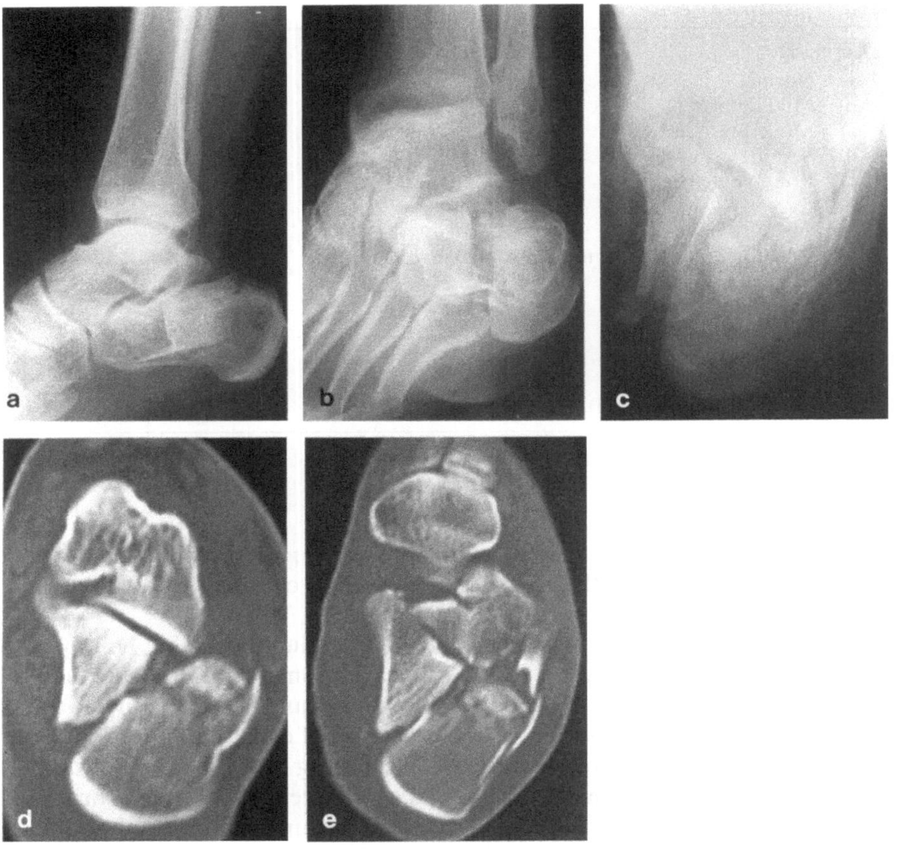

Fig. 2 a–i. Type II fracture treated according to protocol. **a–c** Lateral, internal rotation, and Harris axial view. **d, e** Coronal and axial CT scans. **f–i** see p. 183

articular reduction with damaged cartilage. There were two near-anatomical articular reductions: one of these required a subtalar fusion. There were no approximate reductions. Five cases developed a partial wound dehiscence. Four of these subsequently healed with wet to dry dressing changes and whirlpool therapy. The fifth case required a below-knee amputation after failure to control the wound dehiscence, two failed free flaps and the development of uncontrolled calcaneal osteomyelitis. Twenty-five patients with isolated fractures and previous occupations were evaluated for return to work. Fourteen returned to their previous occupation, five had changed jobs, and five were disabled. Despite an anatomical reduction in 94% of the cases, a good–excellent result was present in only 71% (24/34). Figure 2 shows an example of a type II fracture treated according to protocol.

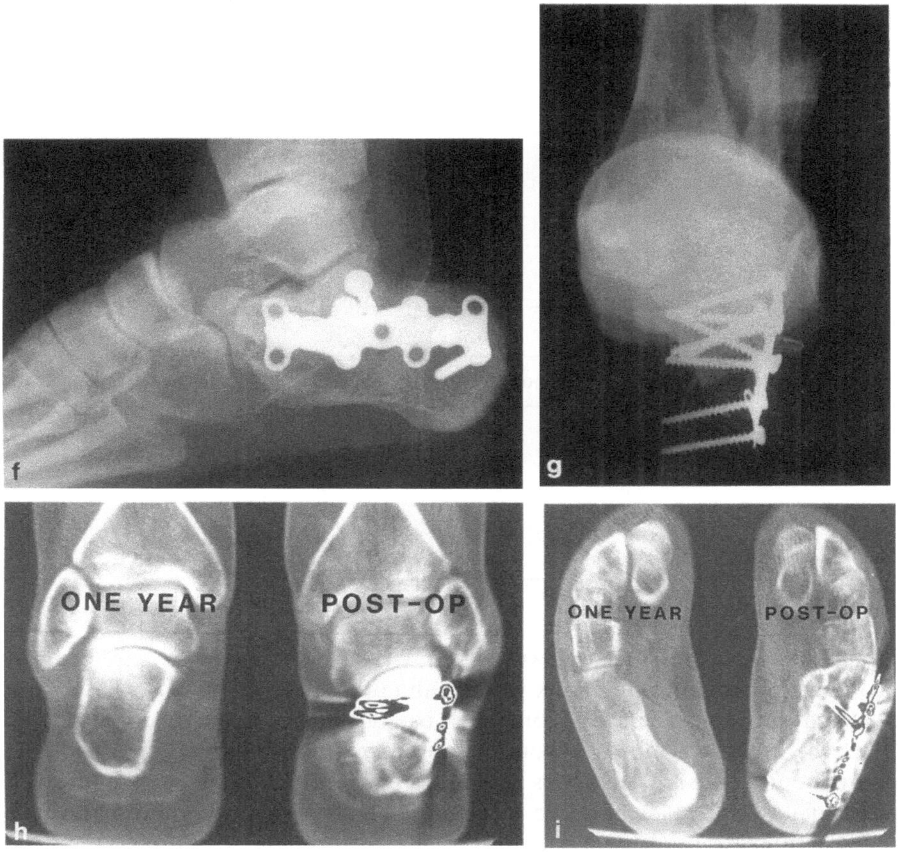

Fig. 2 *(continued)*. **f, g** Postoperative views. **h, i** One-year postoperative CT scans showing excellent alignment and maintainence of both body and joint

In the type III fractures there was only one anatomical reduction (10%). Two cases developed wound complications; one required a free tissue transfer which was successful. Nine fractures were isolated injuries in patients with previous occupations; one returned to work, one changed job, and the remainder were disabled. Clinically there were no excellent results, and the good result did not correlate with an anatomic reductional. Ninety percent of the cases went on to a poor result or failure: seven (70%) of these required a subtalar fusion.

In the type IV fractures, there were two near-anatomical reductions: both subsequently required a subtalar fusion. One patient was diabetic and developed a wound dehiscence requiring a free flap which was successful. Two fractures were so comminuted that they required primary arthrodesis. The remaining two fractures both occurred in the same patient. One was an open

Table 2. Follow-up results of 50 operative cases

Type	Reduction				
	Anatomical	Near-anatomical	Approximate	Total	
I	10	0	0	10	
II	32	2	0	34	
III	1	6	3	10	
IV	0	2	4	6	
	43	10	7	60	
Type	**Outcome**				
	Excellent	Good	Poor	Failed	Total
II	13	11	3	7	34
III	0	1	2	7	10
IV	0	0	0	6	6
	13	12	5	20	50
	25		25		

grade II injury; the other was associated with a severe ankle fracture-dislocation. Both had approximate reductions and ultimately went on to below-knee amputations; one side for uncontrolled osteomyelitis despite a successful free flap, the other for improved comfort and increased mobility.

Six patients (12%) in this series developed peroneal tendonitis which resolved after plate removal, while two patients (4%) developed asymptomatic peroneal subluxations. Twelve patients (24%) had complaints related to the sural nerve; eight had transient paresthesias, three of these had permanent anesthesia. All of these occurred before the modified lateral approach was used.

The 50 surgical cases were evaluated to determine whether functional results correlated with initial degree of articular comminution. The outcomes in type III and IV fractures were too small for statistical comparison; these groups were combined for analysis. When this combined group (III/IV) was compared to with the type II fractures, worsening articular comminution was associated with worse long-term results. This was highly statistically significant ($\chi^2 = 18.02$, $p < 0.0005$).

The data was also analyzed to determine whether an anatomically reduced calcaneal fracture correlated with a better overall result. The probability of successful functional outcome in these cases was also highly statistically significant ($\chi^2 = 37.43$, $p < 0.0005$).

Discussion

Intra-articular fractures require an anatomical reduction with rigid internal fixation to maximize the chances for good joint function. Müller, in his classification of fractures, addressed the question of prognosis after an articular fracture [21]. The more comminuted an articular fracture was, the worse the outcome expected. Until the advent of CT scanning, however, evaluation of the subtalar joint and hence a prognostic classification of calcaneal fractures was not possible.

Previously, many authors noted the type of fracture and the number of fragments present, the scheme of Essex-Lopresti being the most widely used [1, 3, 7, 12, 28, 29]. None of these authors focused on the joint reduction itself, being more concerned with restoration of overall shape and correction of Böhler's angle to prevent disability. As a result, McReynolds and others stressed the importance of a medial approach to reconstruct the shape of the calcaneus [4, 19]. Unfortunately, this approach results in an indirect reduction of the joint surface. As a result, Stephenson employed both a medial approach for body reduction, and a lateral approach for joint reduction [28].

Our study was, by design, limited to the lateral approach. In all but one case reduction of the body with reconstitution of height, width, and length was consistently reproducible, irrespective of the amount of comminution. Additionally, joint reduction, when technically possible, was easy through this approach. We believe, therefore, that a medial approach is only rarely indicated.

A corollary is that on the basis of our data the principal determinant of outcome is the condition of the articular cartilage of the posterior facet (assuming anatomic *body* reduction). In all but one case body reduction was anatomical irrespective of comminution. The majority of type II articular fractures (98%) had an anatomical articular reduction. The only patient that had less than an anatomical result required a subtalar fusion. Poor results in the other fracture types also correlated with a poor articular reduction. Equally important was the fact that five anatomically repositioned type II and one anatomically reduced type III articular fracture required a subtalar fusion. It appears that although an anatomical articular reduction is necessary for a good outcome, it cannot guarantee, it presumably secondary to cartilage necrosis from the original injury.

Reconstruction of the posterior facet requires restoration of rotation as well as height of the superolateral fragment. Intraoperative Broden's views are the only radiographic method we know of that can clearly delineate posterior facet reduction during surgery [24]. In our series, remanipulation of the fracture fragments based on these views was successful in securing an anatomical reduction in 29 of 35 cases (83%). Despite its use in the remaining fractures, an anatomical articular reduction could not be achieved. On the basis of this data we recommend routine use of remanipulation to improve reduction of those joint surfaces that are technically reconstructible.

In our series the calcaneocuboid joint did not pose a problem, either in reduction or in functional outcome. In every case, the postoperative CT scan indicated that the reduction was acceptable, and no patient complained of pain in this region at follow-up. Although the calcaneocuboid joint is frequently involved in these fractures, if reduction is adequate we believe that problems associated with this joint will be minimal.

The use of bone graft in these fractures is still controversial. Palmer was unhappy with internal fixation techniques and therefore did not employ them. Instead, he suggested that bone graft be used to hold up the articular surface [23]. Letournel, using internal fixation, suggested that bone graft was unnecessary because lag screws were able to hold the articular surface together [15]. In our study, no case was grafted and in no case was there a subsequent loss of articular reduction. In type II fractures the articular surface is split and represents two large blocks of bone that can be repositioned and held with lag screws. Consequently, there is little need for bone graft, and in fact the graft can block articular reduction [15, 18]. In type III fractures the fracture includes a centrally depressed fragment, much like a split depression tibial plateau or die-punch distal radius fracture. Difficulty obtaining a reduction is directly related to inability to stabilize this central fragment. Based on our experience we would recommend a bone graft in type III fractures to buttress the central fragment from below.

In type IV fractures the articular surface is extremely difficult to reduce successfully. In addition, the force expended to create this fracture probably results in irreversible damage to portions of the articular cartilage. Additionally, we have encountered avascular necrosis of some of these fragments at the time of subsequent fusion. Based on our dismal results in this group of fractures we would agree with Hall, Gallie, and others, that primary or early subtalar arthrodesis is justified [9, 10, 14, 22].

Primary arthrodesis, however, is not an easy procedure and removal of the joint surface may result in severe heel valgus and pain [9, 14]. Hall has stated that late arthrodesis in a patient with deformity is also technically demanding and results will not be uniformly good [10]. Our approach was to perform a standard reduction and internal fixation in these patients as the initial procedure. Intraoperative assessment of joint reduction then determined the need for subtalar fusion. If fusion was deferred, the reconstitution of calcaneal height, width, and length at least permitted normal shoe wear. Additionally, subsequent arthrodesis was easier. If the joint was severely damaged and primary subtalar arthrodesis was elected, the initial reconstitution of bony anatomy made this straightforward. Typically, cartilage resection and fusion using large 6.5 mm AO cancellous screws was performed. If excessive subchondral bone was resected, a subtalar distraction bone block fusion as described by Carr et al. was employed [6]. At this time we are no longer performing delayed fusions in type IV fractures, and would recommend that the above technique be used in these cases to insure satisfactory hindfoot contour.

Fernandez stated that soft tissue damage at the time of surgery was a significant problem not commonly addressed in the literature [8]. Minimal soft tissue, peroneal, and sural nerve complications occurred in our patients. We believe this is a direct result of the modified Kocher incision and the "no-touch" technique, both of which limit soft tissue handling and protect the peroneal tendon sheath and the sural nerve [8].

Despite these precautions, wound dehiscence was seen in 16% and calcaneal osteomyelitis in 4% of our cases. Should these problems arise we would recommend the following management protocol. Whirlpool therapy, with wet to dry dressings changes are begun on a daily basis. If this is unsuccessful, a free flap must be used to salvage the extremity. Once an infection has occurred, repeat debridements are performed. If the infection is superficial, the plate and screws may be retained. After the wound bed is deemed clean, a free tissue transfer combined with 6 weeks of intravenous antibiotics is used. If osteomyelitis exists, the hardware must be removed together with all necrotic and infected bone. After repeated debridements and 6 weeks of culture-specific antibiotics, a fusion or amputation based on the amount of remaining calcaneus is performed. If limb salvage is to be attempted, free tissue transfer should be scheduled after the wound is clean, no later than 2 weeks after initial debridement.

Many authors emphasize that subtalar joint motion is important to overall functional outcome [7, 15, 16, 23, 27, 28]. Stephenson compared the results of Palmer and McReynolds with those of his own series and showed that early postoperative motion resulted in significantly improved long-term subtalar motion [28]. That this motion is important is not in doubt. Our ability to evaluate this parameter, however, was difficult at best. Inman's method was laborious to perform and results were inconsistent [13]. Results using the Morrey jog test were tester-dependent and only slightly better [20]. Functionally, the majority of our excellent to good results had little difficulty with uneven terrain, while those with poor results were unable to mow the lawn, walk on the beach, or negotiate irregular sidewalks. On the basis of these findings subtalar motion would be better evaluated by functional assessment than actual range of motion.

A fault of our classification scheme is that it is a two-dimensional representation of a three-dimensional problem. Thus, the fracture lines seem to shift depending on the CT cut evaluated. Understandably the method is crude and arbitrary, but we believe we have shown it to have prognostic significance. Carr has recently demonstrated three-dimensional CT scanning of the posterior facet to be inadequate for articular evaluation [5]. Until three-dimensional imaging is detailed enough for routine use, we would recommend the use of two-dimensional CT scanning to classify these fractures and evaluate operative results.

Conclusions

To evaluate the results of an operative protocol for the treatment of intra-articular calcaneal fractures, a new CT fracture classification was developed based on standardized coronal and transverse CT scanning of both feet. The fractures were categorized according to three vertical fracture lines (A, B, C) which separated the posterior facet into a maximum of four fragments: the sustentaculum, a medial, central, and lateral column. Articular fractures were classified as type I (non displaced), type II (two-part or split fractures), type III (three-part or split depression fractures), and type IV (four-part or highly comminuted joint fractures). Postoperatively a repeat CT was obtained to assess reduction. Results were evaluated using the Maryland foot score and repeat CT scans.

We believe that this CT scan classification of intra-articular fractures of the calcaneus is prognostic, and should be utilized to aid the surgeon in determining surgical treatment and outcome. Although the position of the fracture line does not influence results, it is important in preoperative planning. The use of intraoperative Broden's views for all fractures with B and C lines is highly recommended. Type I fractures are nondisplaced, require nonoperative treatment, and can be expected to have an excellent result. The majority of intra-articular calcaneal fractures are type II split fractures. They are amenable to operative intervention. Good results and return to work can be expected. Type III split depression fractures are less frequent, have a worse prognosis, and should be bone grafted to prevent late collapse of the central fragment. Patients should be counseled that disability and the possible need for a subtalar fusion may occur. Type IV highly comminuted fractures are fortunately rare injuries. They should be internally fixed, primarily to restore calcaneal shape, and then undergo immediate or delayed subtalar arthrodesis.

References

1. Aitken AP (1963) Fractures of the os calcis. Clin Orthop 30:67–75
2. Bèzes H, Massart P, Fourquet JP (1984) Die Osteosynthese der Calcaneus-Impressionsfraktur. Unfallheilkunde 87
3. Böhler L (1931) Diagnosis, pathology and treatment of fractures of the os calcis. J Bone Joint Surg 13:75–89
4. Burdeaux BD (1983) Reduction of calcaneal fractures by the McReynolds medial approach technique and its experimental basis. Clin Orthop 177:87–103
5. Carr JB (1989) Three dimensional CT scanning of calcaneal fractures. Orthop Trans
6. Carr JB, Hansen ST, Benirschke SK (1988) Subtalar distraction bone block fusion for late complications of os calcis fractures. Foot Ankle 9/2:81–86
7. Essex-Lopresti P (1952) The mechanism, reduction technique, and results in fractures of the os calcis. Br J Surg 39:395–419
8. Fernandez DL (1984) Transarticular fracture of the calcaneus. Arch Orth Trauma Surg 103:195–200
9. Gallie WE (1943) Subastragalar arthrodesis in fractures of the os calcis. J Bone Joint Surg XXV/4:731–736
10. Hall MC, Pennal GF (1960) Primary subtalar arthrodesis in the treatment of severe fractures of the calcaneum. J Bone Joint Surg [Br] 42:336–343
11. Harding D, Waddell JP (1985) Open reduction in depressed fractures of the os calcis. Clin Orthop 199:124–131
12. Hermann OJ (1937) Conservative therapy for fractures of the os calcis. J Bone Joint Surg XIX/3:709–718
13. Inman TV (1976) The joints of the ankle. Williams and Wilkins, Baltimore
14. Kalamchi A, Evans J (1977) Posterior subtalar fusion. J Bone Joint Surg [Br] 59/3:287–289

15. Letournel E (1984) Open reduction and internal fixation of calcaneal fractures. In: Spiegel P (ed) Topics in orthopedic surgery. Aspen, Baltimore, pp 173–192
16. Leung K, Chan W, Shen W, Pak P, So W, Leung P (1989) Operative treatment of intraarticular fractures of the os calcis. J Orthop Trauma 3/3:232–240
17. Martinez S, Herzenberg JE, Apple JS (1985) Computed tomography of the hindfoot. Orthop Clin North Am 16/3:481–496
18. Maxfield JE, McDermott FJ (1955) Experiences with the Palmer open reduction of fractures of the calcaneus. J Bone Joint Surg [Am] 37/1:99–106
19. McReynolds IS (1982) The case for operative treatment of fractures of the os calcis. In: Leach RE, Hoaglund FT, Riseborough EJ (eds) Controversies in orthopedic surgery. Saunders, Philadelphia, pp 232–254
20. Morrey BF, Weideman GP (1980) Complications and long term results of ankle arthrodesis following trauma. J Bone Joint Surg [Am] 62/5:777–784
21. Müller ME, Nazarian S, Koch P (1987) Classification AO des fractures. Berlin: Springer, Berlin Heidelberg New York
22. Noble J, McQuillan WM (1979) Early posterior subtalar fusion in the treatment of fractures of the os calcis. J Bone Joint Surg [Br] 61/1:90–93
23. Palmer I (1948) The mechanism and treatment of fractures of the calcaneus. J Bone Joint Surg [Am] 30/1:2–8
24. Sanders RW, Dipasquale T (1989) Intra-operative Brodén's views in the operative treatment of calcaneal fractures. Orthop Trans 13/3
25. Smith RW, Staple TW (1983) Computerized tomography (CT) scanning technique for the hindfoot. Clin Orthop 177:34–38
26. Soeur R, Remy R (1975) Fractures of the calcaneus with displacement of the thalamic portion. J Bone Joint Surg [Br] 57/4:413–421
27. Stephenson JR (1983) Displaced fractures of the os calcis involving the subtalar joint: the key role of the superomedial fragment. Foot Ankle 4/2:91–101
28. Stephenson JR (1987) Treatment of displaced intra-articular fractures of the calcaneus using medial and lateral approaches, internal fixation, and early motion. J Bone Joint Surg [Am] 69/1:115–130
29. Thoren O (1964) Os calcis fractures. Acta Orthop Scand Suppl 70

Classification and Results of ORIF of Calcaneal Fractures

P. Regazzoni, P. Mosimann, and D. Calthorpe

Introduction

The optimal treatment of calcaneal fractures remains controversial [2–4, 6–11, 14, 18, 19, 23, 24]. During the last few years an increasing number of surgeons have reported encouraging results of internal fixation for displaced intra-articular fractures of the calcaneus [2, 6, 12, 15, 17, 20, 22, 26–28]. The prerequisites for open reduction and internal fixation are: good general condition, good soft tissues, an interval of less than 3 weeks after injury, no arterial occlusive disease, and a reliable patient. In contrast functional treatment is indicated for patients in bad general condition, for unreliable patients, those with severe arterial occlusive disease or with severe soft tissue problems, when there has been an interval of more than 3 weeks since the injury, and in cases of undisplaced or completely "smashed" fractures.
Differences in the techniques of internal fixation still exist [2, 4, 12, 15, 17, 18, 20, 21, 24, 26, 27], but there is increasing acceptance that the principles for the treatment of articular fractures can also be applied in calcaneal fractures [2, 12, 15, 20, 21, 27, 28].

Technique of Internal Fixation

On the basis of the technique described by Bèzes [2] we have developed our own standard technique and have used it in more than 110 operations. The details of the procedure and the encouraging results of our first series have been published elsewhere [20, 21]. The relevant steps are:

1. A long incision
2. A subperiosteal dissection up to the subtalar joint (the branch of the sural nerve as well as the peroneal tendons are well protected in the resulting full-thickness flap)
3. Reduction of the articular surface, and reconstruction of width, length, and height of the calcaneus
4. Preliminary fixation with Kirschner wires
5. Cancellous grafting, if necessary
6. Screw fixation of the articular fragments
7. Buttressing of the lateral wall with a plate (comminution with lack of bony buttress at the sinus tarsi sulcus) or staples.

Classification

Many different classifications of calcaneal fractures have been proposed [3, 7, 12, 17, 20, 28]. It is therefore difficult to compare the results of different types of treatment. Standard plain radiographs might give adequate information in extra-articular fractures, but are undoubtedly not sufficient for intra-articular fractures [1, 5, 16, 25]. Thus, all the recent classifications are based on CT imaging [12, 17, 20, 28].

The old Essex-Lopresti classification (or modifications of it) remains useful for a rough differentiation. Closed extra-articular fractures are a special entity, as are completely smashed or open fractures. Basic differentiation of intra-articular (= transthalamic) fractures into tongue-type and joint-depression-type is no longer sufficient or acceptable.

Ideally, a classification should allow an adequate definition of the fracture pattern, help in the choice of the treatment and have a certain correlation with prognosis.

According to our experience with open reduction and internal fixation (ORIF) of more than 100 calcaneal fractures imaged with biplanar computed tomograms we have developed a new classification based on the principles of the AO classification of long bones. The three main types (A, B, C) differentiate peripheral fractures from those involving the subtalar joint alone, and from those with both subtalar and calcaneocuboid joint involvement. Within each type three groups (1, 2, 3) indicate an increasing complexity (Table 1).

Results

From a limited senés ($n = 50$) the validity of this classification seems promising. It was evaluated with regard to indication of increasing injury severity against a three-dimensional deformity index, and with regard to prognosis against the

Table 1. Classification of calcaneal fractures

A. Peripheral
- A1. Peripheral, extra-articular
- A2. Avulsion of the sustentaculum
- A3. Anterior process (alone), intra-articular

B. Subtalar joint
- B1. Posterior facet, simple fracture
- B2. Posterior facet, multifragmentary
- B3. Sinus tarsi and/or middle and/or anterior facet

C. Subtalar and calcaneocuboid joint
- C1. Both joints, simple fracture
- C2. One joint multifragmentary or sinus tarsi
- C3. Both joints multifragmentary

Table 2. Correlation of three-dimensional deformity index with clinical result and pain

	Clinical result[a]		
	Very good	Good	Fair
Three-dimensional deformity index (triple index)	68	71	118
	Pain		
	None	Moderate	Severe
Triple index	56	72	111

[a] Modified Merle d'Aubigné Scheme.

clinical results (modified Merle d'Aubigné Scheme). The results are shown in Table 2. A correlation exists with the overall clinical results, particularly concerning pain and gait. Larger series are needed to allow a final judgment.

Conclusion

The optimal treatment of calcaneal fractures remains controversial. A consensus classification does not exist. A morphological and prognostic classification was developed based on standardized biplanar computed tomography and on experience with over 100 calcaneal fractures which had been internally fixed utilizing a standard technique.

References

1. Bauer G, Mutschler W, Heuchemer T, Lob G (1987) Fortschritte in der Diagnostik der intraarticulären Calcaneusfrakturen durch die Computertomographie. Unfallchirurg 90:496–501
2. Bèzes H, Massart P, Fourquet JP (1984) Die Osteosynthese der Calcaneusimpressionsfraktur. Unfallheilkunde 87:363–368
3. Böhler L (1963) Die Technik der Knochenbruchbehandlung. Maudrich, Wien
4. Buch J (1980) Bohrdrahtosteosynthese des Fersenbeinbruches. Aktuel Chir 15:285–296
5. Crosby LA, Fitzgibbons T (1990) Computerized tomography scanning of acute intra-articular fractures of the calcaneus. J Bone Joint Surg [Am] 2:852–859
6. Eberle C, Landolt M (1986) Ergebnisse nach Osteosynthese von intraarticulären Calcaneusfrakturen. Z Unfallchir Versicherungsmed Berufskr 79:125–128
7. Essex-Lopresti P (1952) The mechanism, reduction technique and results in fractures of os calcis. Br J Surg 39:395–419
8. Giachino AA, Uthoff HK (1989) Current concept review intra-articular fractures of the calcaneus. J Bone Joint Surg [Am] 784–787
9. Harding D, Waddell JP (1985) Open reduction in fractures of the os calcis. Clin Orthop 199:124–130

10. Hörster G (1988) Indikation zur konservativen-operativen Behandlung der Fersenbeinfraktur. Unfallchirurg 91:502–506
11. Järvholm U, Körner L, Thores O, Wiklund LM (1984) Fractures of the calcaneus. A comparison of open and closed treatment. Acta Orthop Scand 55:652–656
12. Johnson E (1990) Intraarticular fractures of the calcaneus: diagnosis and surgical management. Orthopedics 13:1091–1099
13. Kempf I, Touzard RC (1978) Les fractures du calcanéum. J Chir (Paris) 115:377–386
14. Knopp W, Neumann K, Vogelheim P, Kayser M (1988) Kann die operative Therapie von Fersenbeinbrüchen Spätfolgen verhindern? Hefte Unfallheilk 200:449–450
15. Leung KS, Chan WS, Shen WY, Pak PPL, So WS, Leung PC (1989) Operative treatment of intraarticular fractures of the os calcis: the role of rigid internal fixation and primary bone grafting. Preliminary results. J Orthop Trauma 3:232–240
16. Lowrie IG, Finlay DB, Brenkel IJ, Gregg PJ (1988) Computerized tomographic assessment of the subtalar joint in calcaneal fractures. J Bone Joint Surg [Br] 70:247–250
17. Mutschler E (1988) Der Fersenbeinbruch – detaillierte Diagnostik, Klassifikation und Konsequenzen für die Therapie. Unfallchirurg 91:486–492
18. Poigenfürst J, Buch J (1988) Behandlung der schweren Brüche des Fersenbeines durch Reposition und perkutane Bohrdrahtfixation. Unfallchirurgie 91:493–501
19. Pozo JL, Kirwan E, Jackson AM (1984) The long-term results of conservative management of severely displaced fractures of the calcaneus. J Bone Joint Surg [Br] 66:386–390
20. Regazzoni P (1991) Behandlung von Calcaneusfrakturen. Basler Beitr Chir 3:49–62
21. Regazzoni P (1988) Technik der stabilen Osteosynthese bei Calcaneusfrakturen. Hefte Unfallheilk 200:432–439
22. Ross SD, Sowerby MR (1985) The operative treatment of fractures of the os calcis. Clin Orthop 199:132–143
23. Russe OJ, Russe F (1989) Klinische und radiologische Nachuntersuchung von 149 Fersenbeinbrüchen nach percutaner Aufrichtung und Fixation. Hefte Unfallheilk 200:445–448
24. Schellmann WD (1988) Technik der Bohrdrahtosteosynthese. Hefte Unfallheilk 200:426–431
25. Segal D, Marsh JL, Leiter B (1985) Clinical application of computed axial tomography scanning of calcaneal fractures. Clin Orthop 199:114–123
26. Stephenson JR (1987) Treatment of displaced intraarticular fractures of the calcaneus using medial and lateral approaches, internal fixation and early motion. J Bone Joint Surg [Am] 69:115–130
27. Zwipp H, Tscherne H, Wülker N (1988) Osteosynthese dislozierter intraarticulärer Calcaneusfrakturen. Unfallchirurg 91:507–515
28. Zwipp H, Tscherne H, Wülker N, Grote R (1989) Der intraarticuläre Fersenbeinbruch. Klassifikation, Bewertung und Operationstaktik. Unfallchirurg 92:117–129

Comparison of Open Versus Closed Reduction of Intra-articular Calcaneal Fractures: A Matched Cohort in Workmen

R.E. Buckley and R.N. Meek

Introduction

The treatment of intra-articular calcaneal fractures has been very controversial because of good results claimed with and without operations [12, 14, 19, 36, 37]. Intra-articular fractures in other weight-bearing joints are routinely treated with anatomical reduction and rigid fixation. No good prospective, randomized studies exist in this area of fracture surgery. Paley, in a review in 1989, saw the lack of standardization in fracture classification and evaluation protocol to be the main reason for the lack of progress in the literature in definitive calcaneal fracture surgery [25].
The purpose of this study is to compare clinical results in operative versus nonoperative treatment of displaced, intraarticular calcaneal fractures.

Patients and Methods

From March 1978 to May 1987, 19 displaced intra-articular fractures of the calcaneus in 16 Workers' Compensation Board (WCB) patients were surgically treated by the senior author.
Follow-up was obtained on 17 of the 19 surgically treated fractures of the calcaneus in 14 WCB patients (three bilateral fractures). Two patients could not be found for follow-up. Only WCB patients with follow-up of longer than 2 years were included.
For each operatively treated calcaneus fracture, a WCB patient with a conservatively treated, displaced intra-articular calcaneal fracture was carefully matched. These conservatively treated patients had not been treated by the senior author but were located through extensive WCB records. Sixteen patients with 17 fractures (one bilateral) were selected for matching before actual patient follow-up. Criteria for selection and subsequent matching involved type of fracture, age at time of injury, occupation, and year of injury. The Essex-Lopresti classification was used for determining fracture type (Fig. 1) [7]. All fractures were either moderately or severely displaced. All 34 calcaneal fractures had occurred in male laborers or tradesmen who had fallen. The average age of the operatively treated group was 37 years (range 23–57 years). The average difference in age between matched pairs was 4.5 years. Pairs were matched in regards to year of injury, with follow-up averaging 6.3 years (range

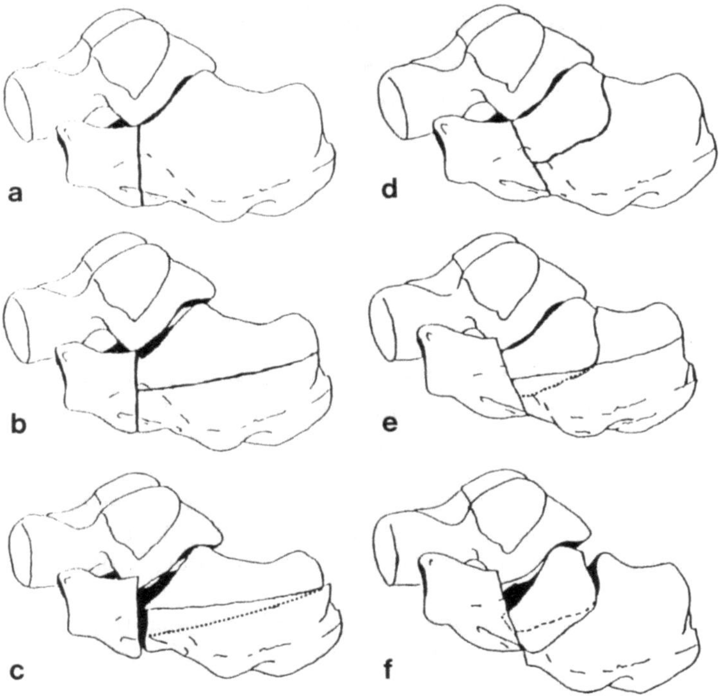

Fig. 1. a Undisplaced intra-articular fracture. **b** Mildly displaced tongue-type fracture. **c** Markedly displaced tongue-type fracture. **d** Undisplaced joint-depression fracture. **e** Mildly displaced joint-depression fracture. **f** Markedly displaced joint-depression fracture. Only categories **b, c, e** and **f** were included in the study

2.5–11.5 years) for the operatively treated fractures and 5.4 years (range 3.3–7.7 years) for the conservatively treated fractures.

The indications for surgical treatment in the operative group were a displaced intra-articular fracture and incongruity of the articular surface of the posterior facet joint. This was initially investigated with plain radiographs and tomography, but in the later years of the study CT was used adjunctively. All fractures treated operatively showed a diminished or reversed tuber-joint angle (average 16° change from normal foot).

A lateral approach was used with a tourniquet. The sural nerve was protected, the peroneal tendons were retracted, and the calcaneofibular ligament was detached [23]. The posterior facet was elevated and reduced and held with Kirschner wires or AO screws. Radiographs were taken at this time to ensure adequacy of reduction. The lateral wall was subsequently reduced and held with a plate and screws, Kirschner wires, or AO screw fixation. If the fracture extended into the calcaneocuboid joint, this was also reduced and fixed. Iliac crest bone graft was used in 3 of 17 fractures.

Anatomical reduction was achieved in 7 of 17 calcaneal fractures. A small step, of greater than 1 mm but less than 2 mm, was left in 9 of 17 fractures. One open reduction resulted in a very comminuted gapped joint surface with a defect greater than 2 mm. Early active postoperative range of motion was initiated and patients were allowed partial weight-bearing at 6 weeks, progressing to full weight-bearing as tolerated.

Four of 17 operatively treated feet had early postoperative wound sloughs. None of these required grafting or antibiotics and all healed primarily. Sural nerve lesions occurred in 5 of 17 feet, but all recovered sensation except one patient. Sensory loss and neurological pain continued in this patient postoperatively, resulting in his undergoing a sural neuroma resection. He was no better after this second procedure. In total, 9 of 17 operatively treated feet had a surgical complication, while the nonoperative group had no such complications.

The nonoperative group had all been treated without a closed reduction and with initial elevation of the foot and non-weight-bearing. Eight patients had casts and 8 patients (one bilateral) had no immobilization. Weight-bearing was started at 6 weeks and progressed as tolerated. The patients from both operative and nonoperative groups were treated at the same WCB rehabilitation facility.

Follow-up of the 34 calcaneal fractures involved three components: (1) clinical history and physical examination of the feet, (2) plain radiographs (lateral calcaneal view and axial view of subtalar joint), and (3) CT scans (axial and coronal cuts of the calcaneus and subtalar joint with computer-generated sagittal reconstruction). The clinical evaluation was performed by one examiner (R.B.) who had not been involved in the treatment of any of the patients. The matching was unknown to the evaluator until the completion of all patient examinations. A detailed history was obtained about presence, intensity, and location of pain. The preinjury and postinjury occupations were scored (light, moderate, heavy labor) for each patient. This scoring was based on the amount of labor performed and the ability of the patient to perform it. Patient self-evaluation of personal results was scored (satisfied, reserved, dissatisfied). Days to return to work were obtained from WCB charts. A clinical scoring system was utilized to evaluate each patient regarding clinical subjective criteria [31] (Table 1). Objective parameters that were measured included subtalar range of motion (as determined by the McMaster technique [21]) and tuber-joint angle. Plain radiographs and CT scans were viewed by two radiologists to ensure initial patient matching was accurate.

Results

All but 3 of 34 feet had residual discomfort after 5.9 years average follow-up (Table 2). Of the 3 patients with no pain, 2 had had open reductions and one had been treated conservatively. Universally, the patient's discomfort was located deep in the calcaneus or over the lateral subtalar joint in the operative

Table 1. Scoring system (max. 100 points)

1. Pain (30 units)	
None	30
Exercise	25
Mild (daily living)	20
Pain with weight-bearing	10
Pain at rest	0
2. Activities: walking (20 units)	
Normal	20
Restricted on rough ground	15
Moderate restriction	10
Able to walk short distances	5
Unable to walk	0
3. Work (20 units)	
Able to perform usual occupation	20
Some restrictions on usual occupation	15
Substantial restriction or change of job	10
Partially disabled; selected jobs	5
Unable to work	0
4. Gait (10 units)	
Normal	10
Mild (exercise-induced) limp	8
Moderate limp	5
Severe limp	0
5. Appliances (10 units)	
None	10
Insole	8
Special shoe	5
Cane or crutch	0
6. Medication (10 units)	
None	10
Some activities	5
Daily	0

and conservative groups. Surpriginsly, no patients claimed to have significant pain in the heel pad region. Two conservatively treated patients had constant pain necessitating subtalar fusions (at 10 and 12 months; they were scored clinically at their prefusion level). No other late reconstructive procedures were performed on any patients. Most patients in both groups acknowledged continued lessening of pain after the fracture until approximately 2 years, after which no or very slow improvement occurred. No patients had worsening symptoms except the 2 who went on to early subtalar fusions. When comparing matched pairs of feet for pain (Table 3), there was no indication that those patients with an open reduction had less pain than their matched conservatively treated counterparts (mean 2.24 vs. 2.41; Wilcoxon matched-pairs signed-ranks test two-tailed, $p=0.31$). Walking on rough or sloped ground caused discomfort for all patients except 3 of the 34 patients who had no pain on follow-up. As part of the evaluation, analgesic use was documented. Analgesics were used by one patient in each group but infrequently (less than once per week). The majority of patients advocated wearing good-quality athletic footwear, but personal preference led to many different types of shoes and insoles being worn for work and leisure.

A change of occupation or degree of physical workload (light, medium, heavy) occurred in 16 WCB laborers. Fourteen laborers did not change their basic physical workload. Most patients returned to work at "light" duties and progressed from there. All patients returned to work. There was no significant difference between the conservative and operative groups in their ability to return to work. The operatively treated patients returned to work in an average of 236 days (range 90–540 days). The conservatively treated patients returned to work in an average of 306 days (range 42–960 days). This was a subjectively measured statistic as patients returned to work at different levels of workload. Statistically, the matched groups showed no difference between groups (paired *t*-test, $p=0.26$).

In all 34 feet the motion of the subtalar joint was measured at follow-up by the McMaster technique [21]. The average motion was 52% of normal (range 0–85%) for the nonoperative WCB patients. The average motion was 47% of normal (range 0–90%) for the WCB patients who had an operation. The 2 patients with a subtalar fusion had no motion, as was also the case with one of the operatively treated patients. This patient had had the poorest intraoperative joint surface reduction. No difference existed between matched patients regarding subtalar motion (paired *t*-test, $p=0.46$).

The overall clinical score given to each patient was judged to be the most important criterion of clinical patient evaluation as it combined all aspects of patient function. The conservatively treated patients had an average score of 75.5 (range 30–100). The operatively treated patients had an average score of 77.8 (range 40–100) (Table 2). There was no significant difference between matched pairs of WCB patients (paired *t*-test, $p=0.66$). Two operatively treated patients and one conservatively treated patient had perfect scores.

The adequacy of fracture reduction did correspond with clinical score (Table 4). Anatomically reduced fractures achieved a higher clinical score (83.9 average) than those operatively reduced with a step (greater than 1 mm; 74.7 average). Nonoperative treatment, despite major joint incongruency, gave as good a clinical result (75.5 average) as operative treatment if the joint surface was left with a step. Those patients whose calcanei were anatomically reduced had a statistically significantly better clinical score than their matched conservatively treated counterparts (paired *t*-test, $p<0.01$).

Discussion

The controversy regarding treatment of this difficult problem has continued for many years since Böhler, in 1933, started operative reduction of calcaneal fractures [3]. In 1984 the nonoperative treatment of 21 intra-articular calcaneal

Table 2. Follow-up results

Pair	Study arm[a]	Age	Fracture class[b]	ORIF[c]	Year	Reduction[d]	Pain	Change work[e]	Pain level[f]	Subtalar motion (%)	Satisfaction[g]	Work return (days)	Clinical score (max. 100)
1	1	39	2	1	1982	4	1	0	3	63	2	180	68
	2	40	2	2	1978	1	2	0	1	71	1	220	100
2	1	43	2	1	1984	4	1	1	2	36	1	260	78
	2	39	2	4	1985	2	1	1	3	33	2	285	68
3	1	35	2	1	1984	4	1	0	3	67	2	300	83
	2	33	2	3	1986	1	1	0	3	27	1	540	78
4	1	46	2	1	1982	4	1	1	2	43	1	425	78
	2	42	2	4	1983	2	1	1	3	50	1	165	76
5	1	30	2	1	1982	4	1	0	2	64	1	97	78
	2	24	2	4	1982	2	1	1	2	88	1	255	78
6	1	41	2	1	1985	4	1	0	2	33	2	365	83
	2	39	2	2	1985	2	1	1	2	33	1	285	83
7	1	57	2	1	1985	4	2	0	1	60	1	150	100
	2	54	2	2	1986	2	1	1	2	67	1	180	83
8	1	36	1	1	1985	4	1	2	2	86	1	460	78
	2	39	1	2	1980	2	1	2	3	43	2	180	40
9	1	37	2	1	1986	4	1	0	2	60	1	225	81
	2	37	2	3	1987	1	1	1	2	75	1	255	70
10	1	25	2	1	1983	4	1	0	2	67	1	300	88
	2	34	2	2	1983	1	1	0	2	70	1	210	88
11	1	25	2	1	1983	4	1	0	2	67	1	300	88
	2	34	2	4	1983	2	1	0	3	40	1	210	71
12	1	24	2	1	1985	4	1	1	2	44	3	120	73
	2	35	2	2	1982	1	1	0	2	66	1	105	90
13	1	48	2	1	1986	4	1	0	2	71	1	42	83
	2	43	2	3	1985	1	1	1	2	30	1	90	83

14	1	29	2	1	1984	4	1	1	4	0	3	960	35
	2	27	2	4	1985	1	1	2	2	50	1	120	78
15	1	52	2	1	1985	4	1	1	3	80	2	365	76
	2	48	2	4	1981	2	1	1	2	20	1	515	63
16	1	33	2	1	1985	4	1	1	4	0	3	365	30
	2	43	2	3	1985	3	1	1	3	0	2	90	63
17	1	23	1	1	1982	4	1	0	3	50	2	300	83
	2	21	1	2	1979	2	2	0	1	38	1	315	100

[a] Study arm: 1, conservative; 2, operative.
[b] Fracture class: 1, Moderately displaced fracture; 2, severely displaced fracture.
[c] ORIF (open reduction, internal fixation): 1, none; 2, screws; 3, Kirschner wires; 4, combination.
[d] Reduction: 1, anatomical; 2, Step (1–2 mm displacement); 3, Poor (>2 mm displacement); 4, None.
[e] Change work: 0, no change; 1, heavy to medium or medium to light; 2, heavy to light.
[f] Pain level: 1, none; 2, exercise-induced; 3, moderate; 4, constant.
[g] Satisfaction: 1, satisfied; 2, reservations; 3, dissatisfied.

Table 3. Level of pain in 17 pairs of patients with calcaneal fractures

Pain level[a]	Conservatively treated	ORIF
1	1	2
2	10	9
3	4	6
4	2	–
	17	17

[a] Pain level: 1, none; 2, exercise-induced; 3, moderate; 4, constant.
The average pain level was 2.41 in the conservatively treated group, 2.24 in the ORIF group.

Table 4. Fracture reduction versus clinical score in 17 pairs of patients with calcaneal fractures

Fracture reduction	Clinical score	No. of patients
Anatomical	83.9	7
Step (1–2 mm)	74.7	9
Poor (>2 mm)	63.0	1
None	75.5	17

fractures was critically reviewed by Pozo et al. who found 67% good results after at least 8 years follow-up [29]. The authors had classified all calcaneal fractures and looked at those that were displaced and involved the posterior subtalar joint. On the other hand, Stephenson, in 1987, reported 77% good results with operative treatment of intra-articular calcaneal fractures with an average 3-year follow-up [36]. Congruity of the joint surfaces was thought to be very important for the end result.

In a retrospective study comparing open versus closed treatment of calcaneal fractures, Jarvholm, in 1984, found that overall results were equal in 39 patients with 4-year follow-up [18]. Numerous authors have compared the success of different treatment modalities for fractures of the calcaneus but no definitive conclusions can be drawn [1, 2, 4–6, 8, 9, 11, 13, 20, 22–24, 27, 28, 30, 31, 33–35, 37].

Two reviews in 1989 [9, 25] found that no surgical studies in the literature had included CT scans of calcaneal fractures. CT is a very valuable tool in radiological investigation of calcaneal fractures [6, 10, 15–17]. It can also be used for evaluating old calcaneal fractures [38] and should be the basis of a new classification for these fractures because it provides very detailed three-dimensional information. Pain is the most important outcome variable leading to a poor result. This study shows no difference between nonoperative and operative treatment regarding pain (Tables 2 and 3). Jarvholm found similar results in a comparative study of open and closed treatment of calcaneal fractures [18]. He concluded that results were equal regarding pain and disability. We had 2 patients in the nonoperative group with lateral subtalar pain necessitating subtalar fusion. Both of these initially had a markedly flattened Bohler's angle measuring –12° and –13°. These were two of the most displaced fractures of the study. Their matched operative cohorts had better results despite having similar displacement preoperatively. Yet overall statistically, no significant difference was demonstrated between the pairs. There was no difference between these two groups of patients in their ability to return to preinjury workload. Those in the nonoperative group returned to their original job more often but this was not statistically significant. More patients would be needed in a larger study to determine an answer to this question, but results here are not dissimilar from those of other studies [13, 18, 19, 29].

Subtalar motion was not different when the matched pairs were compared. Leung's 64 patients had an average return of 81% of subtalar motion with an operation [19]. Sclamberg [33] claimed that 80% of his operatively treated patients had no or slight limitation of subtalar motion. Stephenson [36] had a return of 75% of subtalar motion in his 22 operatively treated patients. Eighty percent of patients treated nonoperatively by Pozo et al. [29] had less than 50% of normal subtalar motion. Yet Harding and Waddell [13] reported that 50% of his operatively treated patients had less than 50% subtalar motion. Obviously, there is variation between studies, yet we found no connection between subtalar motion and functional outcome.

Return to work is the goal with a laborer after an injury, but this study shows no statistical difference in this outcome measure between treatment methods. Isolated data on WCB patients is rare, but Salsbury, in 1962, stated that 281 days (average) was needed for return to work of a patient with a comminuted intra-articular calcaneal fracture (data from the 1940s and 1950s with multiple treatment modalities) [32]. This was based on a larger study looking at all types of calcaneal fractures (333 in all) in WCB patients. Our data concurs with these numbers. Leung, in 1989, reported that after operative treatment of 64 intra-articular calcaneal fractures average time to return to work was 158 days [19].

Rowe devised an objective scoring system that was used for evaluating subjective outcome criteria in calcaneal fracture patients [31]. A version of Rowe's scoring system was used in this study (Table 1). We believe that this provides us with the most important statistic in this study. The analysis of this data includes all of the clinical information that determines overall outcome. The matched WCB pairs demonstrated no difference between treatment modalities. Two nonoperative patients that eventually underwent subtalar fusions were very dissatisfied despite solid fusions. Many authors [20, 23, 34] have reported ungratifying results with late subtalar fusion after calcaneal fracture.

Among the operatively treated fractures, anatomical reduction of an intra-articular calcaneal fracture corresponded with a better clinical score than no reduction or a less than adequate reduction (Table 4). The number of patients in this study is not large, but we believe in a perfect anatomical reduction of the joint surface. However, Harding noted that patients with seemingly perfect anatomical and radiographic results intraoperatively, evolved into patients with disabling symptoms postoperatively [13]. Jarvholm claimed that despite reducing the intra-articular step in the operative group of calcaneal fractures, this had no significance for the development of osteoarthrosis [18]. He stated that an equal number of conservatively treated patients developed osteoarthritic disability. From our study it can be seen that a reduction that was less than perfect corresponded with an overall clinical score that was the same as that for patients who had not had an operation.

Conclusion

This matched study of displaced intra-articular calcaneal fractures in workmen demonstrates that there is no difference in pain, return to work, and subtalar motion between those treated operatively and those treated nonoperatively. There is, however, a better overall clinical score in the small group treated operatively in whom anatomical reduction could be achieved. Our experience with these difficult fractures leads us to believe that certain intra-articular calcaneal fractures should be operatively reduced. We feel that patients with relatively little comminution of the posterior facet joint benefit from open anatomical reduction, rigid internal fixation, and early range of motion. Those patients with marked comminution of the posterior facet joint are not helped by surgery.

References

1. Aaron DAR, Howat TW (1976) Intra-articular fractures of the calcaneum. Injury 7:205–211
2. Barnard L (1963) Non-operative treatment of fractures of the calcaneus. J Bone Joint Surg [Am] 45:865–867
3. Böhler L (1931) Diagnosis, pathology and treatment of fractures of the os calcis. J Bone Joint Surg 13:75–88
4. Burdeaux BD (1983) Reduction of calcaneal fractures by the McReynolds medical approach technique and its experimental basis. Clin Orthop 177:87–103
5. Cassebaum WH (1965) Open reduction of os calcis fractures. J Trauma 5:718–725
6. Colburn MW, Karlin JM, Scuran BL, Silvani SH (1989) Intra-articular fractures of the calcaneus: a review. J Foot Surg 28:249–254
7. Essex-Lopresti P (1952) The mechanism, reduction technique and results in fractures of the os calcis. Br J Surg 39:395–419
8. Gaul JS, Greenberg BG (1966) Calcaneus fractures involving the subtalar joint: a clinical and statistical survey of 98 cases. South Med J 59:605–613
9. Giachino AA, Uhthoff HK (1989) Intra-articular fractures of the calcaneus. J Bone Joint Surg [Am] 71:784–787
10. Guyer BH, Levinsohn EM, Fredrickson BE, Baily GE, Formikell M (1985) Computed tomography of calcaneal fractures: anatomy, pathology, dosimetry, and clinical relevance. Am J Radiol 145:911–919
11. Hall MC, Pennal GF (1960) Primary subtalar arthrodesis in the treatment of severe fractures of the calcaneum. J Bone Joint Surg [Br] 42:336–343
12. Hammesfahr JFR (1989) Surgical treatment of calcaneal fractures. Orthop Clin North Am 20:679–689
13. Harding D, Waddell JP (1985) Open reduction in depressed fractures of the os calcis. Clin Orthop 199:124–131
14. Hazlett JW (1969) Open reduction of fracture of the calcaneum. Can J Surg 12:310–317
15. Heger L, Wulff K (1985) Computed tomography of the calcaneus: normal anatomy. Am J Radiol 145:123–129
16. Heger L, Wulff K, Seddiqi MSA (1985) Computed tomography of calcaneal fractures. Am J Radiol 145:131–137
17. Hindman BW, Ross SDK, Sowerby MRR (1986) Fractures of the talus and calcaneus: evaluation by computed tomography. CT J Comp Tomogr 10:191–196
18. Jarvholm U, Korner L, Thoren O, Wiklund L (1984) Fractures of the calcaneus: a comparison of open and closed treatment. Acta Orthop Scand 55:652–656

19. Leung K, Chan W, Shen W, Poh PPL, So W, Leung P (1989) Operative treatment of intra-articular fractures of the os calcis – the role of rigid internal fixation and primary bone grafting: preliminary results. J Orthop Trauma 3:232–240
20. Lindsay WRN, Dewar FP (1958) Fractures of the os calcis. Am J Surg 95:555–576
21. McMaster M (1976) Disability of the hindfoot after fracture of the tibial shaft. J Bone Joint Surg [Br] 58:90–93
22. Maxfield JE (1963) Treatment of calcaneal fractures by open reduction. J Bone Joint Surg [Am] 45:868–871
23. Miller WE (1983) Pain and impairment considerations following treatment of disruptive os calcis fractures. Clin Orthop 177:82–86
24. Nade S, Monahan PRW (1973) Fractures of the calcaneum: a study of the long-term prognosis. Injury 4:200–207
25. Paley D, Hall H (1989) Calcaneal fracture controversies – can we put humpty dumpty together again? Orthop Clin North Am 20:665–677
26. Paley D, Hall H, McMurtry R, Green R (1987) Operative treatment of calcaneal fractures: a long term follow-up; calcaneal protocol; and factors that affect outcome. Trans Orthop 11:484
27. Palmer I (1948) The mechanism and treatment of fractures of the calcaneus. J Bone Joint Surg [Am] 30:2–8
28. Pennal GF, Yadev MP (1973) Operative treatment of comminuted fractures of the os calcis. Orthop Clin North Am 4:197–211
29. Pozo JL, Kirwan E, Jackson AM (1984) The long-term results of conservative management of severely displaced fractures of the calcaneus. J Bone Joint Surg [Br] 66:386–390
30. Ross SDK, Sowerby MRR (1985) The operative treatment of fractures of the os calcis. Clin Orthop 199:132–143
31. Rowe CR, Sakellarides HT, Freeman PA, Sorbie C (1963) Fractures of the os calcis: A long-term follow-up study of 146 patients. JAMA 184:920–923
32. Salsbury CR (1962) A statistical review of fractures of the calcaneus. Can J Surg 5:48–53
33. Sclamberg EL, Davenport K (1988) Operative treatment of displaced intra-articular fractures of the calcaneus. J Trauma 28:510–516
34. Slatis P, Kiviluoto O, Santavirta S, Laasonen EM (1979) Fractures of the calcaneus. J Trauma 19:939–943
35. Soeur R, Remy R (1975) Fractures of the calcaneus with displacement of the tholamis portion. J Bone Joint Surg [Br] 57:413–421
36. Stephenson JR (1987) Treatment of displaced intra-articular fractures of the calcaneus using medial and lateral approaches, internal fixation, and early motion. J Bone Joint Surg [Am] 69:115–130
37. Stephenson JR (1983) Displaced fractures of the os calcis involving the subtalar joint: the key role of the superomedial fragment. Foot Ankle 4:91–101
38. Techner LM, Eannace RJ (1987) Computerized tomography in the evaluation of old calcaneal fractures. J Am Pod Med Assoc 77:243–245

Closed Reduction and Percutaneous Osteosynthesis: Technique and Results in 265 Calcaneal Fractures

M. Forgon

Introduction

The basic principle of any fracture treatment is an exact reduction of the displaced fracture and reliable fixation during the healing period. This is especially true for displaced fractures of the calcaneus. This paper presents details of our conservative method: closed reduction, and percutaneous screw fixation of the reduced fracture.

Not all forms of calcaneal fractures are problematic. Isolated marginal fractures not involving the posterior joint facet are mostly problem-free. All problematic fractures involve the posterior subtalar joint; however, these constitute more than three fourths of all calcaneal fractures. A conservative procedure has been evolved for these fractures at the Traumatology Department of the University Medical School in Pécs, Hungary. The method carries minimal risk, but the good results of our 265 cases prove its considerable usefulness.

Several factors make reduction of calcaneal fractures difficult: the fracture is usually displaced and crushed, the subtalar joint is frequently involved, and the lever arms of the fracture fragments are short. Traction of the Achilles tendon and the ligamentous connections between the fragments also make reduction difficult. For successful reduction several conditions need to be fulfilled: the tuber-joint angle should be restored, the broadened heel should be narrowed, the valgus position should be eliminated, and the step deformity of the subtalar joint should be corrected.

Before reviewing our procedure, it is necessary to make some comments about imaging techniques. There is no doubt that the best information can be obtained by CT. But do we have to cling to CT at any price? If there is metal in the calcaneus, CT is usually not very useful. But a reduced fracture needs to be fixed somehow – mostly with screws, wires, plates, etc. How then can we visualize the reduction without CT? Conventional "axial" radiographs provide little information because of pain on dorsiflexion. We have had very good experience, though, with Broden's simple radiographic technique (Fig. 1). This is the so-called oblique technique [5, 6], which gives very good information on the posterior subtalar joint (see Fig. 7).

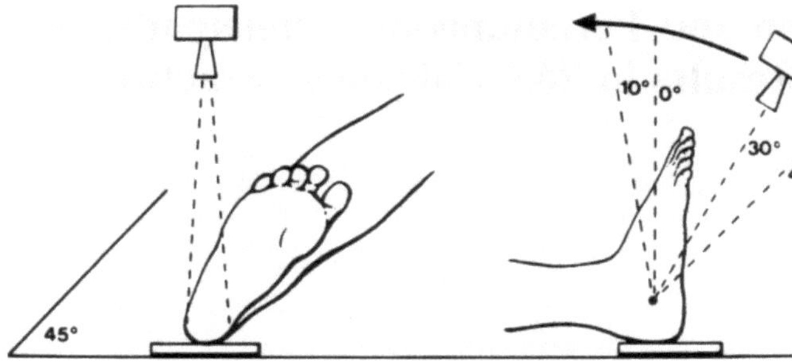

Fig. 1. The "oblique" X-ray technique of Broden gives very good information on the posterior subtalar joint

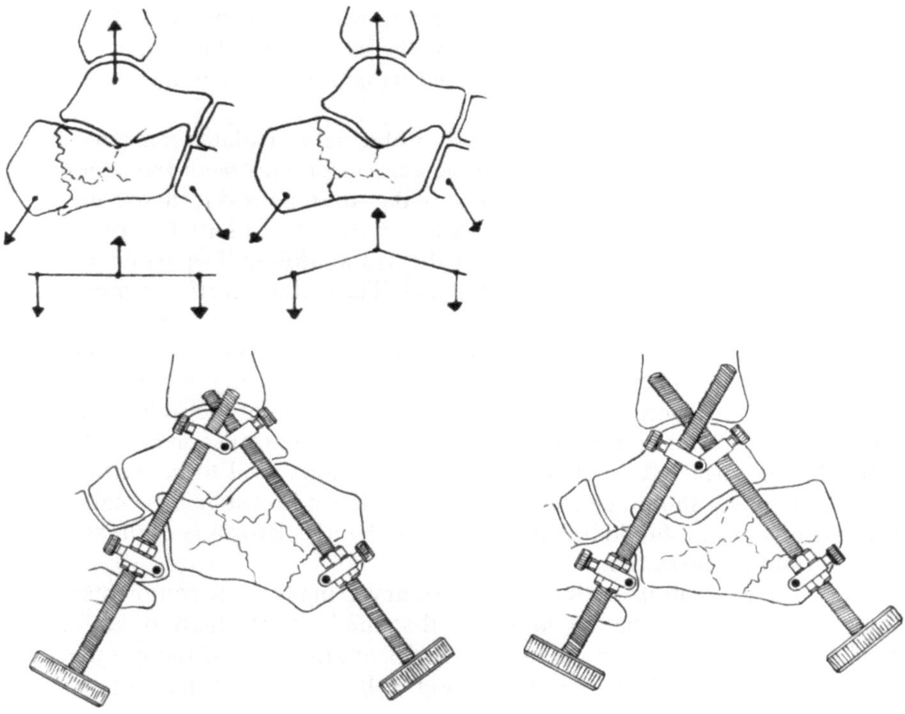

Fig. 2. The device constructed at our institution for reduction of displaced calcaneal fractures. See text for details

Operative Technique

It is important to stress that the reduction should be done early, if possible within a few days of the injury [1, 2]. First the tuber-joint angle is restored, by using a device for the reduction of the displaced calcaneus fractures constructed at our clinic (Fig. 2). The theory behind it is that if distraction is exerted on

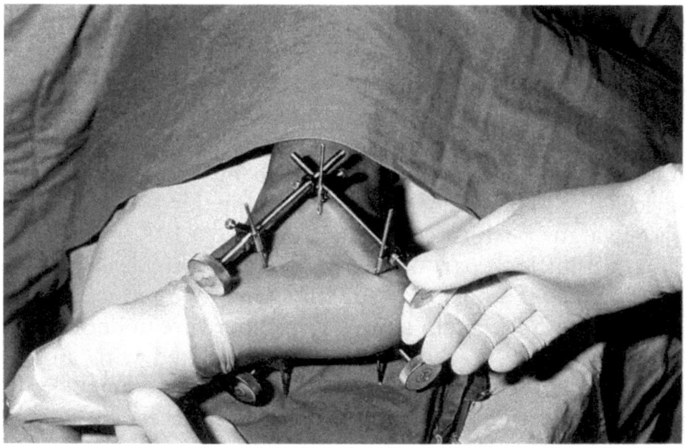

Fig. 3. The shafts of the device are fixed onto the Kirschner wires and a distraction slowly carried out

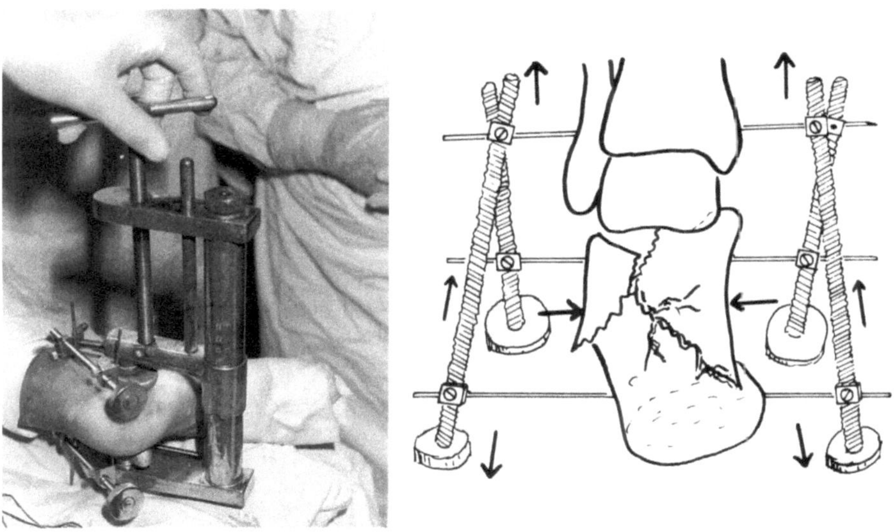

Fig. 4. The broadened heel is narrowed using a Böhler clamp, which can be placed between the shafts of the device

three pints – tuber calcanei, trochlea tali, and os cuboideum – restoration of the tuber-joint angle is fairly easy. The patient lies on his or her side on the operating table during the manipulation. With the aid of an image intensifier three thick Kirschner wires are inserted through the abovementioned three points. The shafts of the device are then fixed laterally and medially on to these wires (Fig. 3). By turning the wheels, slow distraction is achieved between the

Kirschner wires, and the tuber-joint angle is slowly restored, usually within 3–4 min. The reduction can be verified on the image intensifier. The device does not interfere with the visualization of the reduction on the screen.

The second aim, narrowing of the broadened heel, can be achieved by compressing the heel from both sides. A Böhler clamp is suitable for this procedure, its two compressing surfaces being placed between the shafts of the device (Fig. 4). By the same maneuver the third aim is also fulfilled: correction of the valgus position.

The most difficult part of the reduction maneuver is the correction of the step deformity of the posterior subtalar joint. We reduce the depressed calcaneal fragment with the aid of a thick Kirschner wire under image intensifier control (Fig. 5). If this succeeds, the fracture is fixed with an AO malleolar screw inserted percutaneously from the lateral side through a small incision. If there is no step deformity, this maneuver is not necessary.

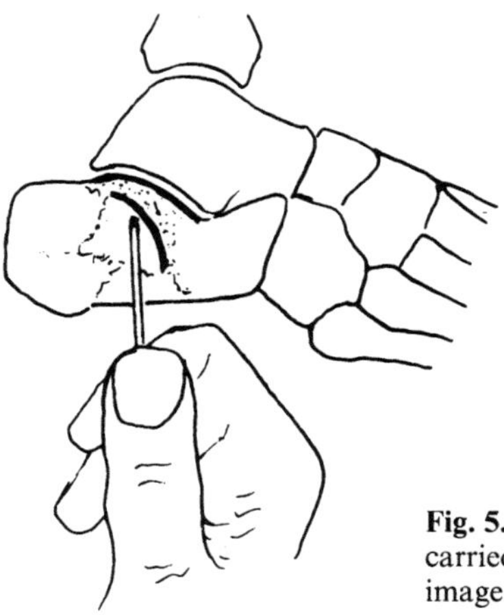

Fig. 5. The elevation of the depressed calcaneal fragment is carried out with the aid of a thick Kirschner wire under image intensifier control

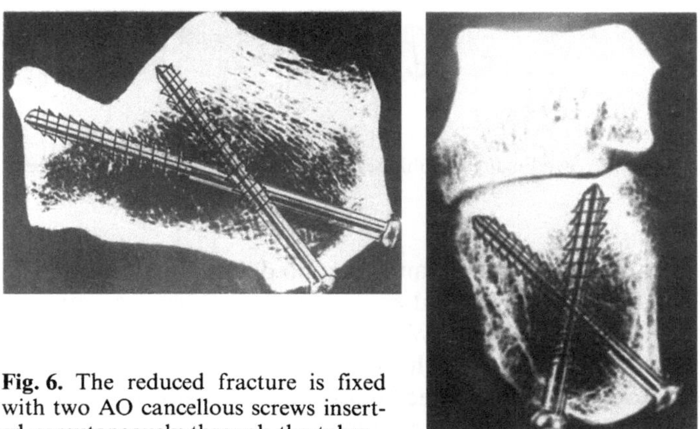

Fig. 6. The reduced fracture is fixed with two AO cancellous screws inserted percutaneously through the tuber

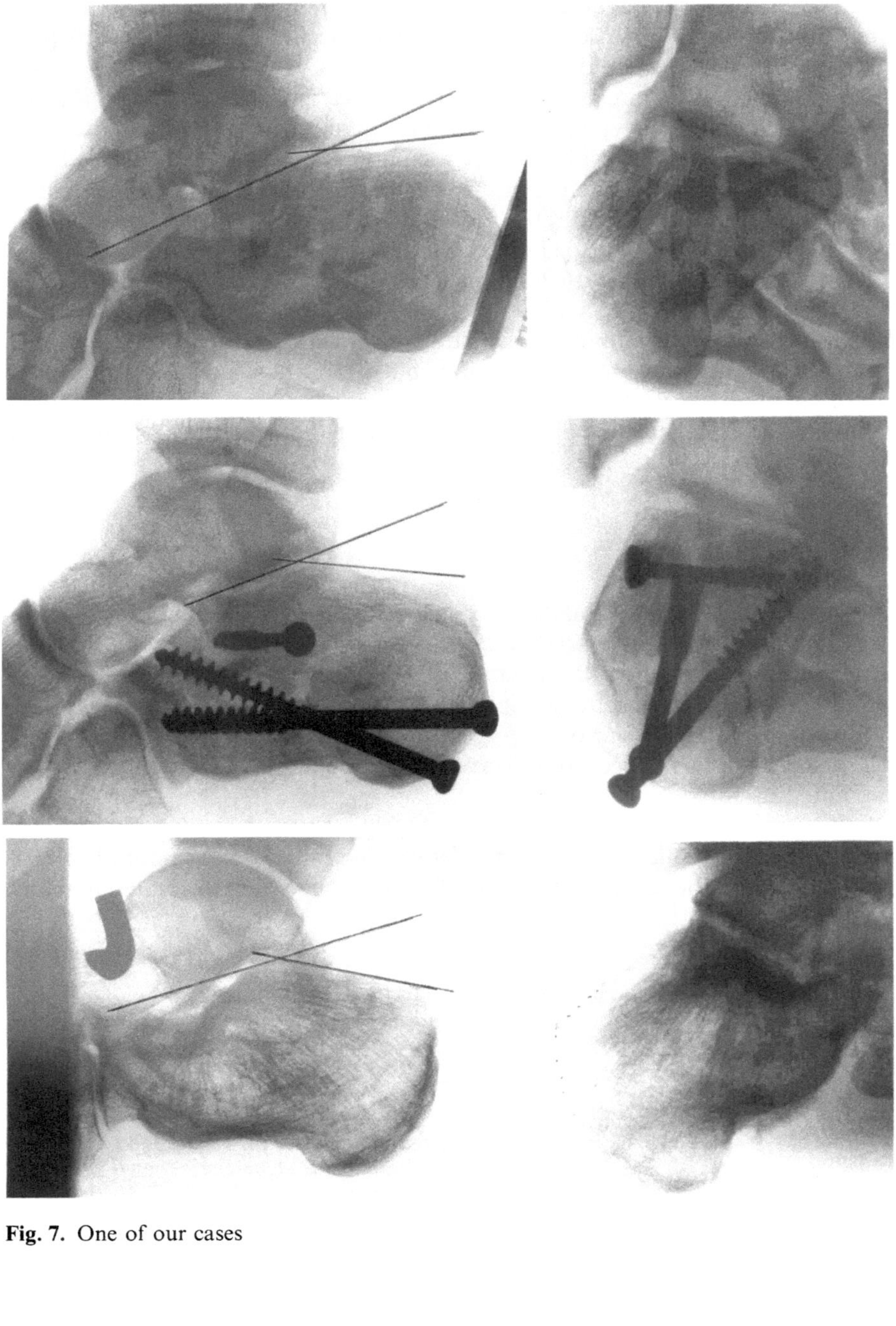

Fig. 7. One of our cases

After a successful reduction the fracture itself is fixed with two long AO cancellous bone screws inserted through small incisions into the heel. If possible the two screws should cross each other (Figs. 6 and 7).
After completion of internal fixation, the device is loosened by turning the wheels back, and removed along with the Kirschner wires. The small incisions on the heel are sutured. After closure a compression bandage is applied.
The stabilization of the fracture in this way makes other fixation unnecessary, and active motion exercises of the foot and ankle can be started immediately. Walking with crutches is also allowed – at first without loading then, after 3–4 days, with cautious, moderate loading. The patient's stay in hospital is usually 8–10 days.
It is not easy to believe that this single fixation with two or three screws will hold the fracture without redislocation, but it is a fact we have established based on our experience with 265 cases. The screws support the strong cortical points of the calcaneus like pillar-supports inserted during the rebuilding of a house (Fig. 6). Figure 7 illustrates one of our cases.

Evaluation of Results

Our results [3, 7] were evaluated retrospectively using a special points system [4] which measures many variables indicative of the state of the foot (Table 1). The maximum score is 100. A score of 80–100 is rated excellent, 70–80 is good, 60–70 is moderate and below 60 is poor.
Follow-up time was 1 year on average. The average age of the patients was 41 years. Return to work occurred on average after 6 months. Complications are presented in Table 2.
Of the 265 cases treated in this way, 42.6% achieved results classified as excellent, 42.7% as good, 7.8% as moderate, and only 2.7% as poor (Table 3). In the literature the results of calcaneal fractures have been evaluated in many

Table 1. The point system used for evaluating results

Pain
Range of motion (in degrees)
Radiograph
Function
Limp
Walking distance
Walking up and down stairs
Walking on a slope
Rising on tiptoe
Running
Use of a stick
Orthopaedic shoe

Table 2. Complications

Complications	Patients	
	Number	%
Redislocation of the fracture	12	4.1
Failure of the technique	6	2.0
Problems in wound healing	10	3.7
Side plate syndrome	15	5.1
Sinus tarsi syndrome	2	1.0
Post-traumatic flat foot	11	4.1
Sudeck syndrome	0	

Table 3. Results

Fracture type	Result			
	Excellent	Good	Moderate	Poor
I	39	35	7	0
II	39	51	12	3
III	35	39	1	4
	113 (42.6%)	125 (47.1%)	20 (7.5%)	7 (2.6%)
	238 (89.8%)		27 (10.2%)	

different ways. It is thus not possible to compare our results with those from other studies. We believe, however, that our closed method, which overall produced 89.8% excellent or good results and only 10.2% moderate or poor results, must be an advance in the treatment of this unfortunate fracture.

References

1. Forgon M, Zadravecz G (1983) Zu den Repositions- und Retentionsproblemen der Kalkaneusfraktur. Aktuel Traumatol 13:239–246
2. Forgon M, Zadravecz G (1984) Our procedure in 207 comminuted fractures of the calcaneus. SICOT World Congress Edition, London
3. Forgon M, Zadravecz G (1987) Unser Verfahren zur Behandlung der Kalkaneusfractur. Hefte Unfallheilk 200:255–256
4. Forgon M, Zadravecz G (1990) Die Kalkaneusfraktur. Springer, Berlin Heidelberg New York
5. Zadravecz G, Forgon M (1982) Radiographic investigation of the subtalar joint (in Hungarian). Magyar Traumatol Orthop Helyreallito Sebesz 25:44–47
6. Zadravecz G, Palkó A (1982) Radiographic examination of the calcaneus: the "oblique" technique (in Hungarian). Magyar Radiol 34:13–20
7. Zadravecz G, Szekeres P. (1984) Spätergebnisse unserer Behandlungsmethode der Kalkaneusfraktur. Aktuell Traumatol 14:218–226

Results of Operative Treatment of Calcaneal Fractures

S.K. Benirschke, K.A. Mayo, B.J. Sangeorzan, and S.T. Hansen

Introduction

The calcaneum is the most commonly fractured tarsal bone, and to date is still regarded as an enigma for orthopaedic surgeons. Therapeutic options are varied, and one can find support for either aggressive or conservative methods of treatment. The controversy between operative and conservative treatment hinges on the patient's clinical result, many facets of which are purely subjective in nature. The resultant disability is difficult to establish, as it depends on the patient's ability to return to premorbid activities. Gait abnormality, pain, and decreased subtalar and ankle range of motion are just a few of the factors that must be considered when evaluating the functional results following these difficult fractures. The confusion regarding treatment options is also the result of inconsistent radiographic methods used to evaluate the fractured os calcis. This paper describes our method of operative treatment of this fracture, with an analysis of the functional results following treatment.

Patients and Methods

A retrospective analysis of 65 patients with 80 operatively treated calcaneal fractures was undertaken in patients treated between January 1, 1985 and December 31, 1988 at the University of Washington, Seattle, WA. Patients were examined in follow-up from 6 months to 54 months, using physical examination to evaluate the range of motion and hindfoot symptoms. Ankle range of motion was measured as degrees less than the motion of the uninjured side. Subtalar range of motion was measured as a percentage of the range on the unaffected side, i.e. <25%, 25%–50%, 50%–75%, 75%, or >75%. Shoewear modification, if used, was noted. Return to preinjury activities was noted. Results of a questionnaire to evaluate patient impressions following surgery are still undergoing review.

Preoperative treatment involved splinting and elevating the ankle in the neutral position, with radiographic evaluation consisting of lateral and axial (Harris) views, along with two-plane CT scans. Fractures were classified according to Letournel's system, based on examination of radiographs, CT scans, and intraoperative findings (Fig. 1–6).

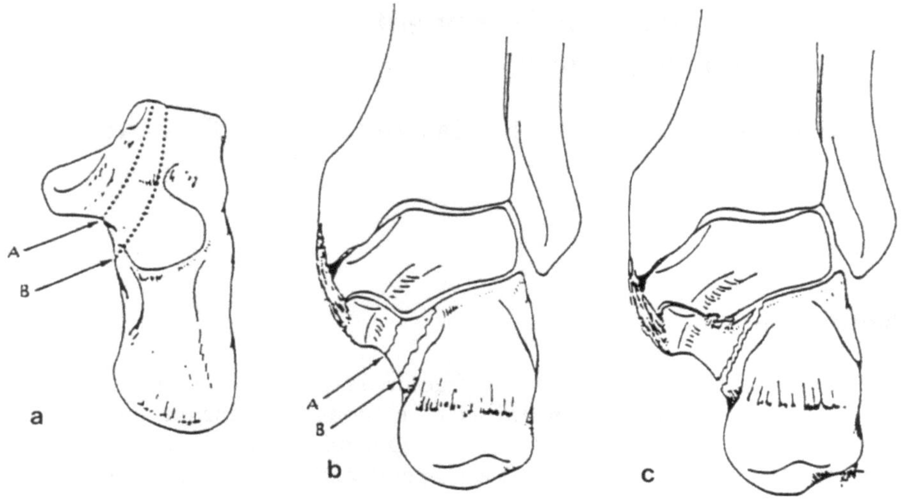

Fig. 1a–c. The constant separation fracture line. **a** The fracture runs through the sinus tarsi behind the interosseous ligament. **b** The fracture intersects the thalamus. **c** A two-fragment fracture without displacement (exceptional)

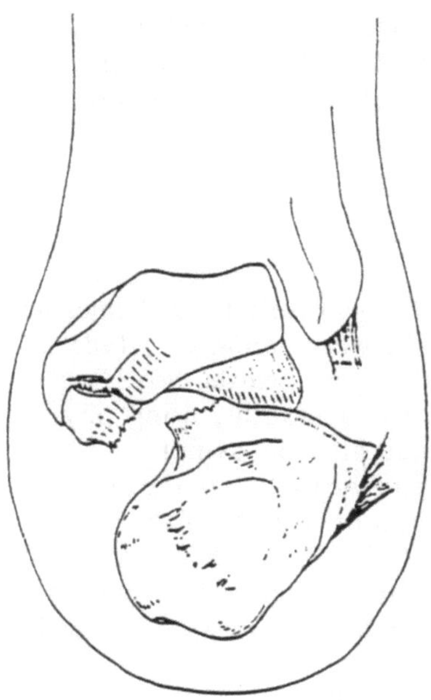

Fig. 2. Two-fragment fracture of the calcaneus. The inner fragment remains connected to the talus. The external one is dislocated outwardly

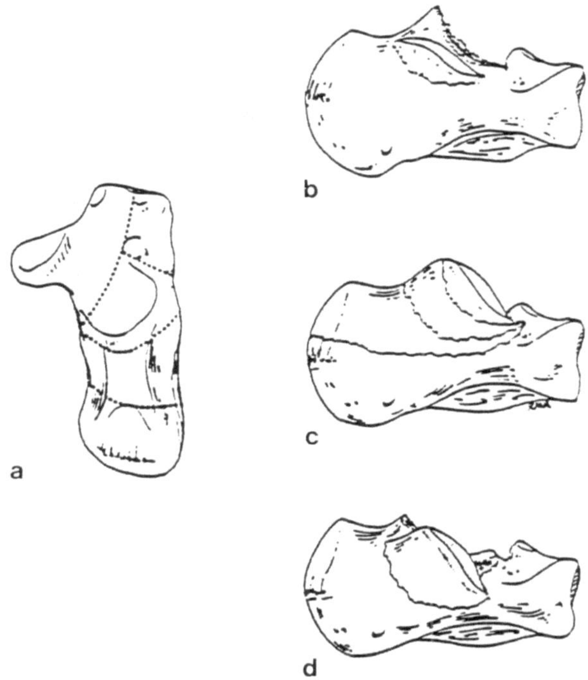

Fig. 3a–d. Three-fragment fractures. **a** Impaction of the thalamus: the various fracture lines seen from above. **b** Horizontal impaction of the thalamus. **c** Possible fracture lines of a vertical impaction. **d** Vertical impaction of the thalamus

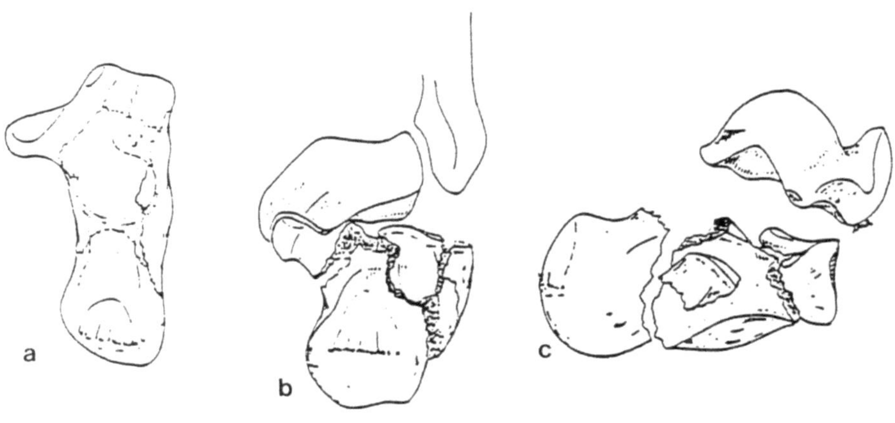

Fig. 4a–c. Complex calcaneus fractures comprising four fragments or more. **a** Fracture lines on the upper aspect of the bone. **b** The fracture seen from behind. **c** Profile of the same case

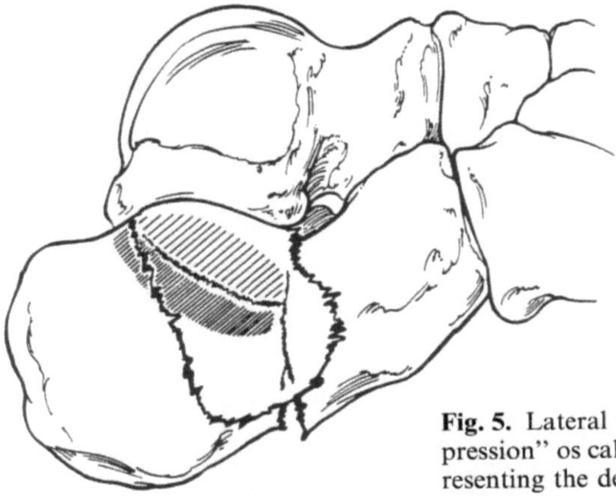

Fig. 5. Lateral view of a typical four-part "joint depression" os calcis fracture, with the *shaded area* representing the depressed segment

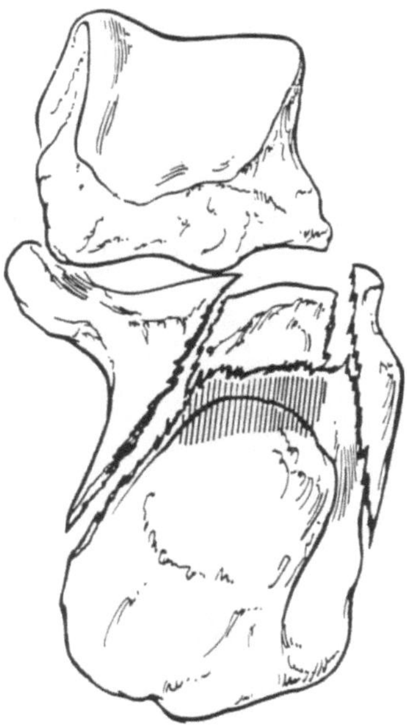

Fig. 6. Axial view (Harris 45° oblique) demonstrating the four components of the fracture: medial sustentacular fragment, central depressed fragment, lateral wall/posterior facet fragment, and tuberosity

Resolution of swelling usually required 3–5 days, but in some instances took as long as 14–21 days, with those fractures often accompanied by fracture blisters requiring debridement. After 10–14 days fracture reduction was often complicated by soft tissue contracture, specifically the triceps surae, and early healing. No fractures were operated on later than 6 weeks after the injury.

All patients underwent open reduction and internal fixation via a lateral approach, with three patients undergoing a simultaneous medial approach. A thigh-high tourniquet was routinely employed. The lateral approach was a modification of that described by Palmer and Letournel. The incision is a "J" shape for the left side or an "L" shape for the right side, with a subperiosteal dissection of the skin flap off of the lateral wall, comprising a periosteal-cutaneous flap (Fig. 7). Exposure in this manner allowed visualization from the tuberosity distally to the calcaneocuboid joint. In our early experience the more gently curving approach of Palmer and Letournel led to wound-healing problems at the apex of the incision, due to a concentration of tension at the suture line upon restoration of calcaneal length and height following reduction. After modification of the approach to the more pronounced "J" and "L" configurations there have been no wound complications with the exception of occasional superficial epithelial loss.

Positioning of the patient for surgery evolved to the patient being in the true lateral position on a beanbag, with care being taken to protect the down-sided brachial plexus and peroneal nerves. This afforded excellent visualization of the fracture anatomy, along with reproducible alignment of the foot for radiographic verification of reduction and implant position. Early attempts to perform the reduction in the supine position were met with frustration and therefore abandoned. The vast majority of procedures were done in the lateral position, with bilateral injuries treated consecutively rather than simultaneously.

Reduction aids included 4.0 and 5.0 mm Schanz pins placed intraoperatively in the tuberosity component of the fracture (Fig. 8). This aided in the manipulation of the tuberosity, so that the subsequent reduction of the articular surface was obtained and held with 0.045 in and 0.054 in Kirschner wires. The anterior process component of the fracture was simultaneously reduced (including those fractures involving the calcaneocuboid joint) and held in a similar fashion (Fig. 9).

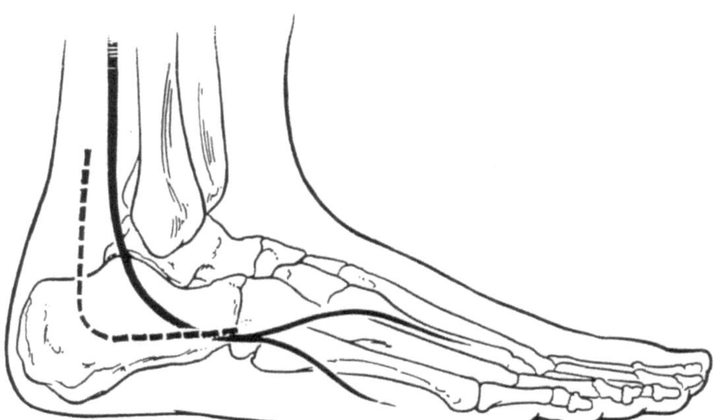

Fig. 7. Surgical approach shown as *dashed line*, with sural nerve shown just above it within the elevated periosteal-cutaneous flap

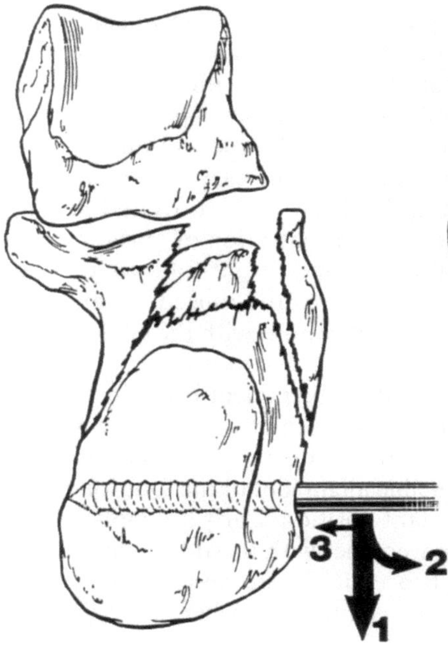

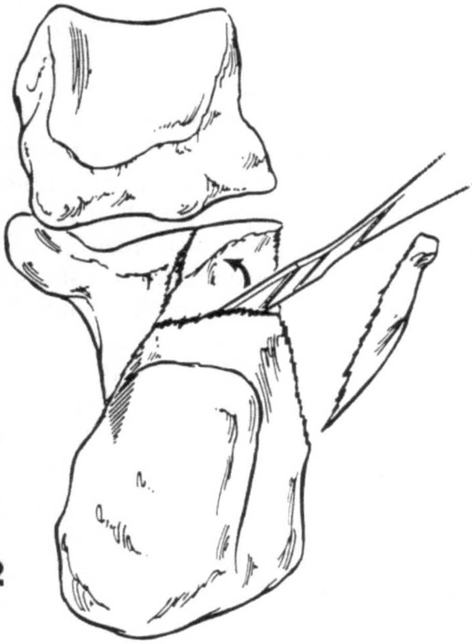

Fig. 8 *(left)*. 4.0/5.0-mm Schanz pin placed laterally in the tuberosity fragment, with vectors of manipulation shown as: *1*, restoration of height; *2*, valgus; and *3*, medial translation, all with reference to the sustentacular fragment. Medial wall reduction is indirect

Fig. 9 *(right)*. Freer elevator being used to reduce the depressed articular segment to the sustentacular fragment/medial posterior facet. The lateral wall/articular segment has been reflected, to aid in visualizing the medial component of the posterior facet reduction

The tuberosity component of the fracture, is routinely malaligned with varus, lateral translation, and shortening, was indirectly reduced to the medial wall and held with axial Kirschner wires. Prior to placement of fixation, true lateral and axial views of the foot were obtained to document reduction.

Internal fixation consisted of a 3.5 mm reconstruction plate, gently curved and positioned on the lateral side, from the anterior process to the tuberosity. Lag screw fixation was used to compress the articular reduction with two screws placed superior to the plate (Figs. 10, 11). Early attempts [10] were made to use the AO Y plate for additional tuberosity fixation, but difficulty in contouring led to the use of the reconstruction plate alone, or in combination with the cervical H plate placed under the reconstruction plate. In areas where screws could not be used, specifically the anterior process, Kirschner wires were placed and impacted next to the plate.

Sixty-two operative procedures incorporated autogenous cancellous bone grafting to the defect remaining after reduction, obtained either from the anterior or the posterior iliac crest. The surgical wound was closed over a 1/8 in. Hemovac drain, using an inverted buried suture of 2-0 Vicryl closing the

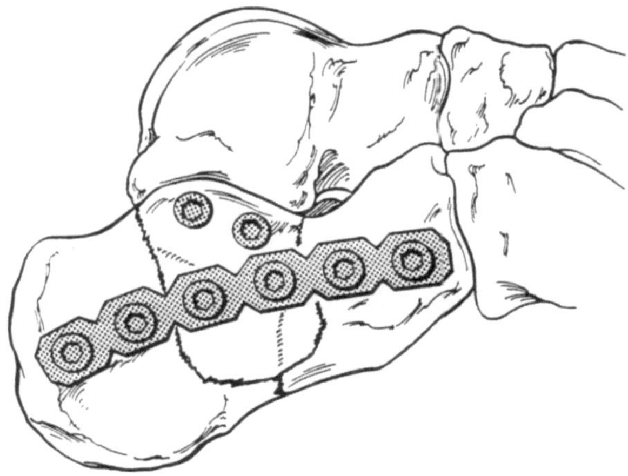

Fig. 10. Lateral view of the reconstruction using a 3.5-mm reconstruction plate extending from the tuberosity to the anterior process, with two separate 3.5-mm lag screws to stabilize the posterior facet

periosteal-subcutaneous layer, with a skin suture of 3-0 Dermalon. All cases were splinted and elevated in the neutral position of the foot and ankle for 72 h. Drains were removed approximately 48 h postoperatively.

Upon removal of the plaster splint, the limb was placed in a removable splint of aluminum lined with sheepskin. When the incision was dry (3–5 days) active range of motion of the ankle and subtalar joints was begun. Sutures were removed approximately 21 days after surgery. Patients were fitted with support stockings to control foot and ankle edema, and encouraged to wear them for at least 6 months postoperatively. Analgesics were generally discontinued 3–4 weeks after surgery, or, if continued, prescribed only for use at night. No non-steroids were used early in the postoperative course.

Non-weight-bearing ambulation was employed for 12 weeks, with active range of motion of the ankle and subtalar joints during this period. Patients with bilateral fractures were confined to bed-to-wheelchair ambulation during this period. Resumption of weight-bearing then ensued according to patient tolerance, with discontinuation of aids by 16–24 weeks. Individuals with unilateral fractures were instructed to weight-bear on the forefoot initially, with gradual resumption of heel-to-toe ambulation.

Patients were encouraged to use shoes with a shock-absorbing (i.e. Vibram) sole. Physical therapy modalities to help regain range of motion and strength were individualized, depending on financial means and patient motivation. If employed, these modalities were used for up to 6–12 months following surgery; thereafter they were found to be of questionable benefit. Hardware was removed in 58 cases as an outpatient procedure, with no restriction in weight-bearing after suture removal.

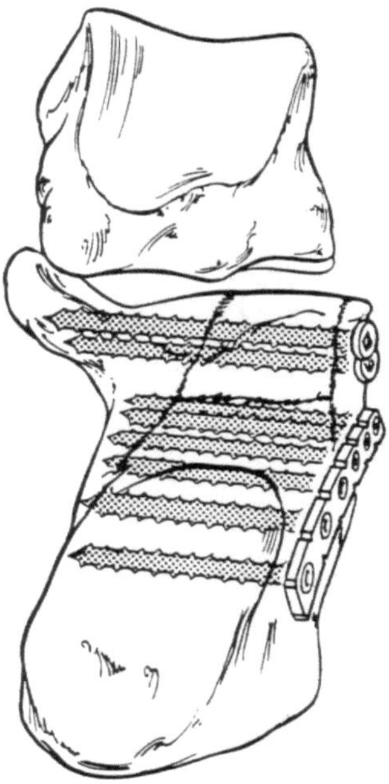

Fig. 11. Axial view of the reconstruction, showing the placement of the posterior facet lag screws into the sustentacular fragment

Results

Sixty-five patients with 80 displaced intra-articular os calcis fractures were reviewed by the authors in a follow-up that ranged from 6 months to 54 months. All but 2 patients had follow-up times longer than 6 months (mean 18 months). Patient age ranged from 13 to 69 years, with a mean of 36 years. There were 27 right, 23 left, and 15 bilateral fractures (19%). All patients with bilateral injuries were male. Of 65 patients studied, 57 were male and 8 were female (12%). Seventy-seven fractures were closed injuries; the 3 open injuries (4%) were medial in location.

Fractures were classified postoperatively on the basis of radiographs, CT scans, and intraoperative findings. They included: 0 two-part fractures (extremely rare), 33 (41%) three-fragment fractures, and 47 (59%) four-fragment and more complex fracture variants (see Figs. 1–4). CT was helpful in delineating tuberosity position, size of sustentacular fragment, and presence/absence of calcaneocuboid involvement. Intraoperative findings often worsened the classification type, due to unrecognized articular injury and/or the discovery of additional fracture fragments.

Injury mechanism involved a fall or jump from a height in 50 patients (77%) and a motor vehicle accident in 13 (16%). One of the remaining 2 patients was injured in a pedestrian vs. car accident and the other had the limb crushed by a car. Thirty-six patients (55%) had their os calcis fracture(s) as an isolated injury. Twenty-nine patients had associated injuries, including spine fractures, closed head injury, pelvic fractures, long bone fractures, and ipsilateral foot trauma. Twelve patients (18%) had spinal fractures associated with their os calcis fracture(s): 3 were incomplete lesions, while the remainder were neurologically intact with respect to their spinal fracture.

All patients underwent open reduction and internal fixation, 79 with a combination of plate(s), screws and Kirschner wires, and the remaining 13-year-old with screws alone. Autogenous cancellous bone grafting was used in 62 cases (77%). Hardware was removed in 58 cases (72%), routinely 12 months after surgery.

Eight procedures (10%) developed wound complications at the apex of the surgical incision necessitating local wound care, with the wound healing in by secondary intention. These were after the use of the approach described by Palmer and Letournel. The "J" and "L" approaches used later did not lead to the apical wound problems seen with the more gently curving approach.

There were five infections (6%), with no early infections secondary to the surgical approach. Three patients developed cellulitis laterally 3–6 months postoperatively; each case resolved upon removal of the hardware and with short-term antibiotics. The three patiens concerned were a chronic alcoholic, a paranoid schizophrenic with incomplete paraplegia, and a patient with a severe closed head injury. A fourth patient, with a grade III B open calcaneal fracture, developed persistent drainage from the medial wound. Drainage ultimately ceased following medial debridement of necrotic bone fragments and lateral hardware removal. The final, deep infection involved a patient who seeded his right subtalar joint 9 months postoperatively, secondary to an intravenous cocaine injection. He was treated with staged debridement, placement of an antibiotic-impregnated methylmethacrylate "spacer," and oral antibiotics until the sedimentation rate returned to normal. Ultimately, 4 months after debridement, he underwent a subtalar distraction bone-block arthrodesis, resulting in a solid fusion with no residual infection.

Three patients underwent subtalar arthrodesis, 2 within the first year. The first patient was discussed above. The second had a compartment syndrome and comminuted calcaneal and talar fractures. Her fixation failed, and she underwent a successful arthrodesis with resolution of her pain. The third patient, with bilateral injuries, underwent a right subtalar arthrodesis 18 months after the injury, for painful arthritic symptoms unresponsive to nonsteroidal medications. All patients had Letournel complex fracture types (more than four).

A decrease in ankle range of motion of $>10°$ occurred in 8 patients, 5 of whom had ipsilateral foot trauma (ankle fracture, talus fracture, compartment syndrome). The remaining patients had $<10°$ loss of ankle range of motion. Patients with bilateral injuries attained at least 40° arc of motion.

Subtalar range of motion was initially quantified in degrees, but due to examiner error and wide patient variability it was than assessed as the percentage of the patient's subtalar range of motion on the uninjured side. This was found to be reproducible and more wieldy as a means of interpatient comparison.

Sixteen patients (20%) had >75% subtalar motion, 15 (19%) had 75% subtalar motion, 34 (42%) had 50%–75% subtalar motion, 11 (14%) had 25%–50% subtalar motion, and 4 (5%) had <25% subtalar motion.
Four patients required shoe inserts or modification for ambulation. The remainder either returned to previous shoe wear or adopted use of a shoe with a shock-absorbing sole (i.e. Vibram). The latter was at the authors' encouragement.
Three patients had symptomatic sural neuromata at the superior portion of the lateral incision. One patient had a transposition of the neuroma at the time of hardware removal; the other 2 are considering operative transposition. No patients were made neurologically worse secondary to operative intervention, with the exception of peri-incisional numbness that had a variable return. Most patients who presented with tibial nerve sensory deficits had partial or complete return of sensation within 4 weeks of injury. More dense tibial nerve deficits took correspondingly longer to resolve (6–9 months), as might be expected.
Twenty patients (30%) had significant activity modifications, involving either a change in work status to a more sedentary occupation, or vocational rehabilitation to achieve the same. The remainder returned to their previous activities, with variable modification in recreational pursuits. Patients followed for more than 2 years noted continued improvement in subtalar symptoms. Patients with the more severely injured subtalar joints developed symptoms sooner.
One patient, a 69-year-old man, died of a myocardial infarction 6 weeks after being struck by a car as a pedestrian. He sustained a right hip fracture, a left Schatzker type III tibial plateau fracture, and a right joint-depression four-part os calcis fracture. He underwent internal fixation of all his orthopaedic injuries, and was mobilized from bed to chair early. Autopsy confirmed severe three-vessel coronary artery disease with acute infarction. This was the oldest patient in our series.

Discussion

Surgical management of intra-articular calcaneal fractures remains a controversial subject. It is routinely one of the few articular fractures that is nonoperatively treated. Patients learn to live with their disability, and are told that a fusion (triple, subtalar) in the hindfoot area can be done as a salvage procedure. Unfortunately, the deformities arising from many conservatively treated calcaneal fractures lead to complex salvage attempts with less than optimal results. Not only is the subtalar joint involved, but the tuberosity malalignment usually results in a short, wide, varus heel. The heel lever is shortened, and the overlying tibiotalar relationships are altered, leading to earlier arthritic spurring of the talar neck secondary to dorsiflexion impingement. This is as a result of the talus being driven down into the calcaneal body at the moment of injury, changing what has been referred to as the "talar-floor" angle from approximately 30° to nearly 0°. Thus, the subtalar relationships and the tibiotalar mechanics are altered. An isolated in situ subtalar fusion does not help to correct the secondary changes seen in the ankle. The distraction bone block arthrodesis is a salvage attempt to correct both the ankle and subtalar problems.

Our enthusiasm for treating calcaneal fractures operatively has been motivated by the problems our foot clinic routinely sees in following os calcis fractures in the long term. We initially gave each patient the option of surgical treatment, if desired and medically safe. The subsequent problems with the more difficult patient population, i.e. those that we had problems with as regards soft tissue management, have led us to be somewhat more selective about this procedure. The process requires a close interaction between patient and surgeon, with patience necessary for both individuals.

The early wound problems noted with the standard approach were very disconcerting, and only after successful modification of the approach and various aspects of the procedure was our confidence restored. Currently we are experimenting with allograft bone grafts rather than autogenous sources of cancellous bone, and have been satisfied with the early results. Perhaps the bone graft is not necessary, as in Professor Letournel's experience, but in our hands delayed collapse has been noted in those patients not bone grafted.

The lack of ankle symptoms following surgery supports our assumption that restoration of calcaneal shape does make a difference. Our aim was to reconstruct the entire bone, in shape and substance, with restoration of articular congruity as part of the process. The development of subtalar arthritis following surgery is viewed not as a failure of management but the sequela of a damaged joint – with a fairly simple solution. Despite the presence of arthritic symptoms in many of our patients, because the rest of the hindfoot has been restored the evolution of disabling symptoms appears lengthier, in our short-term experience.

There is no question that there was a tremendously steep learning curve in our treatment of these fractures. We would not like those individuals interested in treating calcaneal fractures to have to repeat our mistakes in order to gain "experience."

Rather, we hope that our methods can be adapted to suit those wishing to pursue this fascinating area. The patients are extremely grateful, and one learns far more about them in the course of following their progress than one does with the care of other fractures. The fact that they continue to improve years later is very encouraging. The early results are gratifying. However, only long-term results of 5–10 years or more will tell us whether we have altered the course of the natural history of this complex hindfoot injury.

Conclusion

This retrospective review of the operative treatment of 80 intra-articular calcaneal fractures has demonstrated that surgical intervention is a viable alternative to conservative treatment. The lateral approach, with an indirect reduction of the tuberosity position and otherwise direct correction of os calcis shape and posterior facet and calcaneocuboid congruity, is the optimal method for treating these injuries. Careful attention to detail, not only in bony reconstruction but also in the treatment of the soft tissues, can lead to a successful surgical result.

References

1. Aitken AP (1963) Fractures of the os calcis – treatment by closed reduction. CORR 30:67–75
2. Bèzes H, Massart P, Fourquet JP (1984) Die Osteosynthese der Calcaneus-Impressionsfraktur. Unfallheilkunde 87:363–368
3. Böhler L (1956) Treatment of fractures, 5th edn. Grune and Stratton, New York
4. Burdeaux BD (1983) Reduction of calcaneal fractures by the McReynolds medial approach: technique and its experimental basis. CORR 177:87–103
5. Carr JB, Hansen ST, Benirschke SK (1988) Subtalar distraction bone block fusion for late complications of os calcis fractures. Foot Ankle 9/2:81–86
6. Cave EF (1963) Fracture of the os calcis – the problem in general. CORR 30:64–66
7. Essex-Lopresti P (1951) Results of reduction in fractures of the calcaneum. J Bone Joint Surg [Br] 33:284
8. Essex-Lopresti P (1952) The mechanism, reduction technique and results in fractures of the os calcis. Br J Surg 39:395–419
9. Gallie WE (1943) Subastragalar arthrodesis in fractures of the os calcis. J Bone Joint Surg 25:731–736
10. Gilmer PW, Herzenberg J, Frank JL, Silverman P, Martinez S, Goldner JL (1986) Computerized tomographic analysis of acute calcaneal fractures. Foot Ankle 6/4:184–193
11. Gould N (1984) Lateral approach to the os calcis. Foot Ankle 4/4:218–220
12. Hall MC, Pennal GF (1960) Primary subastragalar arthrodesis in the treatment of severe fractures of the calcaneum. J Bone Joint Surg [Br] 42:336–343
13. Lance EM, Carey EJ Jr, Wade PA (1963) Fractures of the os calcis – treatment by early mobilization. CORR 30:76–90
14. LeTournel E (1984) Open reduction and internal fixation of calcaneus fractures. In: Spiegel P (ed) Topics in orthopaedic trauma. Aspen, Baltimore, pp 173–192
15. Maxfield JE (1963) Os calcis fractures – treatment by open reduction. CORR 30:91–99
16. Palmer I (1948) The mechanism and treatment of fractures of the calcaneus: open reduction with the use of cancellous grafts. J Bone Joint Surg [Am] 30:2–6
17. Pozo SL, Kirwan EO'G, Jackson AM (1984) The long term results of conservative management of severely displaced fractures of the calcaneus. J Bone Joint Surg [Br] 66/3:386–390
18. Ross DK (1987) The operative treatment of complex os calcis fractures. Techniques Orthop 2/3:55–70
19. Rowe CR, Sakellarides HT, Freeman PA, Sorbie C (1963) Fractures of the os calcis: a long-term follow-up study of 146 patients. JAMA 184:920–923
20. Sartoris DJ, Feingold ML, Resnick D (1985) Axial computed tomographic anatomy of the foot: 1: Hindfoot. J Foot Surg 24/6:392–412

21. Stephenson JR (1987) Treatment of displaced intraarticular fractures of the calcaneus using a medial/lateral approach, internal fixation and early motion. J Bone Joint Surg [Am] 69:115–130
22. Tanke GM (1982) Fractures of the calcaneus: a review of the literature together with some observations on methods of treatment. Acta Chir Scand Suppl 505:1–103

Dorsoplantar Approach to the Calcaneus

J. Poigenfürst

Introduction

The dorsoplantar approach to the calcaneus combines the possibility of wide exposure with a minimal risk of nervous or vascular disturbance. It makes use of an interneural plane between saphenous and sural nerve and an intervascular plane between tibial and peroneal artery and their concomitant veins (Fig. 1). The line of incision follows the lateral border of the Achilles tendon, crosses the midline of the heel, and runs through the sole of the foot to the tubercle of the fifth metatarsal. All nerves and vessels crossing this line are only part of a network with multiple anastomoses. No harm is to be expected when any of them are severed. It is essential, that the cut goes right down to the bone, the plantar aponeurosis, and the short plantar muscles. If one starts isolating layers of tissue, the vascularity of the overlying skin is at risk.

Surgical Technique

Exposure of the Lateral Surface of the Calcaneus (Fig. 2). All soft tissues are separated from the bone by sharp and blunt dissection. As soon as the crossing of the peroneus longus tendon is visible it is followed retrograde to the lateral ankle. In this way a full-thickness flap with broad base can be raised. If only decompression of lateral impingement is indicated, dissection can at this point be stopped since the peroneal tendons do not have to be exposed any further.

Exposure of the Upper Surface of the Calcaneus. By excising the fatty pad anterior to the Achilles tendon with part of the bursa and the posterior capsule, the upper surface is exposed and access to the subtalar joint is free.

Exposure of the Plantar Surface of Calcaneus (Fig. 3). Plantar aponeurosis, abductor digiti minimi, flexor digitorum brevis, abductor hallucis, and the medial part of flexor hallucis brevis are dissected close to their origin from the tuber, leaving just enough tissue for resuturing. As the nerve supply comes from the medial side and enters the muscles in a retrograde curve, the muscles can be moved medially and distally without risk. The same applies to flexor accessorius (=quadratus plantae). In this way more or less the entire plantar surface of the calcaneus is exposed. In the case of long-standing fractures, protruding fragments can be removed; in more recent injuries the fragments can now be manipulated from the plantar and lateral side.

Exposure of the Medial Surface of the Calcaneus. If a full-thickness flap, similar to the lateral side, is mobilized across the Achilles tendon in the direction of the medial ankle, limited access to the medial surface is possible. If this approach has been planned from the beginning, the entire flap can be kept together with the plantar aponeurosis and short plantar muscles, and all structures can be moved simultaneously.

Exposure of the Subtalar Joint (Fig. 4). With the aid of a Steinmann pin the tuber can be tilted laterally or medially. In this way fractures are mobilized and the subtalar joint can be inspected and cleared of debris.

Indications

We have used this approach in 15 operations, for decompression of lateral impingement, subtalar arthrodesis, together with calcaneocuboidal arthrodesis (Fig. 5), corrective osteotomy in long-standing fractures, removal of post-traumatic plantar spurs, and reduction of long-standing intra-articular fractures (Table 1). Stabilization was achieved by transarticular Kirschner wires (5 cases), screws (9 cases) and a plate (1 case). We have operated on only one fairly recent fracture in this way as we feel it may produce too many devascularized fragments.

Results

In the first 12 operations of our series no infection and no skin necrosis were observed. Among the 15 recent cases that we did there is one deep infection, one partial skin necrosis, and in two cases of temporarily diminished sensitivity at the lateral side of the foot. The patient with deep infection did not develop osteomyelitis and ended up with a foot similar to that seen after a "split heal procedure" [1]. The infection started most probably from the Kirschner wires when the patient was putting full weight on his cast. He does not want excision of the scar. The wound of the patient with partial skin necrosis has slowly

Table 1. Operations using the dorsoplantar approach ($n = 15$)

Decompression of lateral impingement	1
Decompression + subtalar athrodesis	6
Decompression + subtalar + calcaneocuboidal arthrodesis	2
Osteotomy + decompression + removal of plantar spur	1
Reduction and internal fixation (old fractures)	4
Reduction and internal fixation (recent fracture)	1

closed completely and the patient is now back at work in the trade building. The reason for the necrosis may have been too generous a use of electrocoagulation. Neurological disturbances on the lateral edge of the foot are caused mostly by rough treatment of the dorsolateral nerve, which lies in the subcutaneous fat close to the bone. In all other 13 cases the scars on the sole are hardly visible (Figs. 6, 7 and 8) and sensation was not diminished. Along the Achilles tendon the scars are always keloid-like, but the patients do not complain. This is more or less the only disadvantage of the dorsoplantar approach, except for one case where we found it difficult to build up enough tension within the calcaneus to support the lateral joint fragment by a bone graft.
The approach appears to be advantageous, especially since it offers the opportunity to place the osteosynthesis material whereever necessary, not limited by edges caused by small incisions. As the four postoperative complications did not produce any lasting negative effect, we feel that the dorsoplantar approach may be a valuable addition to our repertoire.

References

1. Gaenslen FJ (1931) Split-heel approach in osteomyelitis of os calcis. J Bone Joint Surg 13:759–772
2. Poigenfürst J (1991) Der dorsoplantare Zugang zum Fersenbein. Operative Orthop Traumatol (in press)

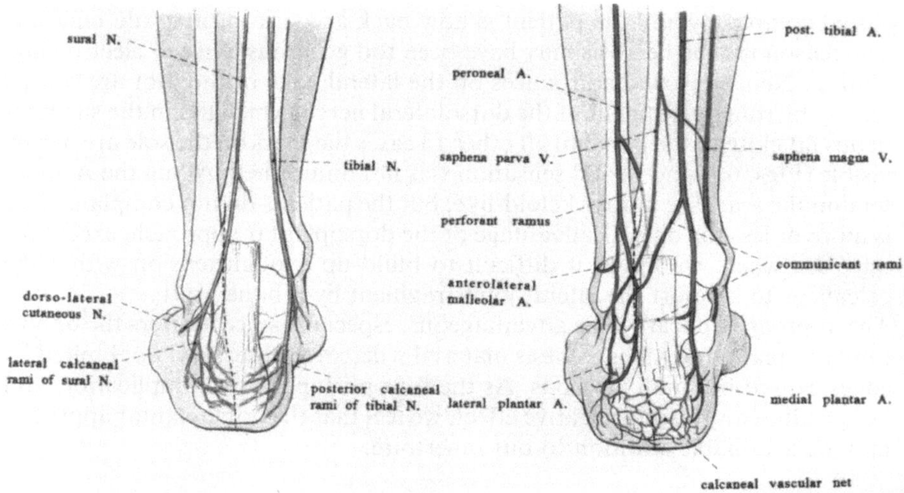

Fig. 1. Nervous and vascular supply of skin around the heel and line of incision. (From [2])

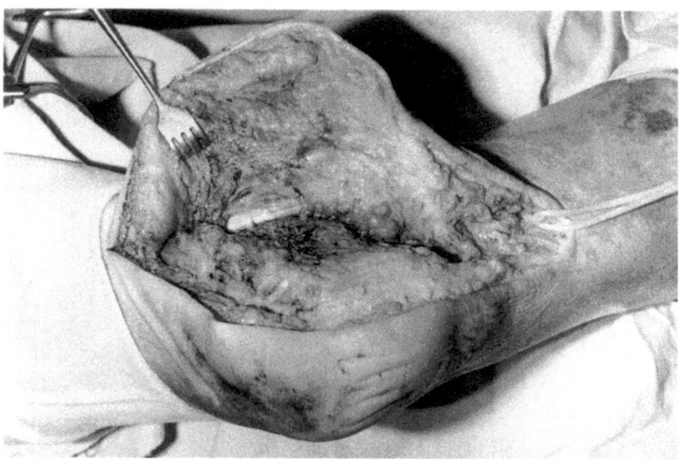

Fig. 2. A full-thickness flap with a broad base is raised from the calcaneus. The crossing of the peroneus longus tendon is visible

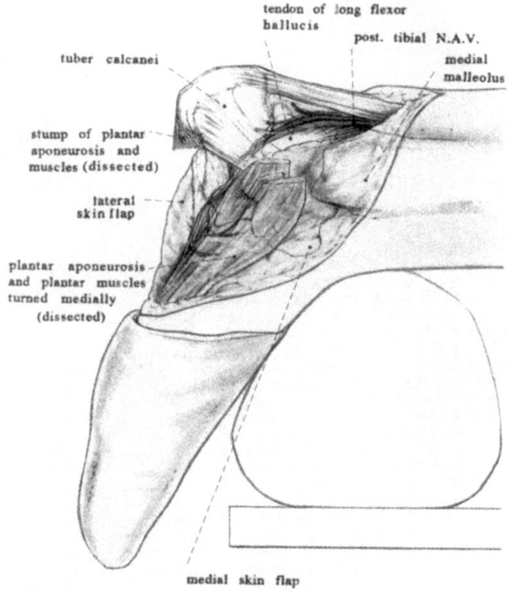

Fig. 3. Anatomical situation after exposure of the lateral and medial side. Plantar aponeurosis and muscles are cut close to their origin from the tuber and retracted medially together with the soft tissue flap. As the nerve supply comes from the medial side and enters the muscles distally, no harm can be done. (From [2])

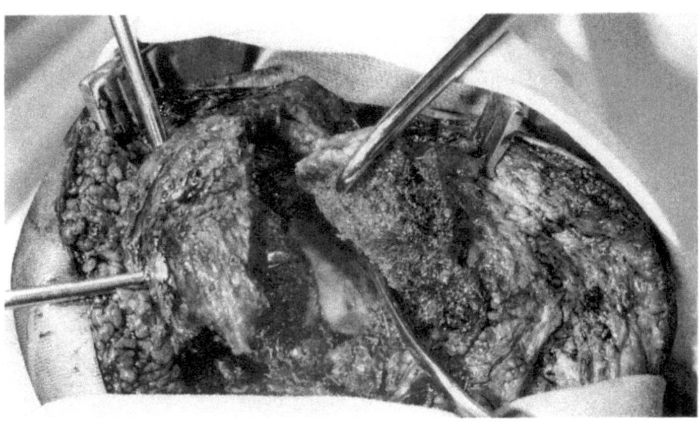

Fig. 4. Fragments are being held aside. The tuber is tilted by means of a Steinmann pin, exposing the plantar surface of the astragulus

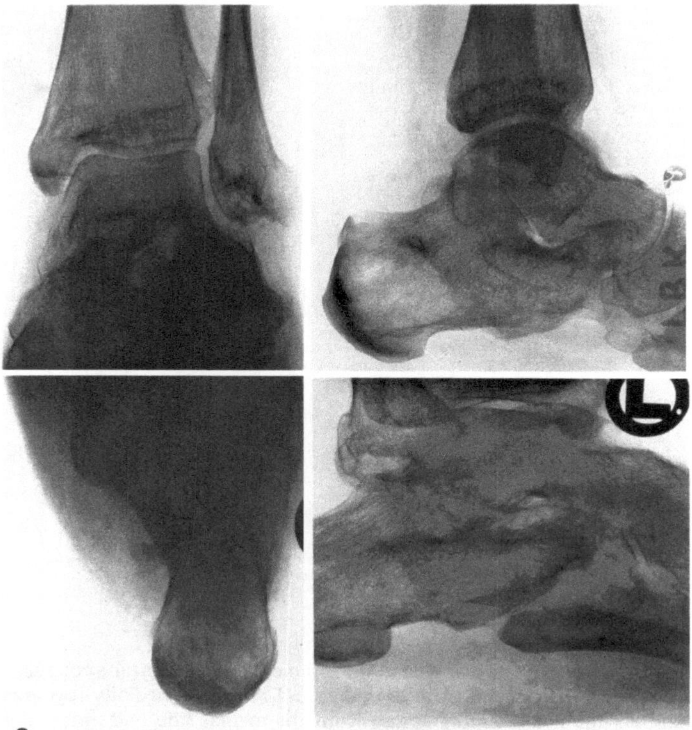

a

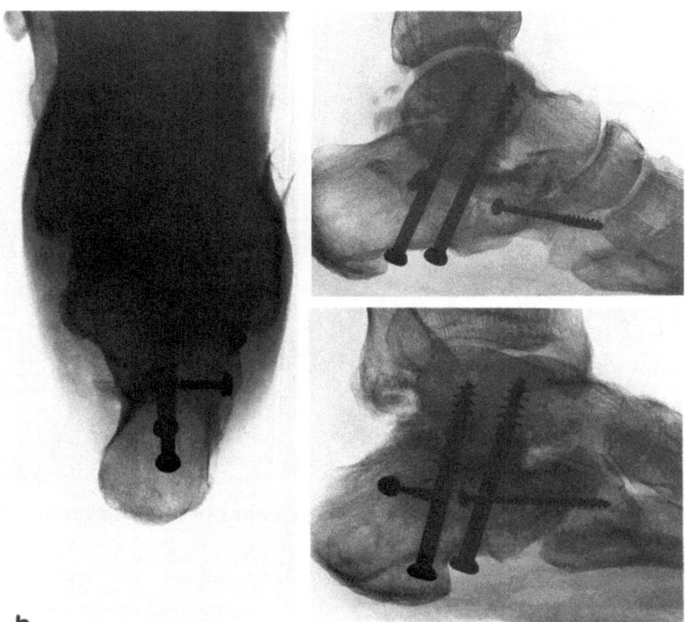

b

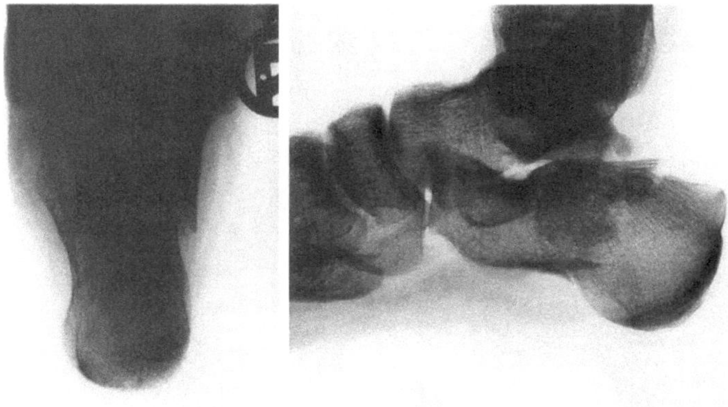

Fig. 6. Fracture of the calcaneus 2 weeks after injury

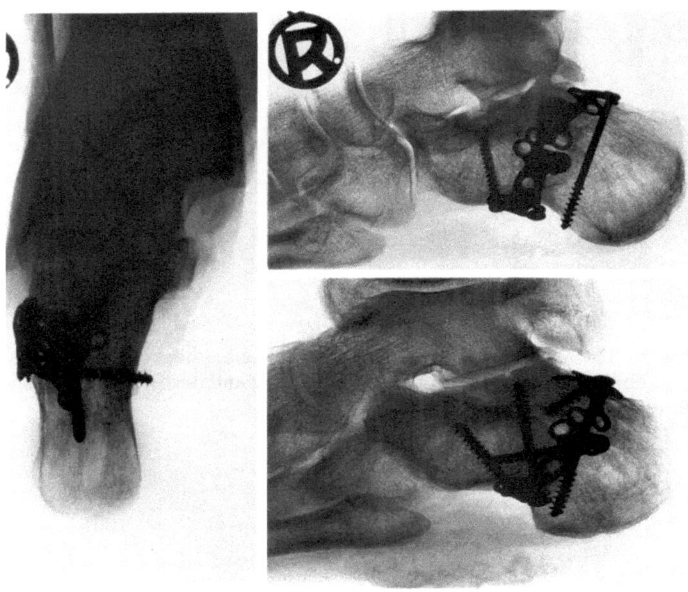

Fig. 7. Follow-up 11 months after open reduction by the dorsoplantar approach and osteosynthesis

◀ **Fig. 5a, b.** Subtalar arthrodesis, decompression of lateral impingement, and fusion of the calcaneocuboidal joint from the dorsoplantar approach after fracture of the calcaneus. (From [2])

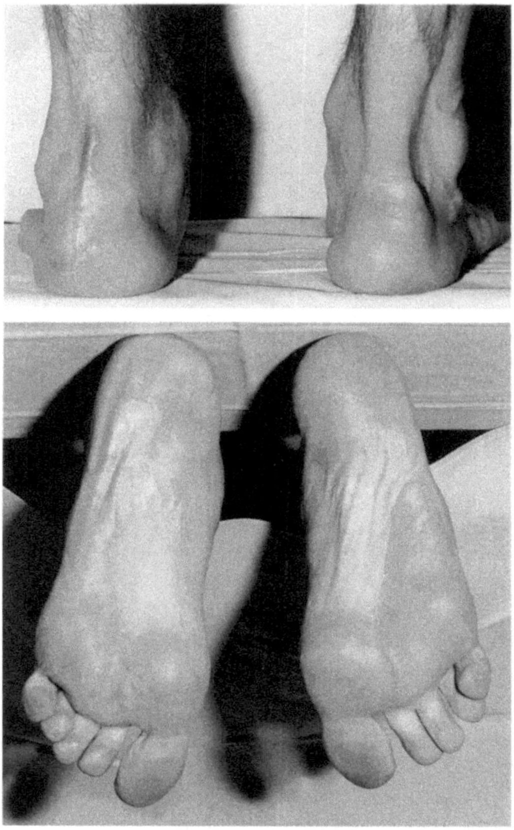

Fig. 8. The scar along the Achilles tendon is keloid like, but does not bother the patient. The scar on the heel and sole is practically invisible and does not hurt. The patient is back at work as an electrical engineer

Subtalar Arthrodesis for Treatment of Late Complications Following Calcaneal Fractures

L. Gotzen and F. Baumgaertel

Introduction

Following a calcaneal fracture many patients complain of symptoms of disability related to the fractured heel. As McLaughlin [8] stated, it must be realized that the subtalar joint is only one of the numerous sources of pain and gait disorders. Pain, mainly in the "outside ankle" region, is the most common symptom. Swelling involves the foot and ankle region, most frequently noted at the end of the day. Many patients complain of stiffness. There remain certain limitations regarding the ability to stand on the toes unaided, to walk comfortably on uneven ground, or to climb ladders. A decreased tuber joint angle up to 0°, producing a flatfooted gait, is not always a serious defect. If there is no osteoarthritis of the subtalar joint or a varus-valgus malalignment of the calcaneus, most patients do well. Some compensatory shortening of the calf muscles occurs and take-off strength gradually improves, but seldom returns to normal. Sooner or later, most patients who have fractured the calcaneus regain the ability to get around with reasonable comfort [8, 10].
Disappointing results with severe disability are related mainly to post-traumatic arthritis, mechanical malalignment, and impingement [1, 4, 6, 7, 9, 11, 13, 14]. Malunited vertical compression fractures are usually characterized by a varus as well as an upward displacement of the posterior half of the calcaneus. The lateral wall is expanded. A chronic stenosing tenosynovitis of the peroneal tendons behind and below the lateral malleolus is likely to result, as well as an impingement of the calcaneus against the fibula. The talus is often dorsiflexed, no longer aligns with the midfoot and forefoot, and is locked into the body of the calcaneus. The subtalar joint is destroyed. There is resultant anterior talotibial impingement and incongruity of the ankle joint.
When nonoperative treatment fails, arthrodesis is indicated as a reliable salvage procedure. The goals of surgical treatment are to relieve pain and to restore talocalcaneal alignment [13]. There is controversy in the literature about whether a triple arthrodesis, a double arthrodesis, or a talocalcaneal arthrodesis alone is the best method of treating degeneration and deformity of the talocalcaneal joint. We agree with those authors who favour isolated talocalcaneal arthrodesis and preservation of the calcaneocuboid and talonavicular joint unless these can be proven to be the source of disabling symptoms [3, 5, 7, 12]. For the majority of patients with a calcaneus distorted by fracture, a subtalar distraction bone-block fusion as advocated by Carr and colleagues [2] is indicated.

Patients and Methods

From 1986 through June 1990 ten talocalcaneal arthrodeses were performed for the treatment of post-traumatic arthritis of the talocalcaneal joint and calcaneal malalignment. Eight fractures had been treated nonoperatively and two fractures operatively with open reduction and internal fixation (ORIF). The time between the calcaneus fracture and the subtalar fusion averaged 18 months (range 7–48 months). The mean age of the patients was 32 years (range 22–62 years). There were 7 men and 3 women.
The common presenting symptoms were a combination of pain in the hind part of the foot, chronic swelling and stiffness in the hindfoot, marked limp, restriction of activities, the need for walking aids or special shoes, difficulty in walking on uneven ground, and limitation of walking distance. The preoperative physical findings included limited or complete loss of motion of the talocalcaneal joint, swelling and tenderness of the hindfoot, painful gait, deformity of the hindfoot, and dysfunction of the gastrocnemius-soleus complex. In all patients the indication for operative treatment consisted of functional disability and persistent incapacitating pain.
In one case an in situ subtalar fusion was done, two cases required a talocalcaneal arthrodesis in combination with a varus correction, and in seven cases a distraction bone-block arthrodesis was performed.

Surgical Technique

The patient is placed in a supine position with a sandbag under the buttock of the affected side and a pneumatic tourniquet on the thigh. A 6–8 cm oblique incision is directed along the lateral aspect of the hind part of the foot, over the region of the sinus tarsi. The sural nerve and the peroneal tendons, lying posteroinferior to the incision, are protected.
In patients suffering from an arthritis of the talocalcaneal joint but with relatively normal overall contour of the heel, heel height, and plane of the subtalar joint, the arthrodesis has only to address subtalar pain and is usually readily accomplished in satisfactory position. After distraction of the talus and calcaneus using a laterally placed distractor, adjacent joint surfaces are denuded of articular cartilage and cortical bone. Removal of the articular cartilage and subchondral bone creates a gap between the talus and the calcaneus that is approximately 5 mm high. The gap is closed with the distractor. For secure fixation, 6.5 mm cancellous bone screws are directed through the tuberosity of the calcaneus into the body of the talus.
A varus heel is badly tolerated by the patients. Even if the heel height is normal and a lateral impingement is not present, a varus deformity produces a poor result. The therapeutic approach is to perform a subtalar arthrodesis with correction of the malalignment. The principle of the varus deformity correction consists of removing a laterally based wedge from the calcaneus, including the joint surface, and resecting the subtalar joint surface (Fig. 1). After closing

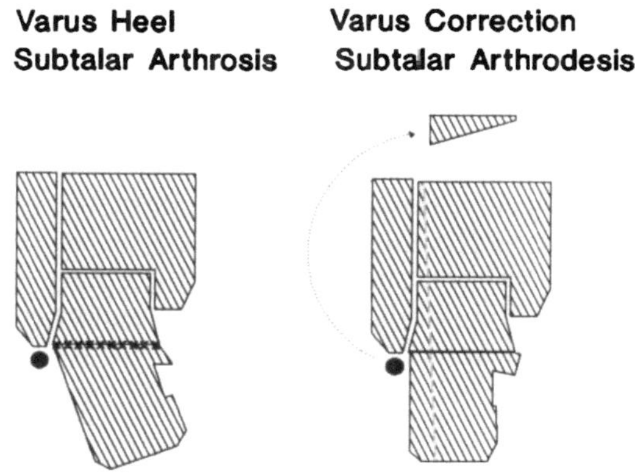

Fig. 1. Principle of varus correction and subtalar arthrodesis for varus heel and subtalar arthrosis

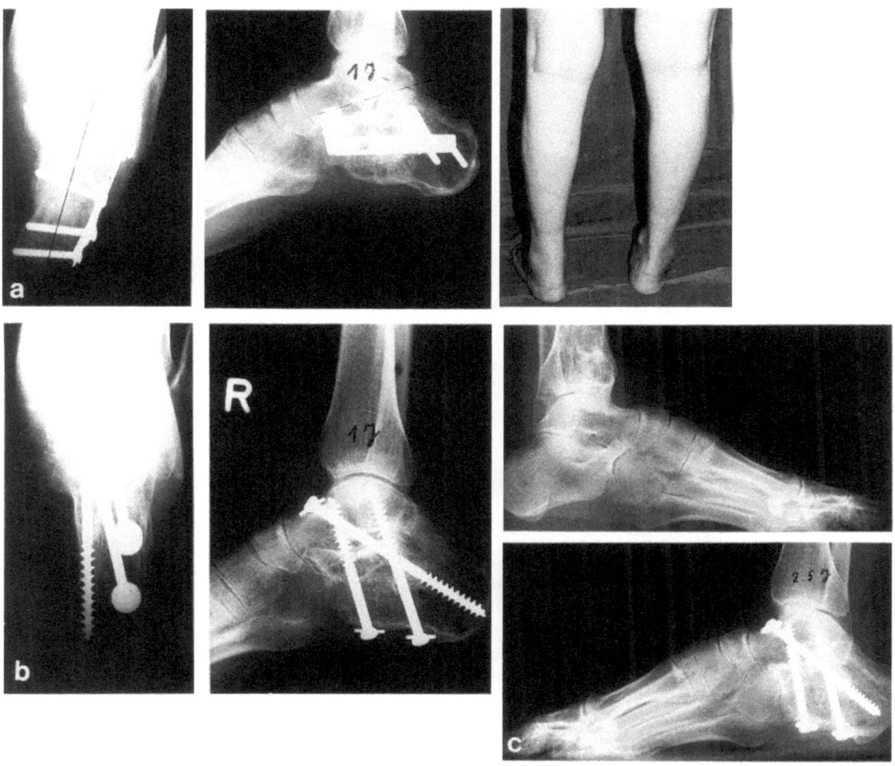

Fig. 2. **a** One year after ORIF of a comminuted fracture of the calcaneus with post-traumatic osteoarthritis and varus malalignment which is more apparent clinically. In addition to the calcaneal fracture the patient had sustained a pilon tibial fracture on the left side. **b** Subtalar screw arthrodesis with correction of the varus deformity at 1 year. Fusion union is solid. **c** Lateral weight-bearing views of both feet at 2.5 years. Note the congruent calcaneocuboid and talonavicular joints at the arthrodesis side without evidence of secondary degenerative changes

the osteotomy gap with the distractor, the position of the hindfoot and contact of the bone surfaces are verified with an image intensifier. Lag screw fixation is done as described above (Fig. 2).

In more complex calcaneal malunion with mechanical malalignment and lateral abutment, a distraction subtalar bone-block arthrodesis is necessary. This fusion technique is designed to restore the anatomical relations of the talus and calcaneus. The realignment unlocks the transverse tarsal joint, restores the heel height, corrects the flatfoot and properly repositions the talus in the ankle mortise. Should the peroneal space still be compromised following distraction of the calcaneus, the expanded lateral wall is removed (Fig. 3).

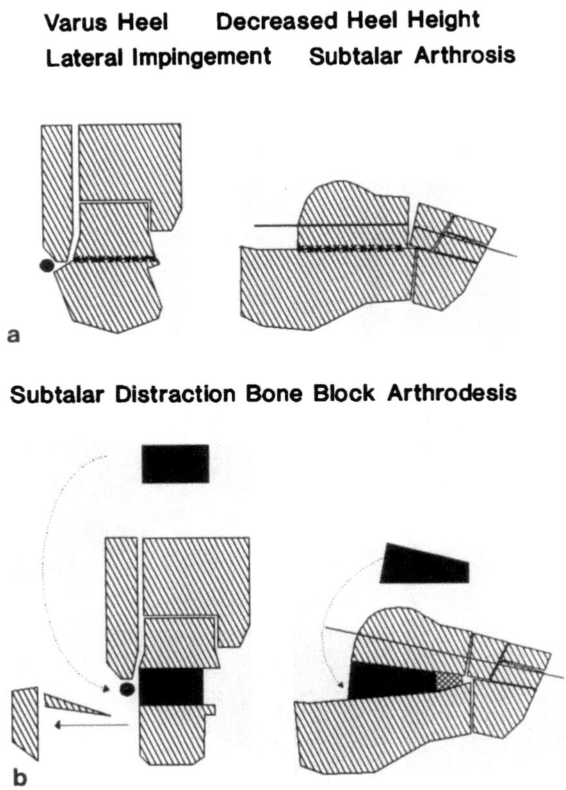

Fig. 3. **a** Composite schematic diagram of an old calcaneal fracture demonstrates that the heel is tilted into varus; the lateral wall of the calcaneus is expanded outward causing fibulocalcaneal impingement and dislocation of the peroneal tendons. The talus is impacted into the calcaneus and has lost its normal declination. The normal plantar arch of the hindfoot is reduced and the heel height is decreased. **b** Distraction bone-block arthrodesis of the subtalar joint. The varus deformity and the hindfoot height are corrected. Simultaneous lateral wall decompression is performed to relieve the narrow peroneal space. The normal relations between the talus and the calcaneus and between the hindfoot and midfoot are restored

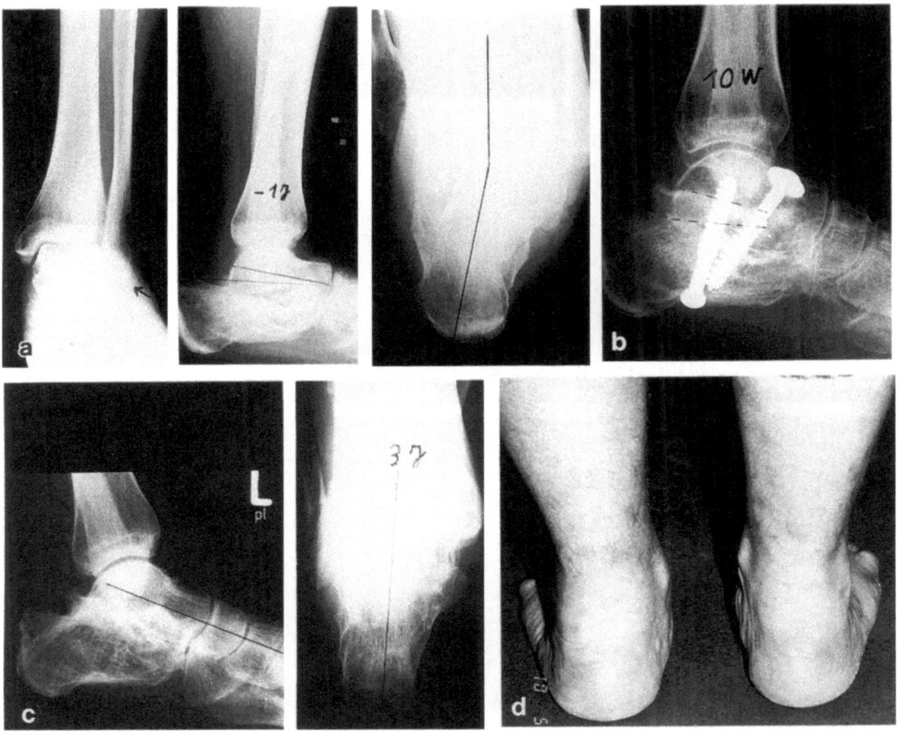

Fig. 4. **a** Radiographs of an old calcaneal fracture demonstrate dorsiflexion of the talus, impaction of the talus into the calcaneus, and valgus malalignment of the calcaneus. **b** The lateral view shows the postoperative status at 10 weeks. A large bone block has been interpositioned between the talus and calcaneus to restore full heel height and correct valgus. **c** Radiographs taken at 3 years show solid union, corrected valgus, and a nearly completely regained plantar arch. **d** Minimal clinically evident valgus of the hindfoot is seen; the biomechanics of the hindfoot are nevertheless restored

We usually use two distractors, one placed medially and one laterally into the calcaneus to distract the subtalar joint and to correct the malalignment. When the calcaneus is distracted back into its normal position and the joint surfaces are resected using an oscillating saw and chisels, a large full-thickness bone block is then inserted into the reopened and repositioned subtalar joint. The technical guidelines given by Carr et al. [2] and Hansen [5] should be strictly followed. A solid bone block taken from the patient's iliac crest is superior to bone bank material. For fixation, fully threaded 6.5 mm cancellous screws should be used instead of lag screws. Both autogenous bone-block material and fully threaded screws are safer in preventing secondary collapse and loss of correction. Figures 4 and 5 illustrate two clinical cases with distraction bone-block fusion.

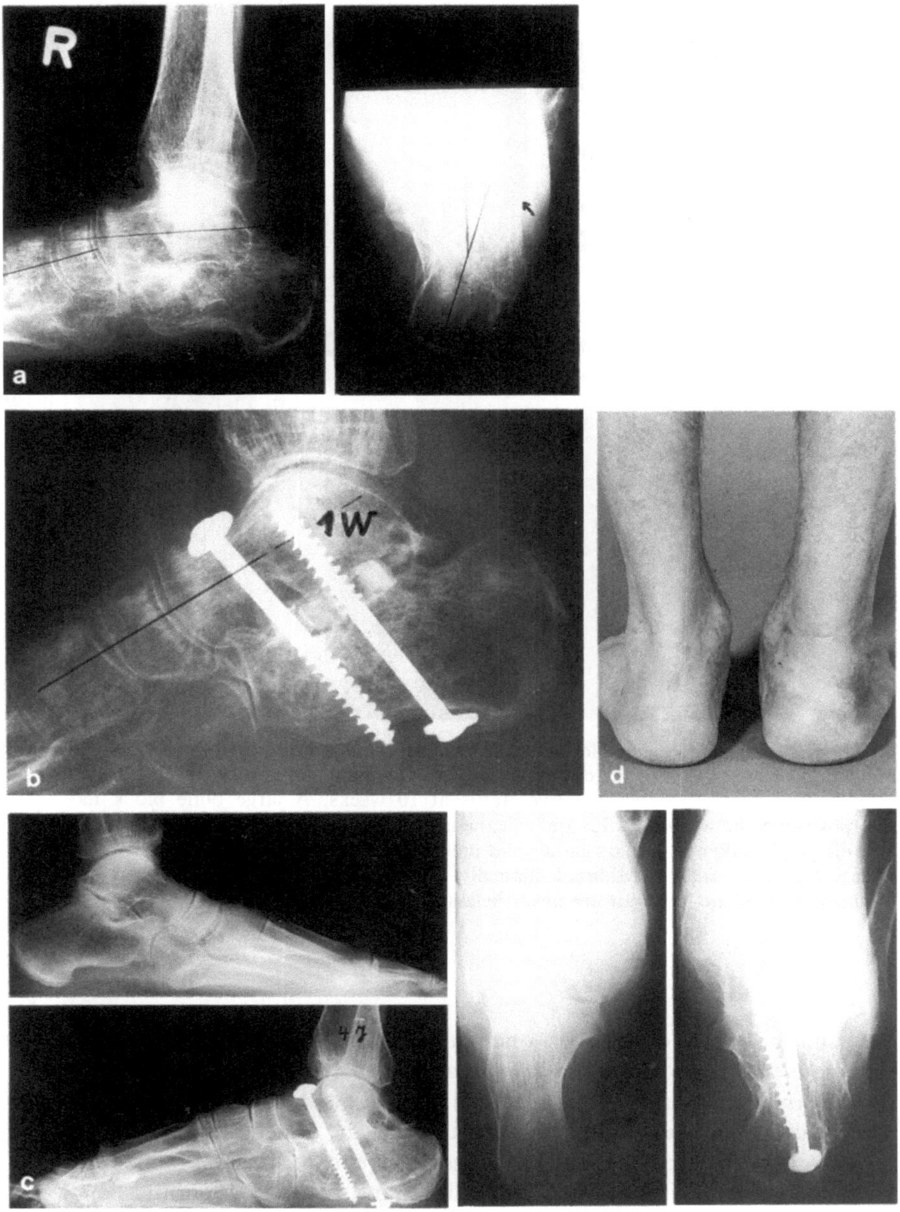

Fig. 5. a Late sequelae of a calcaneal fracture. Note the subtalar arthrosis, flatfoot, and a severe varus deformity of the calcaneus. The bones are osteoporotic. **b** Postoperative radiographs 1 week after subtalar distraction bone-block fusion. Bone material was obtained from the bone bank and fixation done with lag screws.

Results

There was radiographic evidence of union in all ten cases. No foot had progressive degenerative arthritic changes in the ipsilateral talonavicular and calcaneocuboid joints. In three arthrodeses there was some loss of heel height due to collapse of the bone block. In all three cases bank bone had been used and fixation had been done with lag screws.

Nine patients were clinically followed up. The mean follow-up time was 23 months. All patients stated to be satisfied with the result of the operation: four of these were completely satisfied and five had only minor reservations. The five patients with reservations reported having slight difficulty when walking on uneven ground, some restriction of work or recreational activities, and occasional minor pain mostly at the "outside" ankle region. No patient complained of severe pain or severe functional impairment.

Conclusion

Successful reconstruction of the hindfoot for distorted calcaneus following a fracture requires careful analysis of the pathological lesion. In situ subtalar fusion is adviseable only in those cases with painful arthrosis of the subtalar joint but without talocalcaneal malalignment or gross deformity of the calcaneus. When the pathological conditions are mainly related to post-traumatic subtalar arthrosis and varus or valgus deformity of the calcaneus, but heel height and heel width are relative normal, a subtalar arthrodesis with correction of the malalignment is indicated.

In most old fractures of the calcaneus with severe pain and functional impairment, the underlying pathoanatomy consists of post-traumatic arthritis, talocalcaneal malalignment, shortening and widening of the heel, lateral impingement or abutment and incongruity of the ankle joint. For reconstruction, a subtalar distraction bone-block arthrodesis is recommended. The distraction bone-block technique allows the restoration of the anatomical relations of the talus and calcaneus. Leg length, hindfoot height, dorsiflexion of the talus, and malleolar position are corrected. In addition the heel can be narrowed by removing the expanded laterall wall. When using the distracting bone-block

◀ **Fig. 5** *(continued)*. **c** The lateral weight-bearing radiographs taken 4 years after surgery demonstrate solid union, but also some loss of the heel height correction. Note the loosening of the plantar lag screw. The axial view shows the varus deformity nearly completely corrected, but the heel width is still increased because the lateral wall was not resected at the time of surgery. **d** The correct hindfoot alignment and the pathological widening of the heel are also apparent in the photograph technique the guidelines given by Carr et al. [2] and Hansen [5] should be strictly followed. It is important to use autogenous bone-block material and fully threaded bone screws for fixation as recommended by the abovementioned authors, otherwise a secondary loss of correction is likely to occur. Subsequent to subtalar fusion there may be not a complete relief of pain or a full return to activities, but the majority of the symptoms can be markedly relieved compared with the preoperative status.

References

1. Braly WG, Bishop JO, Tullos HS (1985) Lateral decompression for malunited os calcis fractures. Foot Ankle 6:90
2. Carr J, Hansen ST, Benirschke S (1988) Subtalar distraction bone block fusion for late complications of os calcis fractures. Foot Ankle 9:81
3. Cracciolo A, Pearson S, Kitaoka H, Grace D (1990) Hindfoot arthrodesis in adults utilizing a dowel graft technique. Clin Orthop 257:193
4. Deyerle WM (1973) Long-term follow-up of fractures of the os calcis. Orthop Clin North Am 4:213
5. Hansen ST (1991) Posttraumatische Fehlstellung des Rückfußes. Orthopäde 20:95
6. James ETR, Hunter GA (1983) The dilemma of painful old os calcis fractures. Clin Orthop 177:112
7. Johannson M, Harrison J, Greenwood F (1982) Subtalar arthrodesis for adult traumatic arthritis. Foot Ankle 2:294
8. McLaughlin HL (1963) Treatment of late complications after os calcis fractures. Clin Orthop 30:111
9. Miller WE (1983) Pain and impairment considerations following treatment of disruptive os calcis fractures. Clin Orthop 177:82
10. Nade S, Monohan PRW (1973) Fractures of the calcaneus: a study of the long-term prognosis. Injury 4:200
11. Pozo JL, Kirwan OE, Jackson AM (1984) The long-term results of conservative management of severely displaced fractures of the calcaneus. J Bone Joint Surg [Br] 66:386
12. Russotti GM, Cass JB, Johnson KA (1988) Isolated talocalcaneal arthrodesis. J Bone Joint Surg [Am] 70:1472
13. Sangeorzan BJ, Hansen ST (1989) Early and late posttraumatic foot reconstruction. Clin Orthop 243:86
14. Saint-Isister JF (1974) Calcaneofibular abutment following crush fracture of the calcaneus. J Bone Joint Surg [Br] 56:274

Subject Index

Pilon Fractures

Talus Fractures

Calcaneus Fractures

MIX
Papier aus verantwortungsvollen Quellen
Paper from responsible sources
FSC® C105338

FSC
www.fsc.org

If you have any concerns about our products,
you can contact us on
ProductSafety@springernature.com

In case Publisher is established outside the EU,
the EU authorized representative is:
Springer Nature Customer Service Center GmbH
Europaplatz 3, 69115 Heidelberg, Germany

Printed by Libri Plureos GmbH
in Hamburg, Germany